Palliative Care for People with Cancer

Second Edition

Edited by

Jenny Penson MA(ed), SRN, HV Cert, Cert Ed, RNT, Cert in Counselling
Macmillan Nurse/Tutor, North Devon Hospice Care Trust,
Devon, UK

and

Ronald Fisher MA, MRCS, LRCP, FRCA
Lecturer in Palliative Care, and formerly Consultant
Physician in Continuing Care at the first Macmillan Unit,
Christchurch Hospital, Dorset, UK

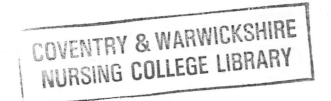

ARNOLD

A member of the Hodder Headline Group
LONDON • SYDNEY • AUCKLAND

Coventry University

First published in Great Britain 1991 by
Arnold, a division of Hodder Headline PLC,
338 Euston Road, London NW1 3BH

First edition 1991

Second edition 1995

Whilst the advice and information in this book is believed to be true and
accurate at the date of going to press, neither the editors, authors nor the publisher
can accept any legal responsibility or liability for any errors or omissions
that may be made. In particular (but without limiting the generality of the
preceding disclaimer) every effort has been made to check drug dosages;
however it is still possible that errors have been missed. Furthermore,
dosage schedules are constantly being revised and new side-effects
recognised. For these reasons the reader is strongly urged to consult the
drug companies' printed instructions before administering any of the drugs
recommended in this book.

British Library Cataloguing in Publication Data
A catalogue record for this book is available from the British Library

Library of Congress Cataloging-in-Publication Data
A catalog record for this book is available from the Library of Congress

ISBN 0 340 61391 2 (pb)

1 2 3 4 5   95 96 97 98 99

Typeset in 10/11pt Ehrhardt. Produced by Gray Publishing, Tunbridge Wells, Kent
Printed and bound in Great Britain by J. W. Arrowsmith Ltd, Bristol

Contents

Part II: Coping Strategies

Preface to the second edition

Since the first edition of *Palliative Care for People with Cancer* cancer remains an indiscriminate and rampant disease. Throughout the world, over 50 million people die of cancer each year. In Europe alone, it accounts for 22 per cent of all deaths. In the UK, one person in three will be given the diagnosis of cancer some time in their lives. Of these, somewhere between one-third and one-half will be cured. Bluntly, this means that at least half of them will need palliative care.

The context in which palliative care takes place has changed greatly. The National Health Service and Community Care Act (1990) which came into being in 1993, results in the purchase of health-care being separated from its providing and funding. Therefore, key elements in further change include business planning, quality assurance, setting standards for care, using models of care and health promotion. Those concerned with providing palliative care services can take heart that, although the changes do have considerable implications, their work continues to be highly valued by government as well as by individuals.

The invitation to produce a second edition has given us the challenge of revising and updating the content and inviting four additional contributions. We have been assisted in this task by the helpful comments of colleagues and reviewers, and by the expertise and professionalism of everyone who has written for us.

It seems appropriate here to acknowledge the particular gifts of Olga Craig, whose chapter 'Reflections' appears as a fitting close to both editions. She brought a wealth of experience and commonsense to her role as a social worker in palliative care where she supported patients, families and staff with great warmth and sensitivity. She was a great character and a very wise woman. She died of cancer in November 1992.

By its nature, palliative care requires a multidisciplinary approach and this is, once again, reflected in the scope of the book.

The increasing emphasis on day care services, which now outnumbers in-patient services in the UK, warrants a more detailed explanation of this essential component of palliative care which has been referred to as its 'spear-head' or 'cutting edge'.

There has been significant advancement in the management of lymphoedema, much of which has been researched and developed by nurses. Therefore, methods of assessment and management of chronic oedema are included.

One often neglected facet of a holistic approach to patient care, is concern with issues of sexuality. This is particularly pertinent to life-threatening and often disfiguring illness, where the need for intimacy and affection may be hampered by poor communication and a lack of understanding.

Palliative care is a professional activity which seeks to set and maintain high standards and to evaluate the quality of the care which is given. The application of these professional issues to palliative care should stimulate much debate.

Doyle (1994) points out that 'it is time for education and training in palliative medicine to be taken seriously'. We hope that this second edition of *Palliative Care for People with Cancer* may make a useful contribution.

Jenny Penson and Ronald Fisher

Acknowledgements

It was not an easy time when we introduced hospice care into the National Health Service but we were inspired by our patients and families and sustained by the dedication and loyalty of those colleagues who pioneered with us. We would like to thank all of them and particularly Frances Alders, Mary Brookes, Olga Craig, Henry Garnett, Charles Hall, Gill Hambling, Maurice Harker, Julia Hopper, Pat Jones, Anne Newbury, Penny Mogg, Margaret Rapson, Pat Rushton, Sue Stone, Elaine Walker and Ronnie Whitlock-Smith.

We also thank profoundly those who have contributed to this book for their wise words and amenability.

Finally, we thank our families for their love and support and patience, without them little would have been achieved.

Jenny Penson
Ronald Fisher

A Physician [or Nurse] does not violate etiquette even if, being in difficulties on occasions over a patient and in the dark through inexperience, he [she] should urge the calling in of others in order to learn by consultation the truth about the case and in order that there may be fellow workers to afford abundant help. For when a diseased condition is stubborn and the evil grows, in the perplexity of the moment most things go wrong.'

Corpus Hippocraticum

List of contributors

The Editors

Jenny Penson MA (Ed), SRN, HV Cert, Cert Ed, RNT, Cert Counselling
Jenny Penson began her involvement in palliative care in 1975 when she became a Macmillan nurse, attached to the first Macmillan unit which was at Christchurch, in Dorset. She has written extensively on many aspects of palliative care and been involved in research on the care of relatives and on bereavement issues. Her other main interests are in complementary approaches to care and in the use of helping skills. She has contributed to conferences and courses all over the UK and abroad, working with many different professional and volunteer groups.

She has recently returned to the palliative care field, as Macmillan Nurse/Tutor at the North Devon Hospice Care Trust, after several years working in multi-disciplinary education in general and nurse education in particular.

Ronald A. Fisher MA, MRCS, LRCP, FRCA
Lecturer in Palliative Care, and formerly Consultant Physician in Continuing Care at the first Macmillan unit, Christchurch Hospital, Dorset.

Ronald Fisher introduced hospice medicine into the National Health Service at Christchurch Hospital in January 1975. This included the first NHS home-care service for cancer patients, the forerunner of the present Macmillan Nursing Service, and a support and advisory team for the district general hospitals. In 1977 a day care service was started.

From 1977 to 1980 he was Chairman of a Select Committee of Experts at Strasbourg at the invitation of the Council of Europe to study 'Problems related to death'.

He has been long associated with Cancer Relief, was its Honorary Consultant, and is now a Vice President of that charity.

The Contributors

Sally Anstey RGN, Dip N (Wales)
Nurse Teacher and Practitioner, South East Wales Institute of Nursing and Midwifery Education, Cardiff, UK

Caroline Badger BA (Hons), RGN
Macmillan Nurse Consultant in Lymphoedema, St Catherine's Hospice, Crawley, West Sussex, UK

Ray Corcoran FRCOG
Consultant Medical Director, Hayward House, Macmillan Palliative Care Unit, City Hospital, Nottingham, UK

Olga M Craig SRN, SCM, Dip Soc Studies (Edinburgh), Cert Child Care (Birmingham)
Formerly Senior Medical Social Worker and a Lecturer at the Macmillan Unit, Christchurch Hospital, Dorset, UK

Ilora Finlay FRCGP
Consultant in Palliative Medicine and Medical Director, Holme Tower Marie
Curie Centre, Penarth, South Glamorgan, UK

**Dawn Foxley RGN, DN Cert, NBS PSll (Care of the Dying), Dip Counselling
and Psychotherapy (PCT Britain)**
Macmillan Nurse Manager, Fife Macmillan Team and Person Centred Therapist, UK

Charlette Gallagher-Allred PhD, RD, LD
Nutritionalist for Kobacker House Hospice at Riverside, Columbus, Ohio, USA

**Elizabeth Grigg MA. Post Grad Dip (Education), BA, SRN, Certs. FPA,
Midwifery, Intensive Care Nursing**
Education Manager, Tor and South West College of Health, Tone Vale Hospital,
Taunton, UK

Denise Hodson SRN, RSCN
Clinical Nurse Specialist, Regional Paediatric Oncology and Haematology Unit,
St James's University Hospital Trust, Leeds, UK

Tim Hunt MD, DSc, MRCP
Consultant Physician in Palliative Medicine, Arthur Rank Home, Macmillan
Continuing Care Unit, Cambridge, UK

Bill Kenny
Psychiatric Social Worker, Formerly Head of Department, Nursing and Social
Service, Dorset Institute of Higher Education, Dorset, UK

Pearl McDaid
Formerly Senior Nurse, Day Care, Department of Palliative Medicine, Michael
Sobell House, Mount Vernon Hospital, Middlesex, UK, now Day Care Organiser,
Luton and South Bedfordshire Hospice, Bedfordshire, UK

Kathryn Mannix MBBS, MRCP
Senior Registrar in Palliative Medicine, The Royal Infirmary and Saint Oswald's
Hospice, Newcastle upon Tyne, UK

Pat Mathers BSc (Hons), PhD, C Biol, MI Biol
Hon. Research Fellow of Health and Community Studies, Institute of Health and
Community Services, Bournemouth University, Dorset, UK. Formerly Senior
Lecturer in Biological Sciences

Ann Newbury SRN, SCM, NDN Cert, FAETC
Team Leader, Home Care Services, Macmillan Unit, Christchurch Hospital,
Dorset, UK

**Morna Rutherford BSc (Soc Sc/Nurs), RGN, DN Cert, Cert Oncol, Dip
Counselling and Psychotherapy (PCT Britain), BAC accred.**
Macmillan Sister, West Lothian, UK and Trainer, Counselling Unit, Strathclyde
University, UK

Hilary Salway BEd, SRN, Cert Ed, RNT, RCNT, Dip Research
Nurse Consultant and Researcher in Palliative Care.
Formerly Nursing Director of St Peter's Hospice, Bristol. Research and Nurse
Consultant in Palliative care

The Reverend David Stoter
Senior Chaplain, Queen's Medical Centre, Nottingham and Manager, Bereavement
Centre, Queen's Medical Centre, University Hospital, NHS Trust

1

Introduction: palliative care
– a rediscovery

Ronald A. Fisher

'There are indeed two things, knowledge and opinion, of which the one makes its possessor really to know, the other to be ignorant.'

Corpus Hippocraticum

The words 'terminal care' are the most insensitive ones in our medical jargon. They obscure rather than clarify, they mislead, they are inadequate. So why add to the distress of patients and families by using such ill-chosen words?

'Words are the vehicles of thought and feeling, the wires that stretch between us', said the late Lady Violet Bonham-Carter when addressing the Royal College of Physicians (Lloyd-Roberts, 1951). 'I love words', she said, 'because words used properly can make a blank sheet of white paper glow with all the colours of a Turner sky – because they can fill the air with music in a silent room.'

These two words that we use – terminal care – are drab and discordant and diminish the care we are trying to give. The expression 'palliative care' is far more acceptable and carries with it a hint of hope. And yet doctors and nurses, and others associated with cancer, add to the confusion by using both phrases as if they are synonynmous.

I appreciate it can be argued that since incurable cancer is a terminal disease then the care given must also be terminal. But to carry this argument to its logical and perhaps ridiculous conclusion then all care is terminal since life is made up of partial deaths and we begin to die from the moment we are born:

'death borders upon our birth and our cradle stands in our grave.'

Joseph Hall, Epistles (1608) 3.2

We are destined to die, it is a fact of life. Death, as the philosopher Martin Heidegger (1889–1976) said, is the culminating point of both pathology and normality. But too much logic bores, so let us not

'starve the best parts of our minds by leaning on logic'.

J. B. Yeats

So let us accept that palliative care and terminal care are *not* the same, and focus on rehabilitation and control of symptoms.

Palliative care is a broad band of care of indeterminate length which could start the moment the cancer is diagnosed, or even before when there is a gleam of apprehension in the patient's eye. I would suggest that it is at this point that the district nurse should be introduced to the family concerned, even though the care required initially might only be intermittent. Terminal care is only a part of the palliative care programme and comes at the end of life, that is in the last hours or days. Perhaps 'ultimate care' would be a better expression.

Sir Thomas Browne, a 17th century physician of some repute, said 'death is the cure of all diseases' in which case doctors and nurses always lose-out in the end. If we accept this, it follows that our endeavours should be to increase the quantity and improve the quality of the proceeding years. If we now re-arrange those words in the context of the patient with advancing malignant disease and say that our endeavours should be to improve the quality of the preceding days, weeks, months and years, and by so doing quite possibly increase the quantity of those weeks, months and years, then we have an acceptable philosophy for palliative care. We can now go on to define palliative medicine as being 'to relieve suffering when cure is impossible, suffering which can be physical, psychological, social and spiritual and which involves both the patient and the family'. A more precise but still acceptable definition is

> 'to do away with the sufferings of the sick, to lessen the violence of the disease'.
>
> *Corpus Hippocraticum*

The reader may be surprised to know that this was written before the birth of Christ, probably by Hippocrates, but then as it says in the book of Job: 'with the ancient is wisdom'.

It is not inappropriate to enrich these definitions with the words of Barbara McNulty, who was once the nurse in charge of the home-care service at St Christopher's Hospice in London. In the early 1970s I was privileged to accompany her on her round in the community. She taught me so much.

> 'In caring for the dying patient one cannot separate his needs from those of his family – they are a unit whose individual members interact; what affects one will react upon another. One cannot treat a dying patient's physical symptoms and ignore his emotional needs. The home with all its problems, the patient with all his fears and pain are the objects of our concern'.
>
> *Barbara McNulty (with permission)*

I have already pointed out that palliative care may well start the moment the patient is informed of the diagnosis of cancer. Peter Maguire has written that the emotional upheaval that occurs at this time often goes unrecognised (Maquire and Faulkner, 1988). Consequently there is no psychological intervention and the psychiatric morbidity goes untreated.

It should not be forgotten either

> 'that death from cancer is never instantaneous. It occurs in stages, it is a process, and there are variations in the rate at which the final point approaches. Total final death is merely the last in a series of functional organic partial deaths, since although the organs live together they die separately.' (Fisher 1980).

What I am suggesting is that dying from cancer can be a prolonged affair which means the period of palliative care can be very variable in length. Nor should it be forgotten that medicine is not an exact science, we are not always sure what will happen next, therefore a miracle is always possible. Like other colleagues, I have cared for patients with established cancer over periods ranging from one to three to five and even nine years. By improving the quality of a patient's life by, helping the patient to *live* through his or her cancer, every so often a '*little*' miracle happens. Janet McCusker of the University of Massachusetts reviewed 2989 patients dying of cancer during the years 1976–1978 and showed that the length of the 'terminal care period' varied from 1 month to over 4 years (McCusker, 1983). One must again question the appropriateness of the blanket use of the label 'terminal care'. An interesting observation arising out of McCusker's study is the relationship between the length of time that elapses from the diagnosis to the death of the patient and the place of death. As the length of the survival period increased so did the percentage of patients dying at home.

It is encouraging also to know that in Britain, 90 per cent of the last year of life of the patient with cancer is spent at home, and, according to a survey of 703 patients by Derek Doyle, during that year surprisingly 14 per cent are bed-bound for less than 1 week, 27 per cent for 1–4 weeks, 10 per cent for 3 months, and only 4 per cent of the dying are in bed for 3–6 months (Doyle, 1982, 1986). As drug therapy improves we can be cautiously optimistic that these figures will improve and though cure may not be achieved the progress of the disease will be slowed and life prolonged. So we should always give hope as long as it is reasonable to do so. Hope, not for the cure of the cancer, but to enable the patient to achieve goals and live a life full of meaning in whatever environment that patient may be. Without hope there is no endeavour.

Medical historians will report in due course that it wasn't until well into the second half of the 20th century that the fortunes of the chronic cancer patient began to improve. Until then many patients with advancing malignant disease had suffered unnecessarily. For example, millions had unalleviated cancer pain and many tragically died in pain. This is now generally accepted with regret, but then history is full of regrets. Why was this? Why has this been such a neglected area of medicine?

It has been said the fault lies with the education nurses and doctors have received or have not received. An education that has been orientated to cure, so that when we failed to cure we did not know how to cope with our failures and tended therefore to retreat from the situation. What I call the 'Eeyore Syndrome' takes over: (with apologies to A. A. Milne)

> *Said Eeyore*: I make it seventeen days come Friday since anyone spoke to me.
> *Said Rabbit*: 'I was here myself a week ago'.
> 'Not conversing' said Eeyore. 'Not first one and then the other. You said "Hallo" and *flashed past*'!
>
> *A. A. Milne*

Life-sustaining treatments ranging from antibiotics to organ transplants, it is argued, have caused us to concentrate on the disease rather than on the patient. Ivan Illich, the philosopher, calls it 'the medicalisation of life', and the opening sentence of his book *Medical Nemesis* rather startlingly states 'the Medical Establishment has become a threat to life' (Illich, 1974). By this he means health-care professionals have taken over so completely that the patient loses his or her independence. Professor Ziegler of Switzerland, also commenting on the omnipotence of doctors, has coined the word 'thanatocrats' who have the power to prolong life or terminate it.

Another interesting thought is that doctors and nurses have inherited this attitude of neglect over the centuries, that it is a 'hangover' from the past. Is this theory so wild? After all we have inherited and accepted much that is in the *Corpus Hippocraticum* (Hippocratic collection). Hippocrates is universally known as the 'father of medicine' and many of the clinical observations in use today are all there, clearly stated in these ancient manuscripts. As W. H. S. Jones writes

> 'there is within the corpus the work of a medical genius, perhaps the greatest genius among all the physicians whose writings have come down to us. He inherited much from his predecessors but either personally or through his pupils he bequeathed far more to his successors. Whether or not his name was Hippocrates the inheritence is still ours'. W. H. S. Jones (1945).

Over the centuries contributions by Galen, William Harvey, John Hunter, Edward Jenner, Joseph Lister, Alexander Fleming, Frederick Banting and Charles Best, Richard Bright, Thomas Addison, William Osler, Florence Nightingale, Cicely Saunders, to name but a very very few, have added to that inheritance to create medicine as it is today.

Let us now look at a part of that inheritance; at one of the bequests.

> 'First I will define what I conceive Medicine to be. In general terms it is to do away with the sufferings of the sick, to lessen the violence of their disease, *and to refuse to treat those who are overmastered by their disease realizing that in such cases such medicine is powerless.*'
>
> *Corpus Hippocraticum*

We have totally accepted the first half of that definition, but did we not also accept the second half and is it not until recently that we have begun to reject it?

Fascinating though these theories are, the fact remains – we were ignorant of what could be done.

> 'Wisdom is prevented by ignorance and delusion is the result.'
>
> *Bhagaradgta, 5 tr P. Lal*

And delusion certainly was the result because generations of nurses and doctors deluded themselves into believing that nothing could be done for the patient with an incurable cancer with the result that we took refuge in those all too familiar statements 'We have done all we can' or 'There is nothing more to be done'.

In retrospect I suppose we should be grateful for such delusions because if there had been no doubts there would have been no questioning, and if there had been no questioning there would have been no enlightenment. And so we had a neglected area of medicine. Health services world-wide were failing to improve the care of these unfortunate patients, failing to satisfy their physical, emotional, social and spiritual needs. It wasn't until we were alerted by Dr Cicely Saunders to this famine of care that hospices and continuing care units began to appear in this country. We (the editors) were privileged to introduce hospice care into the National Health Service in January 1975 at Christchurch Hospital in Dorset. At the same time we started a home-care service which was the prototype of today's Macmillan nursing service and a peripatetic 'support team' for the hospitals in the district. Two years later we introduced day care.

From these specialist units with their growing expertise and scientific approach was born palliative medicine, now recognised by the Royal College of Physicians as a speciality. The emergence of palliative medicine is one of the best things that has happened to medicine in the 20th century.

When lecturing in the early 1970s I used to remind audiences that since dying is part of living then *care of the dying is care of the living*. It is a vital statement which follows the aphoristic style adopted by the early Greek philosophers. An aphorism is capsulated wisdom, a device used 'to arrest attention and assist the memory'. *Care of the dying is care of the living* – an aphorism which is totally acceptable today, but in those earlier days there was much more talk of helping people to die well, to die with dignity, to have a good death. To my puzzled mind this thanatological terminology was deceptive, full of promise but signifying very little. Better surely to speak of 'a tranquil death'. Nursing care of the dying patient is care for the patient who is still living, it is helping that patient to live his or her life to the fullest whether at home or in hospital. It is care that is not just centred on the individual but includes members of the family. The nurse in a palliative care team, whether in the community or hospital is just as important as the doctor. He or she is in the unique position of being able to spend most time with the patient and the family and, by virtue of this intimacy, acquire a wide knowledge of the patient. This knowledge can be shared with other members of the caring team and in this way the patient and the family receive total harmonious care. As Lisabeth Hockey (1989) says, the nurse is the main communicator between the patient, the relatives and the doctors and has the function of not only giving care but of coordinating the care of others.

I remember saying in 1974, prior to the opening of the Macmillan Unit at Christchurch, that I considered we were a short-term concept in a neglected area of medicine and that a measure of our success would be when we had made ourselves redundant. Obviously I have modified this view over the years but I still believe that if all nurses, whether working in a hospital or the community, receive adequate education in palliative care then most patients, most of the time, can be cared for by the family doctor and family nurse and the hospital team. The relief of cancer pain is an excellent example of this because there are now standard procedures of pain control, that are well within the scope of any nurse or doctor. Surveys have demonstrated that total or acceptable relief can be achieved in 71–97 per cent of patients (Twycross, 1989).

What then is the role of the specialist unit and the specialist nurse? Both are of vital importance. They are there to advise on difficult problems, to take over the care of the patient if necessary, preferably on a temporary basis, to research and evaluate, and to teach. Given the tools, the community and hospital nurses will be able to play their natural roles. It is important that as far as the 'family nurse' is concerned, this role should not be stolen from them. After all, nurses have worked in the community for some considerable time, in fact from 1859 when that socially conscious philanthropist William Rathbone started the District Nursing Service in Liverpool (Hardy, 1981). There is a wealth of 'know-how' inherent in this service.

This book is primarily for nurses. The contributors have tried to look at the problem through the nurses' eyes and then give the information which will enable them to give the comprehensive care which will satisfy the needs of the patient and the family, and indeed their own needs should the occasions arise. Doctors, medical social workers, physiotherapists, medical students, occupational therapists, teachers, administrators and others will also find much to interest them. The contributors are all experts in their various fields and are, or have been, associated with palliative or continuing cancer care over many years. Their involvement in undergraduate and particularly post-graduate education has been extensive. We have tried to include the more important aspects, but inevitably there will be omissions in a book of this size. Ethical issues, symptom control-confusional states, communication, counselling skills, bereavement, nutrition and complementary therapies have all been highlighted.

I will conclude with yet another telling passage from the *Corpus*, hoping that I have made the point that apart from technology, there is little that is new in our medical philosophy.

> 'With regard to disease, the circumstances from which we form a judgement of them are
> * by attending to the general nature of all, and the peculiar nature of each individual, to the disease, the patient, and the applications;
> * to the person who applies them, and that makes a difference for better or for worse;
> * to the patients habits, regimens and pursuits;
> * to his conversation, manners, taciturnity, thoughts, sleep or absence of sleep, and sometimes his dreams.
> * to his picking and scratching.
> * to his tears, alvine discharges, urine, sputa and vomitings, and to the changes of disease from the one into the other;
> * to the deposits, whether of a deadly or critical character;
> * to the sweat, coldness, rigor, cough, sneezing, hiccup, respiration, erudation, flatulence, whether passed silently or with a noise;
> * to haemorrhage and haemorrhoids;
> * from these and their consequence, we must 'form our judgement'.
>
> *Corpus Hippocraticum*

We must indeed and we cannot be more holistic than that!

It should be remembered also that palliative care does not necessarily end with the death of the patient. Until life begins to glow again some surviving relatives may need support during the bereavement period. Likewise for those patients whose disease has been controlled as a result of treatment, there may be a transition period during which the family nurse and the family doctor will need to 'map the middle ground of survivorship and provide psycho-social support' (Loescher *et al.*, 1989). As Mullen (1985) reflects 'there is no moment of cure but rather an evolution from the phase of extended survival into a period when the activity of the disease or the likelihood of its return is sufficiently small that the cancer can now be considered permanently arrested'. It is only then that palliative care can end.

I cannot close without these final and relevant words of advice from our 'Father':

> 'The Physician (and Nurse) must have a certain degree of socialability, for a morose disposition is inaccessible both to those who are well and those who are sick'.
>
> *Corpus Hippocraticum*

How true!

References

DOYLE, D. (1982). *Journal of the Royal College of General Practitioners* **32**, 285–91.
DOYLE, D. (1986). Domiciliary care – a doctor's view. In: *International Symposium on Pain Control*, pp. 61–7. Royal Society of Medicine.

FISHER, R. (1980). European Public Health Committee. Problems Related to Death: Care of the Dying. Report of the European Public Health Committee, Council of Europe Strasbourg. Chairman of Committee and Editor of Report.

HARDY, G. (1981). *William Rathbone and the Early History of District Nursing.* G. W. & A. Hesketh, Ormskirk.

HOCKEY, L. (1989) Medical education. In: *The Edinburgh Symposium – Pain Control,* pp. 3–15. Royal Society of Medicine International Congress – Symposium Series.

ILLICH, I. (1974). *Limits of Medicine: Medical Nemesis.* Penguin, Harmondsworth.

JONES, W. H. S. (1945). Hippocrates and the *Corpus Hippocraticum.* In: *Proceedings of the British Academy,* Vol. XXXI, communicated 6 June 1945. Geoffrey Cumberledge, Amen House, London.

LLOYD-ROBERTS (1951). The power of words. Lecture at the Royal College of Physicians, November 1951. Reported in *The Lancet,* 1 December 1951.

LOESCHER, L. J., WELCH-MCCAFFREY, D., LEIGH, S. A. *et al.* (1989). Surviving adult cancers. Parts 1 and 2. *Annals of Internal Medicine* 111, 411–32, 517–24.

MCCUSKER, J. (1983). Where cancer patients die: an epidemiological study. *Public Health Reports* March–April 1983, 98(2), 170–6, University of Massachusetts.

MAGUIRE, P. and FAULKNER, A. (1988). How to communicate with cancer patients. Part 2. Handling uncertainty: collusion and denial. *British Medical Journal* 297, 972–4.

MILNE, A. A. (1928). *The House at Pooh Corner.* Methuen, London.

MULLEN, F. (1985). Seasons of survival: reflections of a physician with cancer. *New England Journal of Medicine* 313, 270–3.

TWYCROSS, R. (1989) Medical education. In: *The Edinburgh Symposium – Pain Control.* Royal Society of Medicine International Congress – Symposium Series.

From cure to care: the role of the nurse

2

Ethical issues

Tim Hunt

'One must have studied much to know that one knows little.'

Anon.

Nurses and doctors are entrusted with caring for the sick; this is a privilege. Today, in a hectic world, there is little time to think and nurses and doctors are under growing pressu.e to make decisions. They find themselves faced with increasing and conflicting demands in attempting to give good care and, balance the economy of health-care. They may forget what is right and what is wrong and this may result in forgetting their duties to both their patients and to their professions. Such considerations introduce thoughts on the ethics and morals of patient care. Ethics can be considered as the theory of morals. There are many approaches to outlining the principles of ethics; one simple outline or pattern is to consider three broad principles:

  (i)   justice and fairness;
 (ii)   autonomy – respecting the choice of the patient;
(iii)   beneficence – kindness to patients.

Justice and fairness

The practice of justice and fairness may depend on political decisions, often at government level. For example, should limited funds be directed to the care of the elderly or to transplant surgery? But the carer may also need to make difficult decisions. Does the carer give more time and effort to one patient at the expense of another patient? Which patient should be expected to pay for a private night nurse when there is only one Marie Curie nurse and two patients with equal need? Frequently there is no way of being fair because the carers efforts are constrained by matters outside their control. Nevertheless, these principles are pertinent to patient care.

Autonomy – respecting the choice of the patient

In an ideal world each person ought to have complete personal freedom to decide how they want to be looked after. However, this is seldom possible. At one extreme there is the comatosed, confused or demented patient; these patients cannot express their wishes. At the other extreme is the articulate patient who is very able and knows what he or she wants but his or her requirements cannot be fitted into the rigid system of care. If the principle of autonomy is recognised then problems do arise in considering the wish of any patient who wants to die.

Beneficence – kindness to patients

It is fundamental to a caring profession that the carers are beneficent; their aim is to do good, to be kind and charitable in feeling. If the need for doing good is accepted then maleficence, that is the doing of evil or ill-will to another, must be prevented. Even when a patient or his or her relatives are displeasing, aggressive or do not want to follow the advice which has been given, carers must refrain from being spiteful or acting with vengeance. When speaking to patients doctors and nurses should not frighten them or abuse their position of apparent authority.

In looking after patients with advanced cancer, while many of the problems are different from those seen, for example, in obstetrics or intensive care units, the principles of ethical and moral thought remain the same. There are three areas which provoke much thought in the care of the patient with advanced cancer:

  (i)   what to tell and not to tell the patient and relatives;
 (ii)   not striving officiously to keep a patient alive; and
(iii)   euthanasia.

What to tell and not to tell

'What a distance there is between what people say and what they think.'
Jean Racine (1639–1699)

There is no doubt that a decade ago patients were given limited information about their illness and this, especially, was the case with patients with cancer. With immense social and educational changes, no longer is it embarrassing to discuss disease and death; these topics feature frequently on radio and television and in print. Therefore, public awareness about illness and cancer is considerable. In the United States the present trend is to disclose nearly every possible aspect of a disease, and although this is not yet evident in Europe, the caring professions must take into account such trends when communicating with patients and their families. The fundamentals to help decide on what to tell and not to tell are first, the autonomy or rights of the patient; and second, kindness and beneficence to the patient.

The earlier approach of being frugal with the truth was considered kinder to the patient. The arguments in favour of this policy may be on the following lines. If an ill person is given unfavourable or disturbing information, the problems for that already troubled person are increased. Further, it may be felt that telling the truth will remove the often underlying hope that the disease will regress or that treatment will bring about a complete cure. Hope is a necessary requirement for survival, so that if the hope of the patient is removed or diluted, so too may the will for survival be removed. These considerations rest mainly on being kind to the patient, they do not consider truth. Here there is a conflict between kindness and truth, and what may be meant by truth is difficult to define as will be mentioned later. There are examples where the carer, in telling the truth, can be unkind; a frequent criticism of busy out-patient clinics is that honest information is given to patients but in a hurried and seemingly cold and curt manner. This may impart truth but cannot be condoned as it violates the principles of beneficence. Therefore, in certain situations, if truth negates beneficence then truth may not be of such importance.

There are other areas where truth may underline ethical consideration for the patient. For example, a patient may enter a state of denial, rejecting what he or she has been told about his or her illness. Some carers cannot accept this and strive to breach this denial because they believe that denial does not help the patient. But denial may be a normal coping mechanism for some people and if a patient wishes to continue denial then that wish should be respected. To force information on a patient against their wish is contrary to the principles of autonomy and beneficence.

> 'Before you tell the "truth" to the patient, be sure you know the "truth", and that the patient wants to hear it.'
>
> *Richard Clarke Cabot (1868–1939)*

In broad moral terms the importance of truth cannot be denied, but it is the application of truth as an obligatory principle that is often unclear. The professional carer cannot speak in terms of absolute or whole truth because they often do not know what is happening and what will happen to a patient. When they think they are speaking the truth to a patient what they are expressing is an opinion based on their experience, and opinion may be some distance from the truth. The logic and thought as to what is truth is a subject of its own with far-reaching consequences, but the carer must be cautious about making claims on the importance of truth and prudent when they think they are speaking the truth to the patient. It will be of value to examine some of the practical issues. Why do doctors and nurses hesitate to give a patient information about his or her own illness?

- It takes both time and patience to explain an illness in terms that can be understood. It may be difficult to create an opportunity which is unhurried so that there is time to answer questions and support the distress that may result in what will be a sensitive discussion.
- Sometimes the carer may find discussion difficult because it requires a mental agility and sensitivity to feel the nuances from the patient. At other times the carer may have become so close to the patient that it is painful to disclose disturbing information because one does not want to further upset the patient. A further reason may be that the discussion may encroach on the personal problems of the carer.
- Relatives often feel that to disclose too much information could be injurious to the mental health of the patient, and may request the carer to filter information given to the patient. Some of the ethical considerations have been mentioned earlier, but carers may find themselves in a difficult position between patient and relative because if they accede to such requests they may remove the autonomy of the patient. Some relatives fear disclosure of information because they do not know how to respond to the patient once additional and more pertinent information is given, and although the ethical principles of the caring profession apply to the patient, carers may have to give equal support to a distressed relative.
- Inter-professional communication problems do arise. For example, if information is disclosed to a patient, will it upset other professionals who are also involved in the case? A patient often asks a nurse about his or her illness; the nurse may vacillate because he or she is uncertain of the views of the general

practitioner, and if pertinent information is disclosed it may fall on the next carer who visits the patient to provide emotional support to help the distressed patient. It is often not possible to avoid such problems but there is a responsibility on each carer to try and enhance communication.

There is no single or correct way to communicate with a patient. Each patient is individual as are carers, but all carers need considerable sensitivity to establish what the patient wishes to know. This will help determine what to tell, when to tell and how to tell. Sensitivity requires flexibility for good communication.

There are a few guidelines to supplement the ethical principles; in general the greater the request for information from a patient the more information should be provided, likewise the greater the patient's ability to understand the greater is the need to disclose information at a depth in keeping with his or her mental ability, and the information given must be within the comprehension of the patient.

Ethical considerations embrace the subject of confidentially, and professional codes have evolved in this subject to help the patient. In simple terms, if doctors and nurses need honest and unrestricted information from the patient then they must provide an implied assurance that the information will not be disclosed. Otherwise the patient will give partial or even misleading information which may hamper correct diagnosis and treatment of an illness. The patient may need to be assured of this aspect.

Problems may arise in considering what to tell and what not to tell relatives. If a patient has a competent mind the carer's duty is to discuss first with the patient his or her illness and plans for his or her care. In practice the first discussion often takes place with the closest relatives. This may be done to try and unravel the thoughts and known wishes of the patient, but no person other than the patient (except in the case of children) has the right to consent or decide on treatment for that patient. Voluntary disclosures about the illness should not be made to a third party without the consent of the patient; third parties, in a technical sense, include relatives and friends. If the patient is denied information and it is given to others, or if relatives are allowed to make decisions, the carer may be removing autonomy from that patient. If patients and relatives are not equally informed there is a risk of considerable misunderstanding. The ideal is to discuss sensitive matters with the patient and relative at the same time.

In recent years there has been much attention to making medical notes available to patients, as under the Access to Health Records Act 1990, and guidelines issued by the Department of Health. But there are instances where disclosures of information to the patient, or others, may cause serious harm to the physical or mental health of that patient. It is the duty of the carer, likewise the health authority, to act at all times in the best interests of the patient, and therefore most careful thought is required before medical or nursing notes are made available to patients. This point is recognised in a legal judgement in 1994. It is erroneous for carers and others to think that notes should be made available routinely to patients.

As professionals, carers need to re-examine what they communicate to a patient. Perhaps they should establish what their patients want to know and what element of truth they require and not tell them what they think they should be told. But this is difficult and often impossible.

Not striving officiously to keep a patient alive

'Thou shalt not kill; but need'st not strive
Officiously to keep alive.'

Arthur Hugh Clough (1819–1861)
The Latest Decalogue

The last decade has heard many voices speaking for the quality of life instead of the length or quantity of life for those patients with advanced illness. This view has been promoted by the hospice movement. Sometimes these doctrines are considered as the quality of life and the sanctity of life and may be the subject of considerable debate. Belief in the sanctity of life would seem very finite and implies, in its strictest sense, that every step should be taken to keep the patient alive; it is thought that this belief stems from early religious codes. On the other hand, the quality of life views are based on subjective and compassionate assessments. Awareness of the need to consider the quality of life came about 30 years ago when studies of patients dying in hospital wards showed that carers should work to enable a patient to die peacefully and to live until he or she dies. Those who have cared for the very sick know that it is possible to maintain a policy of continual and sometimes aggressive intervention, without conviction that it will help, sometimes at extreme psychological and physical distress to the patient and relatives. It is to overcome such suffering that caring trends today are towards the quality of life concept.

At first it may seem that the extreme interpretation of the sanctity of life doctrine is irreconcilable with the quality of life concept. However, in 1957 Pope Pius XII put forward the view that doctors were not obliged to give extraordinary medical measures to keep a patient alive, and in 1977 the Archbishop of Canterbury expressed support for this principle. This brought about discussion as to what are 'extraordinary measures' and related expressions as 'heroic treatments'. It is difficult to make a list of such measures and perhaps every case must be considered on its own, but others may argue that it is impossible to make such distinctions. But extremist views are not only found in religious teachings, because 20 years after the declaration by Pope Pius XII, Lord Hailsham, when Lord Chancellor, said 'The law, at the moment, is perfectly plain; if you have got a living body, you have got to keep it alive, if you can'.

Extending from this discussion as to what professional carers should and should not do to allow an acceptable quality of life in the very sick patient, there has evolved debate on the subtle distinction between carrying out some deliberate act that leads to the death of a patient and not taking action that leads to the same result. In practical terms simple examples include giving a lethal injection or smothering a patient with a pillow with, of course, the intention of killing him or her; not taking some action would be the withholding of treatment as a result of which a patient dies. In moral terms most will regard the first two examples as unacceptable and the third example as acceptable. This concept is referred to as the 'acts and omissions doctrine'. But the apparent distinction between what is an act and what is an omission becomes blurred if the thinking behind the original thought is considered: if treatment is withheld with the intent of killing then this passivity is of the same degree as if the carer had decided to smother the patient.

The concept of acts and omissions is complex and, because it leads to considerable confusion, some argue that it should be rejected partly because of the enormous scope as to what is an acceptable omission. If a person knows that they will benefit from the death of a patient, and if they then fail to treat the patient and he or she dies, this type of omission is as immoral as if the person had smothered the patient. But sometimes omission is because of carelessness, ignorance or laziness and there is no motive to kill the patient. To illustrate the problems that arise in considering the acts and omission doctrine there is the well-known dilemma of the old-age pensioners. If pensioners have insufficient means to keep themselves warm they will die of hypothermia, and society may view this as an omission by those responsible for making available funds to old-age pensioners; but if the same numbers of pensioners were machine-gunned in the streets there would be a very different response from society. Sometimes omissions are unavoidable because carelessness and ignorance will always exist; but most acts can be avoided.

If a person takes on the duty of caring for a patient then that person may be guilty of an offence if they fail to carry out that duty. But in carrying out that duty the problem may be how far should one treat or not treat? The principle of autonomy makes it obligatory to discuss proposed treatment with the patient if he or she so wishes; often patients who have seen many miles of hospital corridors do not wish for further uncomfortable intervention. The carer may have to discuss with the patient what is the aim of further treatment? Will it cause pain or distress? Will it help the extension of life, and will the functioning of that continued life be in any way impaired? The law cannot define the professional carers' precise responsibilities and the carer cannot look for definitive guidelines, but they can consider the principles of justice, autonomy and kindness in each case. But, as professionals, carers may be asked to give their opinion and where they know that there are two of more alternatives on some aspect of treatment then, whenever possible, these should be explained to the patient so as to help him or her to decide on the merits or otherwise of further treatment.

The law does not insist that doctors and nurses should persist indefinitely in treating someone; even in general medicine, following a cardiac arrest, it is not necessary to persist indefinitely in efforts to resuscitate a patient. Where there are cases where the circumstances are changing, it may be that an earlier decision on treatment requires reappraisal. For example, if nutrition is first provided by a nasogastric feeding line and other problems arise in the progression of the disease there is no continuing obligation to continue with such feeding. Therefore there is, in practice, and in general thoughts about this subject, no compulsion to continue with any treatment, but if the carer deliberately withholds what is reasonable and acceptable treatment from the patient then this may be an offence.

The clinical judgement of the doctor is also important. In 1992 the courts ruled that a doctor could not be ordered to carry out treatment against his or her clinical judgement.

There are instances where a competent patient refuses further treatment and, recalling the principle of patient autonomy, the carer should respect this request even if they disagree with it. In these cases there is still a moral obligation to continue to provide care for the patient as required by the principle of beneficence. Of course the duties of the carer may be different if the patient is demented or in some other way unable to comprehend the advantage of therapy, as would be the case if he or she is a danger to him or herself, relatives or other patients. It is good practice to sedate these sad cases by the use of medication. A person's views on when to treat and not to treat must be influenced by their upbringing, spiritual attitude, professional background and private conscience. The aim of care is to provide an optimum living for the remaining weeks or months of the patient's life. Where treatment may cause further mental or physical distress then it must be viewed with circumspection, taking into account the wishes of the patient.

Euthanasia

'Euthanasia is a long, smooth sounding word, and it concedes its danger as long, smooth words do, but the danger is there nevertheless.'

Pearl Buck (1892–1973)

In 1989 an Austrian nurse was charged with the murder of 17 elderly patients in Germany. She admitted using large doses of drugs to provide 'mercy killing'. This nurse may have cared very much for her patients, to the extent that she found their suffering incompatible with living. She decided to practice euthanasia which some may describe as 'mercy killing', but the law in most countries views such action as murder, and we can frequently read about similar cases. Increasingly people are more open in speaking and writing about the suffering of someone they love thereby giving some support to the concept of euthanasia.

What is euthanasia? The word is derived from the Greek – *eu* meaning easy, and *thanatos* meaning death – easy death. But the meaning of the word today is used to describe the hastening of death of a patient to prevent further suffering; and within this broad meaning are a number of terms used to describe different forms of euthanasia, although there is no agreement on the precise meaning of these terms. In general three forms are described – voluntary, involuntary and non-voluntary euthanasia.

Voluntary euthanasia is where the patient has expressed a wish to die and either they or someone else carries out an action to enable this. It is this form that is the basis of attempts to legalise euthanasia.

There is little difference between this and suicide. Whatever views are held by professional carers, there are both legal and professional constraints why they should not encourage a patient to commit suicide. Since the Suicide Act 1961 it is no longer a criminal offence for a person to attempt to take his or her own life, but it is an offence to advise another person on how to set about this.

Involuntary euthanasia is where a competent patient who has the ability to make decisions is not consulted, and his or her life is ended by the action of another person. This is murder.

Non-voluntary euthanasia is where a patient is unable to make a decision, for example he or she may be in coma, and their life is ended by the action of another. The press often describe this as 'mercy killing' and it is this form of euthanasia that causes considerable problems in medical ethics.

There is another distinction in considering euthanasia: this is the use of the terms 'active euthanasia', where death would not have taken place without certain steps being taken as with the giving of a drug, and 'passive euthanasia' where certain steps to prolong life have been discontinued as with the withdrawal of drugs. This is the basis of the 'acts and omissions doctrine' which was considered earlier.

It is difficult to encompass these varied descriptions of euthanasia and one attempt to describe the present meaning of the word was the definition adopted by the Linacre Report in 1981. This report concludes: 'In euthanasia a person's death is brought about on the ground that, because of his present mental condition and quality of life, and sometimes in consideration also of the quality of life of his family, it would be better for him, or at least no harm, if that person were dead.'

Euthanasia has for long been a silent subject and discussion of it is avoided, even among professional carers. Professional carers have all faced the patient who asks for their help to die, and the relatives who challenge why someone should endure such suffering and not be allowed to die. In these conversations carers feel inadequate and may remain silent or move the conversation elsewhere. Why is it awkward to talk about this subject? As with sensitive subjects, the roots of the carers' thinking are difficult to untangle and their thoughts result from professional influences and principles, social concern, respect for life and religious creeds, some of which have evolved over the last 2000 years.

It is no coincidence that the Christian churches, nor indeed the Jewish and Islamic faiths, do not support the taking of ones own life or the lives of others who are in pain or suffering. Probably it is from the early religious teachings that our present thoughts have evolved. Rabbinical teachings forbade the taking of one's life or assisting the ill who wished this. In simple terms, the belief evolved that man was not the owner of his body and that no person should interfere with the natural life span, because to shorten life may prevent receiving absolution which may be given at any time up to the actual moment of death. These early thoughts and teachings probably provided a basis for present religious views on euthanasia, and it was often these views that formulated early civil and criminal laws.

There are examples in early societies where assisted suicide was practised for social or economic reasons. Nomadic tribes, as in the Sudan, could not carry around their very sick, and at times of war and famine the very sick may have burdened the survival of a tribe, and rituals developed to practise some form of euthanasia. In Roman times suicide was sometimes a demonstration of patriotism, and this 'self-sacrifice' is still seen in recent wars and fighting.

What is the present legal situation in Britain? The background to present views dates from 1957 when Dr John Bodkin Adams, an Eastbourne general practitioner, was charged with using excessive doses of drugs to bring about the deaths of some patients. The conclusions of the Adams case should be considered alongside the judgement in the more recent case of Dr Arthur who, in 1981, was charged with the death of a child with Down's syndrome that was given dihydrocodeine. In both cases the doctors concerned were acquitted, but the views of the trial judges provide important guidelines to all carers. First, no person whether a doctor, nurse or other carer is above the law and even a professional code is unable to override the law. Second, it is unlawful for any person to bring about euthanasia or carry out some act with the intention of killing a person. Third, that the proper practice of medicine is to relieve pain and suffering, and adequate doses of drugs may be used to achieve such relief, even if the use of those drugs may shorten life. These views contain important practical considerations.

There are movements for and against euthanasia. In England the Voluntary Euthanasia Society, sometimes known as Exit, was founded in 1935 and now has more than 10,000 members; its counterpart in the Netherlands claims over 36,000 members, while the related organisation in the United States has over 300,000 members. One of the first opinion polls on this subject was carried out in 1969 by Mass Observation and this reported that just over half the population in England favoured euthanasia; in 1976 and 1985 research by National Opinion Poll (NOP) showed 69 and 72 per cent, respectively supporting euthanasia.

In the last few years some important developments have affected attitudes towards expediting the 'natural' life of patients. Some of these have arisen from caring for patients with problems other than cancer and in countries other than Britain, but they have all helped towards understanding a very complex subject.

In the late 1980s there was the case of Nancy Cruzan in the United States. This young lady was for 4 years in a 'persistent vegetative state' (PVS) following an accident, and was kept alive by artificial feeding. Her parents tried to end this treatment, but there was considerable opposition from right-to-life groups and the State of Missouri. The US Supreme Court took the view that individual states could not ignore the express wishes of patients, and when satisfactory evidence was presented on the wishes of Nancy Cruzan the means were withdrawn of keeping her alive. A not dissimilar PVS situation was seen in England in 1992 with the case of Tony Bland who was kept alive for 3½ years by artificial feeding. After requests from his parents there was an application to the Courts which held that it was in the 'best interests' of the patient and 'good medical practice' if artificial feeding was discontinued. It is estimated that there may be over 1000 cases of PVS in England but the Courts have indicated that each case needs to be considered separately.

Both these cases illustrate the importance of recognising the rights or autonomy of the patient, or their appointed representative.

In November 1992 Dr Nigel Cox was convicted of attempted murder at Winchester Crown Court; he received a suspended sentence of 12 months imprisonment. In this case it was claimed that there was no way of alleviating the pain of the patient and he was asked by the patient to arrange for her to die. Dr Cox administered a lethal injection of potassium chloride which killed her. There is no doubt that the media was sympathetic, and when the case came before the General Medical Council considerable tolerance was shown. The professional conduct committee found that Dr Cox acted in good faith, and although in his actions he had 'fallen short of the high standards' expected in medicine he was allowed to continue the practice of medicine. Following this, he was reinstated by his employers with some minor conditions. There can be little doubt that the court, professional body and employing authority, recognised public and media support for actions which a few years previously would have resulted in grave punishment.

It was probably both the Bland and Cox cases that stimulated the House of Lords committee to consider the subject of euthanasia; nevertheless in early 1994 their unanimous report concluded that there should be no change in the law and that euthanasia should not be legalised. It was felt that vulnerable people – the elderly, sick or distressed – would feel pressure, whether real or imagined, to request early death. The committee endorsed patients' rights to refuse treatment; agreed that doctors should not take extraordinary measures to preserve life, and that adequate pain relief should be used even if this shortened life. Special mention was made to increase the use of advance directives or 'living wills' – a document in which people express how they wish to be treated if they become incapable of making or communicating a decision. Such documents are considered important in the United States in directing the care of patients and in England have been the subject of study and promotion by both Age Concern and the Terrence Higgins Trust.

Following many years of national debate, the Dutch Parliament in late 1993 approved a 28-point euthanasia guideline which, if followed, will allow a doctor immunity from prosecution. A request for euthanasia should be made personally by the patient, not by family or friends; the patient must be in unbearable or incurable pain, and be in a clear state of mind and request death repeatedly. The patient need not be terminally ill. The Dutch Parliament has not made euthanasia a statutory right and it remains a criminal offence; it is estimated that over 2000 cases of voluntary euthanasia may take place each year in the Netherlands.

In the United States the campaign to legalise euthanasia has gained enormous momentum, but remains confused. These efforts may be the backlash from the advanced technology that is now available to keep patients alive. There has developed a tacit acceptance of passive euthanasia, but it is in the area of active euthanasia where deliberate steps are taken to end life, that there is the most heated debate. In general philosophers can argue in conceptual terms very convincingly in favour, while medical practitioners are often opposed to active euthanasia. Overlying these debates is the 'slippery slope' argument – if one provides active euthanasia for those who are able to request it, active euthanasia may extend to those who are comatose or unable to express their wishes, and that this may further extend to the senile, the mentally ill and retarded.

In 1991 there was a state poll in Washington to legalise 'aid-in-dying', which despite many problems in the wording of the proposals, resulted in nearly 40 per cent of the voters being in favour of euthanasia. In 1992 the voters of California, by a narrow margin, did not wish to legalise 'doctor-assisted' suicide. At about the same time there was considerable publicity given to Dr Jack Kevorkian, a retired pathologist, who assisted a patient with Alzheimer's disease to take her life using his 'suicide machine' which administered lethal drugs through an intravenous line. Kevorkian later helped more patients to commit suicide in Michigan, a state that does not expressly forbid assisted suicide. This open activity and debate in the United States was further seen in April 1991 when a pro-euthanasia group, the Hemlock Society, published a book listing the types of drugs and dosages that should be taken to commit suicide. Apart from becoming a best-seller it was also recommended in the *New York Times*.

The contortions of the US system are further seen in 1994 where two courts issued absolutely opposite opinions about the constitutional rights to assisted suicide. In the first of these involving a further episode in the Kevorkian saga, a jury failed to convict him of assisting suicide of a patient, despite him clearly breaking a law specifically introduced to stop his activities using his 'suicide machine'! But on appeal the court declared that there is no constitutional right to suicide or assisted suicide. In contrast, the second case, a few days earlier, saw a court in Seattle decide that the state ban on assisted suicide violated the 14th Amendment of the Constitution by restricting a person's liberty.

Living wills were introduced during the 1960s in the United States; California was the first state to recognise these as legally binding documents; in 1992 Pennsylvania was the last state. New importance came in early 1994 when it became known that former President Richard Nixon had signed a living will instructing that he did not wish to be sustained by artificial means. This action seems to have profoundly impressed many of his fellow Americans. While polls show an overwhelming majority of Americans have no wish to be kept alive artificially if they have no hope of recovery, only about 20 per cent have signed living wills.

There is now an increased openness in discussion and debate about euthanasia, but the movement for voluntary euthanasia is not unchallenged; many professional groups remain opposed including major representatives of the hospice movement. Hospice philosophy does not favour euthanasia, and had it done so, it may be that the hospice concept would never have been born, because one aim was that by giving adequate care there would be no requests for euthanasia. But it can be argued that the majority of suffering patients are not looked after in hospices. Further, there are patients even within hospices who request a foreshortening of their life; who find the side-effects of medicines to control symptoms remove their mental faculties and independence, and who feel a weariness and tiredness and want to leave this world. It could be further argued that, because the hospice movement was founded on religious creeds, it follows the views of the main churches which oppose euthanasia, and may not represent the actual views of all those working in the hospice field.

Some of the religious aspects that relate to euthanasia have been mentioned earlier, and while the official doctrines of the main churches oppose euthanasia it is difficult to generalise the contemporary and future views of religious groups. The Papal encyclical *Gardium et Spec* reaffirmed the Vatican's absolute prohibition of euthanasia, but an NOP survey in 1985 suggested that 54 per cent of English Catholics favoured euthanasia. This may reflect the uncertainty whether any official body represents the views of its members. What has become clear is that there is not a religious consensus on this subject, because while only 54 per cent of Catholics in England supported euthanasia, such support was given by 75 per cent of Protestants and 84 per cent of Jews. The opinions of these religious groups 50 years ago is not known but these findings support the view that a person's ethical and moral views are influenced by their religious upbringing and that these views may be changing.

As pressure groups become more active and as more aspects of patient care are debated in public, there will be increased recourse to seeking judicial solutions. These difficulties may be further increased as economic and political policies become more apparent. It is envisaged that the expectations of patients may become more complex when political statements provide rights to patients as seen in the Patient's Charter 1991. Included in this, is that provision should be made so that personal consideration is shown to patients; it may be debated whether this would include a request for voluntary euthanasia.

Professional and other groups are attempting to form consensus views, codes and practices to embrace ethical considerations, but it may be impossible to form an acceptable common view in sensitive areas as the extent of treatment and euthanasia. The reasons for this difficulty is easier to understand if we remember the many complex elements that mould our individual moral codes, which in turn form our ethical principles, and that there are subtle changes in these codes and principles as our experiences are enlarged.

The implications of attempting to legalise euthanasia are immense because the present laws and professional codes are designed to protect everyone. This subject does not concern only the very ill patients with advanced cancer, it also concerns the mentally and physically infirm, those born with congenital abnormalities and even those who have a poor quality of life. In an ideal world it could be argued that care of the living should be so good that euthanasia is unwarranted, but sadly we are not in an ideal world. The problems remain – how can we balance the liberty and rights of a person that we aim to allow throughout life to also extend into their last days or weeks of life? How can the law protect everyone and yet recognise patient autonomy? Can patient autonomy be reconciled with professional ethics and social conscience? Despite differing philosophical standpoints there can be no disagreement that we should be compassionate in out tolerance, intentions and deeds.

Conclusions

Ethical and moral considerations are often the forgotten keystone of professional practice in caring for patients. Perhaps it is easier to overlook such considerations, but those people who are able to embrace this subject will experience a unique insight and a means to examine their own thinking and reasoning in making decisions and, at the same time, recognising the wishes of their patients.

Further reading

BURNARD, P. and CHAPMAN, C. M. (1988). *Professional and Ethical Issues in Nursing.* John Wiley, Chichester.

GLOVER, J. (1977). *Causing Death and Saving Lives.* Penguin, Harmondsworth.

MELIA, K. M. (1989). *Everyday Nursing Ethics.* Macmillan, Basingstoke.

SKEGG, P. D. G. (1984). *Law, Ethics, and Medicine.* Clarendon Press, Oxford.

3

The management of pain

Ray Corcoran

'All pain is subtle, variable and shifting. We are all unskilled in describing our pain. Few patients talk with their doctors, rather doctors and patients talk at each other. Of all health professionals, the nurse is unique in having close, trusted, prolonged contact. This position is one of enormous responsibility and opportunity. At a minimum, the nurse is in the position of translator. . . . At a maximum, the nurse is in a position of a research worker. . . . To liberate this crucial subject, nurses must first educate themselves and then the rest of us.'

Professor Patrick D. Wall, 1987

Introduction

Pain is probably the most feared symptom encountered in advanced cancer. To many people pain and cancer are synonymous. It is a common belief that having cancer means pain is unavoidable and must be accepted. Unfortunately poor management of cancer pain continues to perpetuate this myth. However, nothing could be further from the truth. One-third of advanced cancer patients do not experience pain. Of the remaining two-thirds pain relief can be achieved in about nine out of ten patients simply by applying a number of basic principles. Moreover it must be emphasised that this high degree of pain control can be achieved by the non-specialist. For the small minority in whom the pain persists despite the application of this basic approach, the family or hospital doctor should not hesitate to seek consultative assistance. There will be only a very small group in whom complete pain relief is not possible, but even these patients can be helped considerably so that they are able to cope with any residual pain. Thus cancer pain is neither inevitable nor uncontrollable.

Reasons for failure to relieve pain

There are many reasons but they project a single message – the need to educate and train medical students, doctors and nurses in cancer pain management. As part of an endeavour to educate there may be a need to advocate. If a patient is in pain it may be necessary for the informed carer to point out to other medical and nursing colleagues, in a considerate manner, the need to apply certain measures. The reasons for inadequate pain control include the following.

- *Lack of factual knowledge about analgesics.* The consequence is the prescribing of analgesics that are inappropriate, insufficient and infrequent. Constant cancer pain requires constant analgesia. This must be adequate and given regularly to stop the pain re-emerging. On demand 'PRN' (as required) prescribing only means 'pain relief now and then'.

- *Unfounded fears about addiction, tolerance, respiratory depression.* Too commonly these unnecessary fears mean morphine administration is delayed until the patient is 'really terminal', i.e. moribund. Moreover often it is unappreciated that in cancer pain, morphine doses have no 'ceiling' but must be titrated against the individual's pain.
- *Inaccurate assessment and reassessment.* Accurate assessment and reassessment of cancer pain are central to effective symptom control. Inaccurate diagnosis means inappropriate treatment. Inadequate review can mean inadequate control or unheeded resurgence. In other words, advanced cancer demands the logical approach of careful appraisal and repeated reappraisal.
- *Inadequate use of co-analgesics.* Often it is unappreciated that pains may be only partially responsive or unresponsive to morphine and a patient may need the support of other drugs. Such 'complementary' drugs, although usually having no intrinsic analgesic activity, can greatly help or even replace conventional analgesics in achieving pain control.
- *Inadequate emotional support and communication.* Such deficiencies towards the patient and family may be important reasons for unrelieved pain.
- *Non-use of non-drug measures.* Not all pains are responsive to drug therapy and non-drug interventions have an important role. In particular the use of palliative radiotherapy (see p. 50) and nerve blocks (see p. 51) should be kept in mind.

Assessment – the basis of rational treatment

'Pain' in cancer is a very general term. Most cancer patients have a number of pains. Four out of five cancer patients have at least two or more different pains, while one in three patients have four or more pains. Also, every pain is not a cancer pain. Patients often have pains not directly caused by the malignancy (e.g. dyspepsia, constipation, musculo-fascial pains, osteoarthritis, haemorrhoids, infections, etc.). As already emphasised, unless a considered judgement as to the most likely cause of each pain can be made, then rational treatment cannot be given. It behoves the nurse as much as the doctor to try and differentiate the various pains and to consider the most probable cause of each pain. Thus careful assessment of a patient's 'pain' is a vital part of management. Assessment has four major components.

- A detailed history.
- Accurate measurement.
- Consideration of the patient's 'total pain'.
- Repeated review.

A detailed history

Time spent taking a detailed history is never wasted. The following information should be obtained.

- *The sites of the various pains and their radiation.* These are best recorded on a body diagram (Fig. 3.1). This is especially helpful where there are a number of pains. Completing the body outline in conjunction with the patient can be very rewarding. Its accuracy is affirmed and it is comforting to the patient to see the obvious interest and concern about his or her pains.
- *Duration and frequency.* How long has the pain been present, whether it is constant. If it is intermittent, the frequency and length of each episode.

- *Quality.* Record the patients description of the pain i.e. whether dull, stabbing, aching, burning, etc.
- *Severity.* How severe is the pain? It should be noted that the demeanour of patient and the description of the severity of the pain may not be a reliable guide for a number of reasons. The patient may feel pain is inevitable or may wish to put on a stoic front. He or she may not wish to acknowledge the pain because of its significance (i.e. it indicates the cancer is still present and is progressing) or may fear possible adverse effects if analgesic drugs are prescribed. To obtain a realistic idea the carer should always enquire
  - whether sleep is disturbed
  - whether daily routines or activities have become restricted
  - what drugs have relieved or failed to relieve the pain.

Wherever possible relatives should be interviewed, for their comments may indicate the true level of suffering.

Accurate measurement

The severity of the patient's pain can be measured in a number of ways.

- A popular method is the use of the visual analogue scale (VAS) (Fig. 3.2). The patient is asked to put a mark (or says where a mark should be placed) on

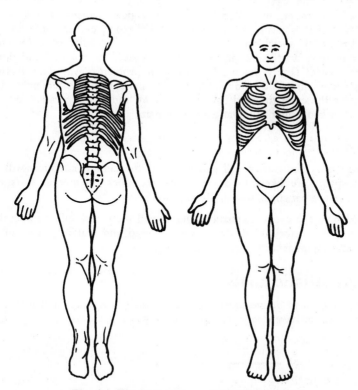

Fig. 3.1 The body diagram (one-third scale).

a 10-cm line according to the severity of the pain, where 0 cm is 'no pain' and 10 cm is 'the worst pain imaginable'. A simple variant of this approach, which most patients have no difficulty in appreciating, is for the carer to draw an imaginary, vertical VAS in the air with their finger and to ask where, between the imaginary 0 and 10, would the patients put their present pain. Some patients become so adept at this that in subsequent assessments they will quote a figure as the carer approaches, without waiting for a prompt!

• Another method is to grade the pain 0–5 according to the description of the pain's intensity i.e. McGill Melzack present pain intensity (PPI) (Fig. 3.3).
• A method that can give patients at home a very real sense of contributing to their management and having some control of the situation is to ask them to keep a pain diary. A set framework can be followed, for example The London Hospital Home Diary (Raiman, 1988), or the format can be personalised according to the individual. Aspects needing evaluation are pain at or over regular intervals; changes in analgesic requirements; sleep disturbances due to pain; and the development of new pains and other symptoms.

All the above methods can be helpful in monitoring the efficacy of any form of treatment but especially drug therapy.

Consideration of the patient's 'total pain'

Pain is an interweaving of physical and psychological elements and it is essential that an assessment is made of the patient's 'total pain', i.e. not only the physical but the emotional, social and spiritual pain. The intensity of such emotional aspects as anxiety, depression, anger, hostility, should be assessed and note taken of the presence of family, financial or spiritual problems. Any such features can lower the pain threshold and intensify the patient's physical pain. It is so important for the carer to stand back and look at 'the whole person' and consider the various components of the patient's total pain.

Repeated review

Almost invariably the cancer will progress and the clinical situation will change. Thus new pains are likely to develop and old ones re-emerge. It is essential therefore that the patient is repeatedly reviewed.

In addition to the above assessment the overall picture should be completed by taking a detailed history of all drugs administered and making a careful note of the physical findings recorded by medical colleagues.

Setting realistic goals

It is always helpful to delineate in one's mind what one wants to achieve. In pain relief it is useful to have a sequence of realistic goals, such as:

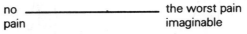

Fig. 3.2 The visual analogue scale (not to scale).

0   No pain
1   Mild
2   Discomforting
3   Distressing
4   Horrible
5   Excruciating

Fig. 3.3 The McGill Melzack present pain intensity (PPI).

- initially to give the patient a pain-free night's sleep;
- then to relieve the pain at rest during the day;
- then to relieve the pain on standing or moving. This form of pain can be a particular problem.

The concept of a 'mosaic of therapies'

Although drug therapy is the mainstay of cancer pain management, alleviation of a patient's pain requires more than just the prescribing of analgesics or co-analgesics. Drugs can never be more than one of a number of approaches needed for pain control. Having stood back and looked at the whole person the carer should choose a combination of measures appropriate for the individual. Keeping in one's mind the image of a 'mosaic' of the measures can be a great help in making this choice. The principal 'pieces' of this 'therapeutic mosaic' comprises the following (Fig. 3.4):

- analgesics;
- co-analgesics;
- psychological approaches;
- physical therapies;
- radiotherapy;
- nerve blocks.

Analgesics

Analgesics are at the centre of any personal group of therapies. The key to effective pain control is to use a few well-known analgesics in a simple sequence of prescribing steps, i.e. an 'analgesic staircase' (Fig. 3.5).

The analgesic staircase

For mild to moderate pain. Start at the bottom of the staircase and prescribe a mild 'non-opioid' analgesic such as regular aspirin or paracetamol. If one of these is ineffective it should not be replaced by the other but by regular administration of a drug from the next 'weak opioid' or 'mild analgesic' step, i.e. codeine, dihydrocodeine or dextropropoxyphene, with or without paracetamol or aspirin. If pain relief is still not achieved with the recommended maximum dose of one of these agents then movement should be upwards to the top 'strong opioid' step and regular morphine commenced. There is no particular advantage in using oral diamorphine rather than oral morphine. Both have similar actions and unwanted effects and diamorphine is rapidly converted into morphine following ingestion.

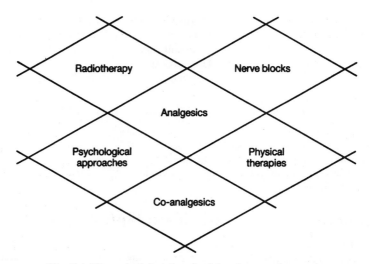

Fig. 3.4 The principle 'pieces' of the therapeutic mosaic.

If the pain is severe. Go straight to the top step and administer a strong opioid from the start.

Duration of the effect of oral morphine solution

Morphine is commonly administered as morphine aqueous solution. The doctor can prescribe it as such or as 'morphine aqueous mixture'. Morphine given orally in this form is relatively well absorbed and peak blood levels are reached after $1^{1}/_{2}$ to 2 h. The clinical effect of a single dose lasts for about 4 h. In general therefore it is illogical to prescribe morphine solution other than every 4 h. Despite this, it

				STRONG OPIOIDS
		WEAK OPIOIDS		Morphine Hydrochloride or Sulphate
		Codeine Phosphate	15–60 mg	Diamorphine Hydrochloride
		Tablets Syrup	4 hrly	
	NON-OPIOIDS	Dihydrocodeine	30–60 mg	
Aspirin	300–600 mg			
Tablets	4–6 hrly	Tablets	4 hrly	
(Soluble form available)		Elixir		
Paracetamol	0.5–1 G.	Dextropropoxyphene	2 tablets	
Tablets	4–6 hrly	and Paracetamol	4–8 hrly	
(Soluble form available)		(Co-proxamol)		

Fig. 3.5 The analgesic staircase. See text for details.

is not unusual to see it prescribed 6–8-hourly. This means for 2 or 4 h the pain will be back, but worse, for it becomes fuelled by spiralling anxiety. Seldom is less frequent administration indicated, although it may be necessary with impaired renal function or if the patient is very old and frail.

Individualisation of morphine dose

Morphine is pre-eminent as an oral analgesic in advanced cancer and, given regularly, will achieve relief in eight or nine out of every ten patients. However, the dose required by any one patient is very variable and the morphine require-ments must be individualised. As has been pointed out, there is no 'ceiling dose'. The dose ultimately required must be attained by titration of the dose against the intensity of the individual's pain. Thus there will be a wide range of doses.

Irrespective of its size each 4–hourly dose can be dispensed by a pharmacist as morphine sulphate or hydrochloride aqueous solution in a volume of 10 ml. This is preferable and safer for most patients at home. It can be very difficult for some patients and relatives to draw up varying volumes of a concentrated morphine sulphate solution into a calibrated dropper.

Dose titration and increment range

Dose titration is central to successful pain control. About seven out of every ten patients will require no more than 30 mg morphine solution 4–hourly. Of the remainder a few will need more than 100 mg 4–hourly. More rarely some individuals will need very high doses. By how much should an individual dose of morphine be increased? There are a number of possible sequences. A commonly used sequence is that suggested by Twycross and Lack (1984), i.e. 5–10–15–20–30–40–60–80–100–120–160–200–240 mg/4–hourly, etc.

The initial dose of morphine solution

The initial dose of oral morphine solution also must be individualised. It will depend on the patient's previous analgesic requirements, the severity of the pain and the patient's age. If the 'analgesic staircase' has been ascended many will require an initial dose of 10 mg 4–hourly: for others 5 mg 4–hourly may be more appropriate. If the patient is elderly, frail or impaired renal function is suspected, an initial dose of 2.5 mg 4–hourly may be adequate. If there is doubt about the magnitude of the initial dose, prescribe a smaller dose and increase this rapidly if it is obvious the pain is not being mitigated. If the pain is controlled by the first dose but the patient is extremely sleepy the next dose should be reduced by 50 per cent.

The bedtime and 'middle-of-the-night' dose

When dose requirements of oral morphine solution have become stabilised often a patient will not need a 'middle-of-the-night' dose, i.e. 2.00 am dose. However, should the patient wake with pain this can be negated by doubling the bedtime (10.00 pm) dose (for those having a dose of 40 mg every 4 h during the day) or increasing it by 50 per cent (for those having a dose of 60 mg or more every 4 h during the day). In some units the augmentation of the bedtime dose is a standard practice. If nightmares or hallucinations should occur with this bedtime increase then routine 4-hourly administrations should be adopted throughout the 24 h.

Controlled-release morphine and mild/moderate pain

Morphine solution can be administered regularly every 4 h without difficulty in the hospice or hospital. In the less well-controlled environment of home the taking of frequent medication on time cannot be guaranteed. For this reason, when analgesia requirements for mild to moderate pain have reached the top step of the staircase many doctors prefer to prescribe twice daily controlled-release morphine (CRM).

CRM is a most valuable form of morphine and has been developed to reduce dose frequency. The various formulations allow the release of morphine over a period of 12 h. Following the taking of a CRM tablet peak plasma concentrations of morphine are achieved after about 2–4 h.

The controlled-release preparation MST Continus has been available for many years. Other CRM preparations that have become available include SRM-Rhotard and Oramorph SR tablets. When a patient is commenced on CRM it is advisable that the various CRM preparations are not interchanged with one another but that the patient is maintained on doses of the particular CRM initially prescribed.

Various strengths of CRM tablets allow wide flexibility in dosage and patient and carer are not faced with an inordinate number of single strength tablets as increasing dosages become necessary. Tablets of 10, 30, 60 and 100 mg are available in all CRM preparations and also 5, 15 and 200 mg tablets are available as MST Continus. For those patients who are unable to swallow tablets or opioid medication has to be administered via a nasogastric tube or a gastrostomy a full range of CRM liquids (MST Continus suspensions) are available in sachets of 20, 30, 60, 100 and 200 mg. The contents of one 20, 30 or 60 mg preparation should be mixed with at least 10 ml of water. The 100 mg sachet should be mixed with at least 20 ml of water and the 200 mg sachet with at least 30 ml of water. The suspensions so formed should be used immediately after preparation. Alternatively the MST Continus granules can be sprinkled onto soft food, e.g. yoghurt.

When the analgesic staircase has been ascended the starting dose of CRM is usually 30 mg 12-hourly. However, as in the case of morphine solution, if the patient is old or frail, or impaired renal function is known or suspected, lower doses may be needed, for example 20 mg 12-hourly or even, very occasionally, 10 mg 12-hourly.

If the pain is not completely allayed CRM dosage should be increased keeping the intervals 12-hourly. At high doses, with many tablets to take, some patients may be given CRM 8-hourly, but this agent should never be given more frequently, otherwise potentially dangerous cumulation may occur.

CRM and severe pain

The slow absorption of CRM and its prolonged action makes this form of morphine unsuitable for the initial treatment of severe pain. The flexibility of morphine solution, given 4-hourly, is needed to be able to rapidly increase the dose to an effective level. However, once the dosage of morphine solution has been stabilised it is usually possible to revert to 12-hourly CRM therapy.

CRM and breakthrough pain

Similarly, CRM is too slowly absorbed to be suitable for treating 'breakthrough' pain. Where pain has been well controlled with CRM twice daily, 'moderate' breakthrough pain on one or two occasions may be treated with dextromoramide given sublingually or orally, or with a single dose of morphine solution. The additional dose of either of these agents may be half or the whole of a single 4-hourly dose of morphine, depending on the intensity of the pain and the magnitude of the regular dose of morphine currently being given. Very severe breakthrough pain will require immediate review of the clinical situation and usually the administration of subcutaneous diamorphine. If frequent exacerbations occur and repeated 'top-up' dose of analgesics are needed to achieve pain control, a new adequate level of regular analgesia must be re-established. This may be accomplished by changing the CRM therapy to 4-hourly aqueous morphine solution and reverting back to CRM later at a different dose when a new effective dose level of morphine solution has been achieved. If the breakthrough pain does not respond to additional opioid the patient's condition needs careful reassessment with consideration of other methods of pain control.

Conversion to CRM

It used to be recommended that when transferring from 4-hourly morphine to CRM the first dose of CRM should be given simultaneously with the last dose of ordinary-release morphine. This is not considered necessary now and the CRM preparation can be commenced 4 h after the last dose of ordinary-release morphine.

Some studies have suggested that CRM (in the form of MST Continus) is equianalgesic mg for mg with diamorphine. Other trials have shown MST morphine to be equianalgesic mg for mg with morphine solution. Although CRM (as MST Continus) has been considered to be better absorbed than morphine solution (having about a fifth greater bioavailability) in practice seemingly this has little or no effect and patients can be transferred from either oral morphine or diamorphine with little or no adjustment of CRM needed (Regnard and Tempest, 1992). In general, the total daily CRM dosage is equated with the total daily dose of morphine solution being taken. The strength of each 12-hourly CRM dose is obtained by dividing the total daily morphine requirement by a factor of two; for example

$$20 \text{ mg morphine 4-hourly} = 120 \text{ mg in 24 h}$$
$$= 1 \times 60 \text{ mg CRM tablet 12-hourly.}$$

Regular 4-hourly morphine at home

One needs to prescribe a preparation that will be easy for patients or for their carers to administer. Also it will need to have wide flexibility of dosing to allow titration. Moreover a tablet form may be preferred to a solution. Prescribing costs also will be a pertinent consideration.

The proprietary preparations available include:

(a) Morphine sulphate tablets (Sevredol) – 10 and 20 mg tablets.
(b) Morphine sulphate solution (Oramorph oral solution) – 10 mg/5 ml.
(c) Concentrated morphine sulphate solution (Oramorph concentrated oral solution)

20 mg/ml. Varying amounts (and therefore doses) may be added to any flavoured soft drink via a calibrated dropper.
(d) Ready prepared unit doses in the form of unit dose vials (Oramorph UDV). Three strengths are available in separate vials 10 mg/5 ml, 30 mg/5 ml, 100 g/5 ml. The dose can be squirted into the mouth or mixed with a soft drink.

A simple 'generic' alternative is to prescribe one bottle of 'morphine sulphate solution' of a set strength, namely the required 4-hourly dose in 10 ml. As suggested by Twycross and Lack (1984) the next increment can be 50 per cent with a possible second increase of 33 per cent before a new supply of morphine is prescribed, i.e. an initial dose of 10 ml may be increased to 15 ml (50 per cent) and then to 20 ml (33 per cent). If this approach is favoured, to avoid anxiety it should be explained to the patient and relatives that a dose 'range' may be necessary from a particular bottle having a fixed initial dose stated on its label.

Whichever preparation is prescribed, clear written instructions should always be given to the patient and family.

Side-effects of morphine and diamorphine

The most common side-effects are drowsiness, constipation, nausea and vomiting.

Drowsiness. Drowsiness when it occurs, is usually transient over 2 or 3 days and this will need to be explained to the patient and family.

Constipation. Constipation almost always occurs in patients taking weak or strong opioids and it is imperative that prophylactic laxatives are prescribed. The preferred approach is the administration of a bowel stimulant with a faecal softener. Such a combination can be prescribed together most conveniently in the form of co-danthrusate capsules (danthron and docusate) or co-danthramer plain or forte liquid or capsules (danthron + poloxamer). Alternatively the combination can be given as two separate products, for example senna + lactulose. The latter softens the faecal contents and stimulates peristalsis, but often with opiates an additional stronger peristaltic stimulant such as senna is required. Sodium picosulphate (Laxoberal) is another stimulant that can be used.

Whether given as a combination or two separate agents, conventional doses often are ineffective in the presence of opiates and the laxative dose must be titrated against the patient's response. Constipation due to the failure to give laxatives prophylactically with opiates is a needless, major problem. It causes so much unnecessary trouble, for example nausea and vomiting, anorexia, and abdominal pain confusion.

Nausea and vomiting. Nausea and vomiting due to morphine therapy is not inevitable. It occurs in about one in three patients. It is more common in the ambulant. Tolerance develops to nausea and vomiting and usually it disappears after 7–10 days. In hospice units anti-emetics are no longer given prophylactically but, in the home, practitioners may feel more comfortable to continue this practice for the first week or 10 days. An antiemetic acting against the chemo-trigger zone (the subsidiary central nervous system emetic centre sensitive to chemical changes) is preferable, for example haloperidol, domperidone, metoclopramide or prochlorperazine.

Confusion and hallucinations. In respect of other side-effects, confusion occurs in about 2 per cent and nightmares and hallucinations in about 1 per cent of patients. If such side-effects do not respond to dose reduction (if feasible) or to an adequate dose of haloperidol, another opioid should be substituted.

Rectal and parenteral administration

Rectal or parenteral administration will be required when oral administration or morphine is impracticable due to the following.

* vomiting;
* dysphagia;
* coma;
* profound weakness.

Analgesic suppositories. Morphine suppositories may be a useful alternative to injections: 15 and 30 mg strength suppositories are readily available but other strengths will be made by the pharmacist. The suppositories may be directly substituted for ordinary oral morphine, i.e. the same dose and same time interval should be used.

Another morphine-like agonist, oxycodone, is available in suppository form. Oxycodone pectinate (Proladone) suppositories can be used at 6–8-hourly intervals. Each suppository is of 30 mg strength and in practice can be considered to be equivalent to about 30 mg oral morphine (i.e. 15 mg morphine solution 4-hourly for two doses). The suppository form now available is not easily divided.

Dextromoramide (Palfium) suppositories in 10 mg strength are also available. These have only a 2–3-hour duration of action and are best reserved for breakthrough pain.

Parenteral diamorphine. When parenteral medication is required, diamorphine is preferred to morphine. Because of its much greater solubility only impressively small volumes of diamorphine are needed for injection. Generally the oral dose or morphine should be divided by three to obtain the equivalent dose of parenteral diamorphine. The oral dose of diamorphine should be divided by a factor of two. Thus the general rule is 3 mg oral morphine = 2 mg oral diamorphine = 1 mg parenteral diamorphine (Fig. 3.6). For morphine alone 2 mg oral morphine = 1 mg parenteral morphine.

The syringe driver

Subcutaneous diamorphine may be given intermittently at regular intervals. If this is favoured, regular administration via a butterfly needle placed *in situ* will obviate repeated piercing of the skin. However, the method of choice for this route is to administer the drug continuously via a subcutaneous butterfly needle from a battery-operated 'syringe driver'. Some care-givers will only use diamorphine alone in the syringe driver; most will use a mixture of diamorphine and other agents as required.

Advice about syringe drivers. Macmillan nurses and colleagues in palliative care units or in pain clinics are always ready to advise about the use of this method. Published information is also readily available (Doyle, 1987; Regnard and Tempest, 1992).

Availability of syringe drivers. More and more general practices and hospital units are obtaining syringe drivers, but they should never be used as a means of convenience and used only when the above indications are present. Some Macmillan nurse home support teams, palliative care units and hospital support teams may loan syringe drivers for specific patients.

Diamorphine and other drugs in the syringe driver. Diamorphine used in a syringe driver can be mixed safely with hyoscine hydrobromide (Scopolamine), hyoscine butylbromide (Buscopan), metoclopramide (Maxolon), haloperidol, methotrimeprazine (Nozinan), midazolam. Cyclizine lactate can react with diamorphine hydrochloride to form an insoluble precipitate. The concentration of each drug has a bearing on the reaction. It is likely to occur if either the concentration of cyclizine or the diamorphine is greater than 25 mg/ml. However, if the concentration of one of these drugs is not greater than 10 mg/ml then the other concentration can be higher than 25 mg/ml.

Sublingual administration

Sublingual administration can be an effective route where doses are relatively low and increases of analgesia are infrequent. On other occasions it can be a disappointing approach. Difficulties may arise due to the following.

- Frequent increases mean an increasing number of tablets to be put under the tongue.
- The increasing taste of the drug in the mouth becomes unacceptable.
- The patient has a persistently dry mouth (common in many patients) so that tablets do not dissolve easily with consequent poor absorption.

Analgesics given sublingually are dextromoramide, phenazocine and buprenorphine. The former two are active if swallowed.

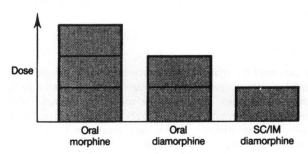

Fig. 3.6 Morphine–diamorphine equivalents.

Other alternative strong analgesics

In the majority of patients morphine sulphate or hydrochloride is effective and acceptable. However, the patient may show an intolerance that necessitates a change to an alternative strong analgesic or a particular opioid preparation may be more appropriate or preferred. Carers who treat advanced cancer patients will need to consider the other strong analgesics available. Some are more potent than morphine and conversion doses will need to be estimated with care.

A strong opioid that has come on to the market recently and is attracting great interest is that of Fentanyl administered transdermally via a skin patch.

The Transdermal Fentanyl 'skin patch' system

Until recently a synthetic opioid analgesic called Fentanyl, which has been in use for over 30 years in anaesthesia and intensive care, was available only in an injectable form. However, now the pharmaceutical company Janssen has formulated this strong opioid into a transdermal skin patch ('Durogesic').

This transdermal system offers a novel alternative administration of a strong opioid in clinical situations where oral therapy is difficult (Zech *et al.*, 1994), e.g. difficulty in swallowing, nausea and vomiting, situations where consistent administration or intake of medicines is difficult, or possibly whether there are significant adverse effects from other opioids. In respect of the latter, although Fentanyl shares the opioid side-effects of morphine, it may well be that this agent causes less adverse actions compared to other opioids (see below).

The Fentanyl transdermal system. The patch or 'transdermal therapeutic system (TTS)' is a rectangular, transparent unit, comprising four functional layers on a protective liner, the latter being removed before application to the skin. The patch or TTS is designed to release Fentanyl continuously into the systemic circulation for 72 h. The release of Fentanyl from a reservoir gel within the patch is controlled by a special release membrane. The amount released (and therefore the plasma concentrations achieved) is proportional to the surface area of the patch. There are four patch sizes available, namely 10, 20, 30 and 40 cm^2, delivering 25, 50, 75 or 100 µg/h of Fentanyl, respectively. The Fentanyl diffuses from within the patch and permeates the outer layers of the skin to reach the subcutaneous zone where it is absorbed into the systemic circulation. The adhesive layer that attaches the patch to the skin is also saturated with Fentanyl and provides the initial loading of the drug. A backing layer forms a protective barrier preventing loss of Fentanyl from the outer surface of the patch.

Pharmacokinetics of the Fentanyl transdermal system. Before diffusing subcutaneously into the systemic circulation, the Fentanyl forms a depot in the upper skin layers. Thus Fentanyl blood concentrations are hardly measurable until 2 h after the application and analgesic plasma concentrations take 6–12 h to occur after the first application. The blood concentrations rise steadily and reach a peak after about 24 h and remain reasonably constant for 72 h. Blood levels can be maintained thereafter by patch replacement every 72 h.

Following removal of a patch the Fentanyl blood concentrations decline only gradually falling about 50 per cent in 17 h (range 13–22 h). This is because there is continued absorption from a reservoir of Fentanyl within the skin and this is only slowly cleared.

Disposal of used patches. Used patches still contain a significant amount of Fentanyl and should be discarded with care. The patient or professional should fold the patch in half with the adhesive side inwards, place it in its original pouch and return it to the pharmacist. Some professionals dispose of the used pouches via their 'sharps' bin'.

Clinical efficacy in cancer patients with pain. A multicentre study (TTS–Fentanyl Multicentre Study Group, 1994) found that the Fentanyl transdermal system provided good pain relief in the majority of patients. It also showed that the system appears to have several advantages compared with oral morphine, for example, improved quality of sleep and morning vigilance, less nausea and vomiting, less constipation, and less breakthrough pain.

Practical details. Although the product can be used in 'strong opioid–naive patients' it would seem prudent until more information is available on use in such patients, that general usage of this product is confined to patients who are already taking strong opioids. Because of the reduced flexibility of dosage, the product is best used in patients with stable, controlled pain, and stable low-to-medium strong opioid requirements.

The initial dose of Fentanyl should be based on the previous 2-h opioid requirements. A recommended conversion scheme from oral morphine is presented in the product's data sheet and also can be calculated from a 'dosage calendar'. For example, a patient using up to 135 mg of oral morphine over 24 h would require a 25 µg/h patch, whereas a patient needing 135–224 mg of morphine over 24 h would require a 50 µg/h patch, and so on. Additional or alternative methods of analgesia should be considered when the patch dose exceeds 300 µg/h.

Because of the delay in analgesic levels of Fentanyl being obtained, ordinary release morphine may be needed for analgesic cover during the first 6–12 h for any breakthrough pain thereafter. The initial dose of patch selected is likely to be adequate in only half or more of patients, so adequate supervision and review is essential. Titration of additional patches generally should be in 25 µg/h steps, based on the patient's response and additional opioid requirements of breakthrough pain during the 72-h application period. Patients using Fentanyl can experience any of the side–effects associated with a potent opioid and it should be remembered that it takes time for Fentanyl plasma levels to decline (i.e. an average 17 h for a 50 per cent reduction in serum levels) and appropriate measures will need to be instituted and maintained for 24 h or more.

As for any opioid drug, initial dosage of Fentanyl and further increments should be considered carefully in the elderly, the frail, or patients with known or suspected renal or liver dysfunction .

Patients who develop fever should be monitored carefully for opioid side–effects since significant increase in body temperature can potentially increase the Fentanyl delivery rate. Exposing the application site to direct external heat source should be avoided.

As with all strong opioids, some patients may experience significant respiratory depression with the Fentanyl transdermal system and patients must be carefully observed for these effects. As mentioned above in respect of adverse effects, respiratory depression may persist after removal of the patch and appropriate treatment may need to be continued for 24 h or more. An opioid antagonist such as naloxone can be administered and repeated doses or a continuous infusion may be required. The incidence of respiratory depression increases as the Fentanyl dose is increased. Consideration of analgesic requirements and careful repeated assessment should be made of patients where analgesic requirements are likely to change, either rapidly, for example after a nerve block, or progressively with time, for example, after radiotherapy for a painful malignant focus.

Skin application of the Fentanyl system. Skin sites should be rotated with each application so as to minimise variations in blood levels resulting in build-up of subcutaneous skin depots. In patients requiring high opioid dosage or patients with skin diseases, it may be difficult to find suitable sites for patch application. The patches should not be applied on broken skin (serum Fentanyl concentrations can be increased 5-fold) but applied to a dry, intact, non-irradiated, and hairless area, preferably over the torso or upper arm. Hairy body areas should not be shaved but clipped. If the site of application needs to be cleaned it should be done with water and not with soap, oils, lotions, or any other agents that might irritate the skin or alter the skin permeability. The skin should be completely dry before the system is applied and patients may require micropore tape to guarantee proper patch adhesion. Since the adhesive layer is impregnated with Fentanyl, hands should be washed after patch application.

Fentanyl patches are contraindicated in patients with known hypersensitivity to Fentanyl or to the adhesive in the system. Local skin reactions such as rash, erythema and itching have been occasionally reported following application of a patch. These usually resolve within 24 h of patch removal.

Future clinical assessment. Increased clinical experience in the use of these patches will determine more fully the significance of any advantages over oral morphine and whether these advantages can justify the increased cost of prescribing this product. Moreover, further clinical experience will help delinate any significant advantages over syringe driver administration of opioids such as diamorphine, especially as so often this route is necessary for the administration of other drugs besides the opioid. Another advantage that has been advanced is that nursing time involved in administering opioids will be reduced. In the community, it has been propounded that district or community nurses will not need to visit so often. It would be unfortunate if this meant the emotional support given to cancer patients and their families at home would be reduced. Hopefully such patients will continue to be visited anyway and the time normally spent in putting out tablets or recharging a syringe driver will be used to give extra emotional support to them as well as to other patients and families.

Additional strong analgesics (Table 3.1)

Some features of other alternatives are as follows:

- Phenazocine (Narphen) can be a useful alternative on occasions. A 5 mg tablet is equivalent to about 20 mg of oral morphine. Although it can be swallowed

Table 3.1 Approximate oral morphine equivalents

Drug	Tablet strength	Duration of action	Four-hourly oral morphine equivalents
Buprenorphine (Temgesic)	0.2 mg	(sublingually) 8 hourly	10 mg
Dextromoramide (Palfium)	5 mg	2–3 hourly	10 mg
Dipipanone+cyclizine (Diconal)	10 mg (+ 30 mg Cyclizine)	3–5 hourly	5 mg
Levorphanol (Dromoran)	1.5 mg	4–6 hourly	7.5 mg
Oxycodone pectinate (Proladone)	30 mg (suppository)	6–8 hourly	15 mg (×2)
Papaveretum	10 mg	3–5 hourly	5 mg
Pethidine	50 mg	2–3 hourly	6 mg
Phenazocine (Narphen)	5 mg	(sublingually) 4-6 hourly	20 mg

the tablet dissolves readily in the mouth and therefore the drug is often used sublingually. A single dose lasts 6–8 h and thus it does not need to be taken as often as morphine solution. Patients may need to be helped to break the small scored tablets when the drug is replacing lower doses of morphine. Sucking a sweet at the same time as the sublingual tablet is under the tongue can mask the bitter taste if this is a problem.

- Dextromoramide (Palfium). This is a valuable agent for breakthrough pain or to cover short-interval pain associated with a practical procedure. Although active orally it is frequently used sublingually. It is rapidly absorbed from under the tongue and as it is not ingested it does not have to pass across the intestinal mucosa or pass through the liver. Both these sites normally metabolise part of the drug (known as the 'first-pass' effect) so by-passing them will result in higher blood levels. This drug acts for only 2–3 h so it should not be used for routine treatment of cancer pain.

- Buprenorphine (Temgesic). This analgesic is a 'partial agonist', i.e. it has a stronger affinity for opioid receptors than a 'pure agonist' such as morphine but evokes less response. The place of the partial agonist in cancer pain management is not fully established (Atkinson *et al.*, 1989). There has been a debate about the use of buprenorphine for a number of years. In the past, authorities have been concerned that because buprenorphine is a partial agonist, it would block or displace morphine from the opioid receptors with impairment of pain control, if they were used together. There is no advantage in using them both simultaneously and no interference has been noted when morphine has been given directly after a patient has been taking buprenorphine (Atkinson *et al.*, 1989).

There has also been concern about buprenorphine's 'analgesic ceiling', i.e. a dose level beyond which no increased benefit occurs. The analgesic ceiling has been stated to occur at a daily dose of about 5 mg, i.e. equivalent to about 50 mg of aqueous morphine 4-hourly (Zenz, 1988). Seemingly the position now is that, if a practitioner felt it necessary to add buprenorphine to the analgesic staircase (see Fig. 3.5), its position is between step two and early step three (Atkinson *et al.*, 1989).

- Methadone. This is cumulative and should not be generally used in the elderly or debilitated. Use in others is best carried out with expert help. Methadone, however, is favoured in 'paradoxical pain' (see below).
- Levorphanol (Dromoran) should be avoided in the elderly. It has been used successfully in younger patients. It is five times more potent than morphine and the duration of action is about 6 h.
- Dipipanone (as Diconal) has very limited use owing to its combination with cyclizine.
- Pethidine. This drug has no role in protracted cancer pain. It has too short an action. Cumulation of the toxic metabolite norpethidine and the number of tablets needed when substituted for morphine also negate its use.
- Pentazocine (Fortral). This is another analgesic agent that has no place in the management of chronic cancer pain. The drug should not be given concurrently with morphine. It has partial antagonistic activity that will reduce the effectiveness of morphine and can intensify the pain.

Paradoxical pain

It has been proposed that there may be some instances of cancer pain in which increasing doses of morphine or diamorphine induces 'paradoxical pain', i.e. pain which is expected to respond to opioids but which ceases to be relieved or is worsened by further administration of the opioid.

It is suggested that such pains may arise because of abnormal metabolism of morphine. Morphine is metabolised in the liver to 3- and 6-glucuronide. 6-Glucuronide is inactive. Thus a patient's analgesic response to morphine appears to depend on the 3-glucuronide:6-glucuronide ratio, the 6-glucuronide being responsible for the analgesic effect.

It has been suggested that paradoxical pain arises when abnormal metabolism of morphine occurs so that there is production of higher than usual quantities of 3-glucuronide and lower quantities of 6-glucuronide. In some patients considered to be exhibiting paradoxical pain such a change in ratio has been found.

Whether such differences are inherent or are induced by disease, drugs or age is not known. The strong opioid methadone does not follow the same metabolic pathways as morphine and so it has been suggested that this opioid may be useful in instances of paradoxical pain. Clinical experience has found it effective in patients who are said to have been experiencing this form of pain.

The concept of paradoxical pain remains a matter for debate but if such a form of pain is suspected, then specialist opinion and advice should be sought.

The Brompton cocktail or mixture

This is the name given to mixtures containing morphine or diamorphine in fixed amounts with cocaine, chlorpromazine and alcohol. There is no longer a place for such mixtures in modern therapeutics. They have no advantages over simple morphine solutions and have decided disadvantages. Increasing the opiate means increasing the chlorpromazine (which does not potentiate the analgesic effect of the opiate) and results in unnecessary sedation. Moreover the cocaine can cause unpleasant hallucinations, especially in the elderly.

Co-analgesia

Co-analgesia is an important part of any therapeutic approach and the co-analgesics are a most varied and interesting group of compounds. Almost all have no conventional analgesic activity but nevertheless their actions may complement or supplant accepted analgesics.

Morphine is an excellent drug but it is not a panacea and there are cancer pains that may be only partially responsive or unresponsive to opiates. Co-analgesics often help allay these pains or support more active procedures such as radiotherapy, nerve blocks, surgery, etc.

The two most widely used co-analgesics are corticosteroids and non-steroidal anti-inflammatory drugs (NSAIDs).

Corticosteroids

Corticosteroids act as co-analgesics by reducing the overall mass of a malignant tumour. Pain from tumour pressure on nerves, brain or hollow organs is thereby relieved. A malignant tumour comprises a central mass of cancer cells surrounded by a non-cancerous zone of chronically inflamed, oedematous tissue. The latter contributes significantly to the total tumour mass. High-dose steroids do not affect the cancer cells but they frequently produce a marked shrinkage of the outer inflammatory zone.

Corticosteroids assist in pain relief in the following situations:

- raised intracranial pressure;
- nerve compression;
- hepatomegaly;
- head and neck tumour;
- spinal cord compression (as an emergency 'holding' effect);
- intrapelvic tumour;
- abdominal tumour.

There are two principal corticosteroids – dexamethasone and prednisolone. Dexamethasone is normally the steroid of choice. It is more potent than prednisolone (2 mg of dexamethasone = 15 mg prednisolone) and hence far fewer tablets have to be taken by the patient. There are 2 mg and 0.5 mg dexamethasone tablets available. It is not always appreciated that these tablets can be dissolved easily in water if desired.

When prescribing corticosteroids as a co-analgesic an initial high dose needs to be given to effect reduction of the chronic inflammatory zone. Thereafter the dosage needs to be reduced progressively to the lowest maintenance dose that controls symptoms, otherwise serious side-effects may occur.

There are various patterns of prescribing corticosteroids, as described below.

- Generally the traditional dose to relieve the headache and other effects of raised intracranial pressure from a brain tumour is 16 mg per day. However, on some occasions, 20–24 mg per day may be considered more appropriate.

- Usually smaller doses, for example 8-12 mg per day, may be given to relieve hepatomegaly, nerve compression, bowel or bronchus compression, etc.
- There are various approaches to reducing the dose of steroids. To obviate serious side-effects most practitioners now favour a relatively rapid reduction over 10–14 days once an initial response has been obtained, for example one method is to maintain the high initial dose for 4–5 days and reduce the dosage thereafter by 2 mg per day every third day to a maintenance dose of 2–4 mg per day. Others may favour a more gradual reduction.
- Response to high dose steroids usually occurs within 24–48 h. If this does not occur generally it is advocated that high doses should be continued for at least a week before it can be said that where has been no response. If there is no improvement after that time the drug can be discontinued.
- The dexamethasone may be given as one or two doses, i.e. in the morning and early afternoon. Sometimes the drug is given four times a day but corticosteroids enhance brain activity and, for some people, later doses may result in insomnia. (Corticosteroids may also stimulate appetite and elevate mood and are often given in small doses to try and produce this effect.)

The nurse will need to become familiar with the patterns of prescribing corticosteroids in his or her own area.

The tumour shrinkage from corticosteroids is temporary. It may last weeks or months. As they have no effect on the actual cancer cells pressure effects will recur as the true tumour mass grows.

Adverse effects of corticosteroids. Corticosteroids are powerful drugs and can give rise to a number of side-effects depending on dosage, duration of therapy and individual response. The adverse effects include the following:

- oral candidiasis;
- fluid retention – leg oedema;
- moon face (cushingoid);
- obese abdomen;
- gastritis, peptic ulceration, with possible perforation or haemorrhage;
- muscle weakness and wasting (myopathy); especially of anterior thigh muscles;
- steroid psychosis;
- steroid diabetes;
- osteoporosis.

Patients on corticosteroids are very prone to develop oral thrush and, whatever the dose being taken, the mouth needs to be inspected regularly and frequently. In respect of steroid diabetes, beware of the patient on corticosteroids who develops polyuria and increasing thirst. Keep the possibility of steroid psychosis in mind if a patient on corticosteroids, especially a high dose, becomes increasingly euphoric, is not sleeping, is paranoid, or is verbose with grandiose ideas.

Non-steroidal anti-inflammatory drugs

NSAIDs are used as co-analgesics particularly to help allay the pain of bone secondaries. NSAIDs have analgesic, antipyretic and anti-inflammatory properties. They probably exert most of these effects by impairing the synthesis of prostaglandins. They inhibit an enzyme called cyclo-oxygenase which is needed for the completion of one of the final steps leading to the formation of prostaglandins.

In many of the bone metastases which are 'osteolytic' (i.e. destroy bone), prostaglandins appear to play an important role in causing the bone destruction and therefore the associated pain. Prostaglandins also sensitise nerve endings making them respond more easily to painful stimuli. Thus the basis for giving NSAIDs to patients with painful bone secondaries is to inhibit the production of prostaglandins by the bone cancer cells.

There are many different NSAIDs available belonging to different chemical categories. Different medical practitioners favour different agents. There is variability in their effectiveness and if one NSAID does not help it is well worth trying another, preferably from a different chemical class. A helpful scheme has been proposed by Mannix and Rawlins (1987). The principal NSAIDs used for painful bone secondaries are listed in Table 3.2.

Adverse effects. Like corticosteroids, NSAIDs are powerful drugs and adverse effects are frequently seen. These include the following:

- dyspepsia: this is common;
- fluid retention with leg oedema: this is common;
- gastrointestinal bleeding (with melaena or frank blood *per rectum*), gastrointestinal ulceration and perforation
- hypersensitivity reactions (asthma, urticaria and other skin rashes);
- blood dyscrasias: rarely.

NSAIDs are to be used with caution in peptic ulceration, allergic disorders (particularly asthma and hypersensitivity to aspirin) and renal and hepatic impairment.

Fluid retention with NSAIDs. The fluid retention associated with NSAIDs is of interest because it is often resistant to ordinary doses of diuretics. Far higher doses than usual may be needed to achieve an effect. The reason is that prostaglandins are necessary within the tubules of the kidney to facilitate excretion of fluid and often this will remain reduced despite conventional doses of diuretics.

The use of the NSAID ketorolac. Ketorolac is a potent analgesic agent of the NSAID class. In general medical use it is indicated for the short-term management of moderate to severe acute post-operative pain. As with many drugs palliative care has adopted this agent for use within its own field and it is especially useful when given by subcutaneous injection in patients presenting with severe pain from bone metastases. The most common approach is to give the drug continuously by a syringe driver. To obviate the risk of serious side-effects (especially gastric or intestinal ulceration and perforation) the total daily dose for the non-elderly is usually restricted to 90 mg and 60 mg for the elderly (patients over 65 years).

Good pain control is obtained in about four out of five patients and in many patients concomitant morphine dosage can be reduced or even discontinued. To obviate excessive opioid effects occurring because pain is so effectively controlled, some units now start at 30 mg of ketorolac per 24 h, increasing to 60 mg per 24 h and then 90 mg per 24 h where appropriate, if the pain is not completely relieved by the initial approach. With some patients the dose of opioid can be reduced by 20–30 per cent every 24–48 h.

Table 3.2 Principal NSAIDs used for painful bone secondaries (grouped into separate chemical classes)

Aspirin	600 mg 4-hourly Aspirin–paracetamol ester (Benorylate) 4–8 g of ester daily (5–10 ml bd)
Ibuprofen	1.2–1.8 g daily in three to four divided doses
Flurbiprofen	150–300 mg daily in three to four divided doses
Naproxen	0.5–1 g daily in two divided doses
Diclofenac	75–150 mg daily in two to three divided doses
Sulindac	200 mg twice daily
Indomethacin	25–50 mg two to three times daily. Max. 200 mg daily
Piroxicam	20 mg daily initially 10–30 mg maintenance in single or divided doses

To reduce further the risks of serious side-effects when giving ketorolac for alleviation of post-operative pain, it is recommended that the maximum duration of parenteral treatment should not exceed 2 days. However, in palliative care faced with chronic cancer pain such a short duration is not usually feasible. In some patients control of the pain by subcutaneous ketorolac administration can be replaced by oral NSAID therapy after 3–5 days but other patients may require subcutaneous ketorolac for 2–3 weeks. In some instances patients have required the treatment for much longer.

The oral formulation of ketorolac has been disappointing. Following discontinuation of the subcutaneous ketorolac practitioners may wish to prescribe the oral NSAID they usually favour.

To protect against NSAID-associated gastric and duodenal ulceration it is important to prescribe routinely the synthetic prostaglandin analogue misoprostol in a dose of 200 μg three or four times daily while the subcutaneous ketorolac is being administered.

Ketorolac should not be used in patients with active peptic ulcer or a history of peptic ulcer. It should not be used in patients with coagulation disorders, those who have shown hypersensitivity to aspirin or other NSAIDs and those having lithium therapy. It should be used with caution in the elderly (>65 years), where there is upper gastrointestinal cancer, in patients on corticosteroids and when given for prolonged periods at high dosage. Ketorolac should be mixed with 0.9 per cent saline to make up the solution to be infused via the syringe driver. Ketorolac may be added to diamorphine in the syringe driver *as long as saline is used*. Ketorolac is not compatible with cyclizine, haloperidol or midazolam.

If administration of ketorolac was contemplated at home the patient and the possible indications for use should be discussed with the Medical Director/Consultant of the local hospice or palliative care unit.

Other co-analgesics

Important other co-analgesics include muscle relaxants, antidepressants, other deafferentation pain co-analgesics, anticonvulsive drugs and antimicrobial agents.

Muscle relaxants. The pain of skeletal muscle spasm has a variable response to opioids and is best treated by measures directed to relax the muscle. Muscle spasm may arise from irritation from an underlying bone secondary or be due to nerve involvement. The spasm may be relieved by massage, relaxation and the use of drugs. Useful agents are diazepam and baclofen (Lioresol).

• Diazepam. Because this drug and one of its active metabolites exert a prolonged effect a single bedtime dose is usually sufficient, i.e. 5–15 mg. Response is often at the expense of drowsiness.
• Baclofen (Lioresol). The dose of this drug should be gradually increased from 5 mg 8-hourly to 15 mg 8-hourly. Again drowsiness often occurs. Nausea and vomiting and confusion are other side-effects.

Muscle pain may not always be due to generalised spasm. The pain can arise from an area of excessive irritability in the muscle or its covering (fascia) caused by strain. This area is called a 'trigger point'. It is a tender, palpable band of muscle fibres. The pain tends to be referred away from the trigger point with a distinctive pattern specific for the muscle involved. The painful condition is called an acute myofascial pain syndrome. The pain can be relieved by application of transcutaneous electrical nerve stimulation (TENS; see p. 49), acupuncture or an injection of local anaesthetic and a corticosteroid (e.g. bupivacaine and depomedrone) to the trigger point area.

Antidepressants. Antidepressants can be effective in relieving pain resulting from the nerve being destroyed by malignant infiltration. This disturbing type of pain, which does not respond to opioids, is called deafferentation pain. Character-istically it is felt in areas of the body supplied by particular spinal nerves, i.e. in the distribution of dermatomes. The pain is felt as a superficial burning or scalding. In many, the lightest of touch can arouse an intense exacerbation of the pain (a phenomenon called allodynia). Stabbing pain is also felt and may be the predominant feature.

Amitriptyline or dothiepin are popular choices of antidepressant. The starting dose of amitriptyline varies from 10–25 mg daily with a slow increase to 50–70 mg daily. Dothiepin is commenced at 50–75 mg daily increasing slowly to 150 mg daily. The drugs can be given as single doses at bedtime. Such drugs produce analgesic effects at doses lower than those used to treat depression. Side-effects are common including sedation, dry mouth, constipation, urinary retention, dizzi-ness and confusion. These drugs are contraindicated in patients with glaucoma.

Other deafferentation pain co-analgesics. Other interesting drugs used to try and mitigate this non-opioid responsive pain include mexiletine hydrochloride and clonidine hydrochloride.

• Mexiletine hydrochloride. This is an anti-arrhythmic agent. It is normally used to treat abnormal rhythms after myocardial infarction or with ischaemic heart disease. Essentially it 'stabilises' nerve cells so they are not so easily stimulated. For this reason it is used to try and inhibit the nerve cells in the spinal cord concerned with pain transmission.
• Clonidine hydrochloride. This drug is normally used against migraine in lower

doses and as an antihypertensive agent at higher doses occasionally it is also used to try and inhibit the nerve cells in the spinal cord involved in pain transmission.

These agents are best avoided for pain therapy if a patient has heart trouble or is hypertensive. The advice of a palliative care specialist or an anaesthetist should always be sought before using these drugs for cancer pain.

Anticonvulsive drugs. Such drugs are used to dampen down the erratic firing of nerve cells. In cancer patients they can be useful in relieving the stabbing pain of nerve compression (which often does not respond to morphine alone) or the lancinating component of deafferentation pain.

Carbamazepine (Tegretol) is a popular choice. A small starting dose is best, for example 100 mg twice daily with a gradual increase. The average dose is 200 mg 8-hourly. Occasionally doses of 400 mg 8- or 6-hourly may be reached. Drowsiness and dizziness may occur, also nausea and vomiting. Rashes may appear after some weeks on therapy. Hepatitis and bone marrow depression are rare adverse effects.

Other anticonvulsants such as sodium valproate or phenvtoin may be favoured.

Antimicrobial agents. The pain from cellulitis associated with ulcerating or fungating cancers, or complicating lymphoedema, can be allayed by an appropriate antibiotic, for example Phenoxymethylpenicillin (penicillin V) 500 mg orally 6-hourly, flucloxacillin 250 mg orally 6-hourly, erythromycin 500 mg orally 6-hourly. Metronidazole 400 mg orally 8-hourly can be added when an anaerobic infection is also suspected.

An additional analgesic approach – the use of ketamine

Ketamine has been in use as a parenteral general anaesthetic agent for almost 25 years. In recent years in palliative care it has been found to be a useful analgesic agent in some patients with intractable pain from advanced cancer where morphine and other approaches have proved ineffective. It is usually administered by continuous subcutaneous injection using a syringe driver in a dosage of 0.1–0.5 mg/kg/h.

Ketamine is a 'dissociative' agent and possibly produces its analgesic effects in two ways.

1. By a depressant effect upon certain groups of neurones (called nuclei) in the thalamus which are responsible for the interpretation and onward transmission of pain impulses to the cerebral cortex.
2. By suppression of pain impulse transmission within the spinal cord.

This agent should be used only in a hospital or hospice setting

Psychological approaches

This piece of the mosaic has many components and these include the following:

- sensitive listening;
- relaxation therapy;

- hypnosis;
- distraction;
- imagery.

Sensitive listening

All carers should aim to be 'good' or sensitive, empathic listeners. Such listening is a disciplined skill. It does not come naturally as one might think and the carer should read and practise appropriate approaches (Nelson-Jones, 1988). Sensitive listening is an essential adjunct to any form of pain therapy. Such listening involves the characteristics given below.

- Not just hearing words, but listening for cues, for example the way the words are said and the implications behind their content.
- Seeing as well as hearing, i.e. perceiving 'body messages'.
- Conveying one's attention, interest and availability ('attending' the patient). This is a powerful way of affirming a patient's worth and reducing isolation.
- Encouraging the patient to talk, so that pent up frustration and anger are released and anxieties are expressed.

Communication skills are discussed further in Chapter 16.

Relaxation therapy

Although there is widespread belief that relaxation helps to relieve pain there is little research to demonstrate its effectiveness, especially in cancer pain. Nevertheless, the benefit to individuals and the knowledge of how pain, anxiety and muscle tension tend to intensify each other, form a reasonable basis for its use. It seems that even if it does not have an effect on the pain, relaxation therapy improves the person's mood and attitude so that he or she can cope better with the pain.

There are many relaxation techniques available and they need to be matched to specific patients and specific situations. Some have an inward focus on the body (e.g. rhythmic breathing, jaw relaxation) and these may not be the best for a patient distressed about body changes. Others have an outward focus, for example pleasant imagery, when one imagines oneself back in a secure and peaceful environment. For those with pent up emotions 'progressive relaxation' may be beneficial, i.e. various muscle groups are tensed, held and then relaxed. For others with prolonged pain a meditation technique may be preferable (see Chapter 15).

Relaxation is a skill that has to be learnt by patients. It is not simply resting or reading a book or watching television. Relaxation therapy for a cancer patient is a helpful adjunct. It can never be a substitute for other therapies such as analgesics. Nurses who are interested may wish to seek suitable education and experience and read appropriate accounts, for example McCaffery and Beeb (1989).

Hypnosis

There are numerous reports about the successful use of hypnosis in reducing cancer pain. The problem again is that much of the published evidence is inadequate, i.e. reports are either on single cases or on small numbers of patients, there are no appropriate controls and pain measurements are variable. Doubters question whether hypnosis is any more beneficial than just the emotional support given by the carer. Nevertheless, there have been impressive responses in certain individuals and these, allied to the other many anecdotal reports, suggest that hypnosis can be of great help to some patients (Wood, 1989).

Once the hypnotic stage has been entered various approaches may be used. These include such highly interesting strategies as outlined below.

• Dissociation of the patient from the pain and from his or her current body state, back to a pain free, enjoyable period. Patients can be taught simple techniques to enter this dissociation state themselves, i.e. auto-hypnosis.
• Suggestion of anaesthesia being generated in the hand and transferring this to the part of the body in pain by touching that area with the hand.
• Suggesting that the pain is a pulsating light which decreases in frequency and intensity and as the light diminishes so does the pain. A train disappearing into the distance taking the pain with it is another imagery form.
• Substituting the pain with a less disturbing sensation, i.e. a tingling sensation or a pressure.
• Displacing the focus of the pain to a less important part of the body, i.e. to a toe or to a thumb with the pain leaking away from its tip.

Distraction

Distraction is drawing the patient's attention away from pain onto other stimuli. All sensory approaches can be used, i.e. hearing, seeing, touching, moving. Distraction strategies may be used against both short episodes of pain (less than an hour) and chronic pain (McCaffery and Beebe, 1989). In all instances the content of the techniques must be individualised. For brief episodes of pain, i.e. from short practical procedures or for pain on movement, a number of techniques can be used. These include focusing on an object (e.g. a flower or picture in a magazine) and describing it mentally or verbally, listening to music through a headset or singing a tune mentally, tapping out a rhythm with the fingers or feet, holding onto or rubbing an object.

For on-going cancer pain the strategy is to improve the level of sensory input so that the patient does not lie in bed or sit in a chair thinking only of his or her pain and impending death. Commitment and consideration are needed by the carer so that a structured programme is elaborated for the patient, including adequate periods of rest. The programme may include such inputs as listening to music or a talking book, craft-work, exercise, conversation with individuals, selected television and video viewing, being taken out for visits, etc. In the home simply putting the bed by a window so a patient can look out and watch the world go by can be a great help. There is a great need for well-planned, individualised programmes for patients. An occasional, single distraction episode is of minimal use.

Imagery

This is another well-known supportive technique which is gaining popularity. Again there is no definitive research data available but individual reports support the benefit of this approach. In this technique the patient is helped to use his or her imagination to develop sensory images to help reduce the pain intensity. If the pain is brief the carer may suggest that the patient imagines the pain is becoming stinging rather than lancinating or a pleasant warmness rather than an ache. If the pain is prolonged then a more lengthy, systematic approach is needed. The patient may benefit from 'guided imagery'. Two examples of the latter approach are given below.

- The patient is helped to imagine the body to be a bag which becomes slowly filled with sand. When full a slit in the bag is imagined and as the sand slowly trickles away so does the pain.
- After an appropriate preamble the patient is helped to imagine that there is a hole in the body close to the painful area. Each time the patient breathes out it is imagined that more and more of the pain leaks out through the hole.

Helpful accounts on the use of imagery are readily available (McCaffery and Beeb, 1989).

Physical therapies

In physical therapies some form of stimulation is applied to the skin and superficial tissues. Stimulating the skin to relieve pain is probably as old as the human race. It is seen in its simplest form in everyday life with the mother rubbing the painful area of the child's arm or leg hurt by a fall. The physical therapies commonly used in practice include the following:

- superficial application of heat or cold;
- superficial body massage;
- transcutaneous electrical nerve stimulation (TENS);
- acupuncture.

Superficial application of heat or cold

Provided they are applied at a comfortable intensity, the application of heat or cold may help bring relief when there is localised pain. Heat may be applied in a variety of forms including via an electrical heat pad, a hot-water bottle (wrapped in cloth to prevent burns), radiant heat, immersion in a warm bath or Jacuzzi. Cold may be applied in various containers wrapped in cloth to prevent tissue damage, for example cold gel pack, plastic bag containing ice and water, a bag of frozen peas (hit gently to separate the constituents).

Application of heat and cold is suitable for the non-cancer types of pain occurring in the cancer patient, for example musculo-fascial strain, muscle spasm, joint stiffness. It is generally suggested that application of heat directly over an area of malignant infiltration should be avoided in case this favours an acceleration of the growth. Cold has a more prolonged pain relieving effect than heat but usually the latter is preferred by patients.

Superficial body massage

Many carers are becoming proficient in the use of superficial body massage. To many cancer patients this is most pleasurable and the relief of physical and mental tensions can help to decrease the pain.

Physical well-being is enhanced, probably by relaxation of muscle tension and by increasing skin circulation. Also a caring touch usually brings comfort and reassurance. In addition, the degree of intimacy afforded by this procedure may give a patient the confidence to talk about underlying fears and other problems.

Extensive body massage is too tiring for most advanced cancer patients and any areas with underlying cancer infiltration need to be treated with caution. However, limited massage of the hands or feet, or a back and shoulder rub, can be most pleasant and comforting. Some nurses may wish to gain the knowledge and skill of superficial body massage and there are appropriate courses available.

A growing interest is developing within palliative care in the use of essential oils and massage (aromatherapy, see pp. 240–1) and in a particular form of massage involving reflex areas in the feet and hands (reflexology).

Transcutaneous electrical nerve stimulation (TENS)

In this technique low-intensity stimulation of large nerve fibres within a painful area is carried out through electrodes applied to the overlying skin. These large nerve fibres rapidly conduct the stimuli along to the spinal cord where they activate an agent called enkephalin. This agent inhibits, or 'closes the gate' on the painful stimuli being conducted from the area at a slower rate along smaller nerve fibres.

The patient wears a battery-powered stimulator and flexible wires conduct the current to electrodes on the skin. The electrodes are applied with a conductive gel and held in place with adhesive tape. The aim is to induce a tolerable tingling sensation. The technique is taught to patients so that it can be self-administered. The patient may need to use the stimulator for a few hours or for the entire day.

It is uncommon for the technique to be useful in severe cancer pain. Beneficial effects have been found in moderate pain in cancer patients, especially for benign musculo-fascial pains, scar pain, post-herpatic neuralgia and phantom limb pains.

A significant limitation of the usefulness of TENS in cancer pain is that its efficacy rapidly declines with time. In some studies (Ventafridda *et al.*, 1979) only 10–30 per cent of patients who obtained initial relief were still using the technique after a month. Another problem is that the positioning of the electrodes in relation to the painful area and the finding of the optimum electrical stimulus can be very time consuming. TENS should be performed by trained personnel, for example physiotherapists, who can explain the technique to the patient in simple terms and who have the skills and patience to correctly position the electrodes and find the optimum electrical stimulus.

TENS should not be used in patients with a pacemaker and the electrodes should not be placed over the carotid sinus.

Although only a few patients with cancer pain have long-term benefit this procedure is simple and safe and it may be worth considering before embarking on more involved therapies.

Acupuncture

Generally acupuncture is not sufficient to relieve severe malignant pain. It is useful for non-cancer pain such as musculo-fascial pain and muscle spasms. Different intensities of acupuncture therapy may be applied varying from passive needle insertion to electrical stimulation.

Palliative radiotherapy

Palliative radiotherapy can be very effective in relieving cancer pain in selected patients. Doctors and nurses should appreciate that radiotherapy is the treatment of choice for metastatic bone pain. Painful bone secondaries should be discussed with the local radiotherapy and oncology service irrespective of whether the patient is at home or in hospital.

For localised bone secondaries usually a single treatment as a day patient can be given and if pain is not relieved, or if it re-emerges, retreatment is possible. For a larger 'field', for example secondaries throughout the bony pelvis, five to ten treatments may be necessary. For painful, more widespread bone metastases 'half body' irradiation may be indicated. An appropriate single treatment is to the upper or lower half of the body. If necessary, irradiation to the other half of the body can be carried out 6 weeks later. Admission to hospital for a short period is required to alleviate possible nausea and vomiting.

Treatment with morphine and NSAIDs should be commenced while radiotherapy is being arranged and continued until the radiotherapy has taken effect. Pain relief commences about 7–10 days after radiotherapy in many patients: in others it may take 3–4 weeks. As increasing alleviation of the pain occurs so it may be possible to reduce drug therapy or even stop it eventually.

Other painful conditions where radiotherapy may be of help include the following:

- painful ulcerating or fungating superficial lesions;
- painful solid growths on the surface of the body;
- severe perineal pain from an unresectable rectal carcinoma left *in situ*;
- painful metastatic liver enlargement not allayed by drugs.

Nerve blocks

It is possible to relieve cancer pain by blocking the nerve pathways along which the pain stimuli are conducted to the central nervous system. Nerve blocks are a valuable approach but patients and procedures need to be selected with care if pain relief without adverse sequelae is to be achieved. Nerves can be interrupted either temporarily or for a long period.

- Temporarily by injecting a local anaesthetic (such as bupivacaine or lignocaine) around the nerve.
- For a prolonged period, by destroying a portion of the nerve by one of several techniques, i.e. local infiltration of chemicals such as alcohol, phenol, chloro-cresol, or by the application of cold (cryotherapy) or heat (thermocoagulation).

These techniques are usually carried out by specially trained anaesthetists. The anaesthetist will always be pleased to see the patient initially in the hospital ward, or at home as a domiciliary consultation. Alternatively, it may be possible for the patient to attend a local centre for pain relief.

Nerve blocks can be carried out at a variety of sites and can be directed at:

- the spinal nerves; and
- the sensory fibres which transmit pain from the organs (viscera) within the body.

These accompany the autonomic nerves.

The spinal nerves

Spinal nerves may be interrupted outside or inside the vertebral column. Outside the vertebral column, the principal sites are as given below.

- As the nerve emerges from the vertebral column, i.e. a paravertebral block. This may be indicated, for instance, in the thoracic region for pain in the thoracic spine or posterior ribs or upper abdominal wall.
- As a single nerve coursing across the body, for example an intercostal block, where a thoracic nerve is interrupted as it runs beneath a rib, to treat rib pain at the side or front of the chest.
- When joined with others as a nerve plexus, for example a brachial plexus block, for pain down the arm from malignant infiltration of the plexus not responding to morphine and corticosteroids. In this situation such a procedure has to be considered very carefully as the nerve destruction (neurolytic) agent will affect motor function leaving the patient with a useless arm. Generally when neurolytic agents are to be injected at any site, initially a block with a local anaesthetic is performed to allow the patient to observe the effects. Only if these are acceptable to the patient is the neurolytic block then performed.

Within the vertebral column the block is directed at the sensory roots of the spinal nerves as they traverse the vertebral canal to join the posterior aspect of the cord. The most common sites for the block are given below.

- In the space between the inner surface of the vertebrae and the outermost layers of the meninges (the dura mater), i.e. the intradural or epidural space. Thus, the procedure is termed an epidural block.
- In the space filled with cerebrospinal fluid, between the inner covering of the spinal cord (the pia mater) and the middle layer of the meninges (the arachnoid mater), i.e. the subarachnoid space. This is termed an intrathecal block.

Epidural block

A common indication for an epidural block in the cancer patient is back pain with nerve root pain, due to malignant bone disease of the spine. Usually an epidural catheter is inserted to administer a regular top-up of local anaesthetic solution alone or to complement an infusion of epidural opiates (see below). Single injections of the corticosteriod depomedrone mixed with a local anaesthetic, also may be given epidurally to reduce local chronic inflammatory changes around a malignant focus and nerve-root compression.

Epidural opiates

This is a route which is becoming widely used. By this method opiates are deposited through a fine catheter into the epidural space. In the UK diamorphine is favoured because of its greater safety and is usually given as a continuous infusion over 24 h via a syringe driver. The opiate is absorbed across the meninges and cerebrospinal fluid (CSF), into the posterior horn of the spinal cord where it stimulates opioid receptors on neurones there and inhibits the onward transmission of pain stimuli. The opiate also diffuses upwards through the CSF to gain access to the brain itself.

Epidural opiates are now used where hitherto a neurolytic block would have been the next approach, for example they are being used in difficult cancer pain problems such as intractable back pain and intrapelvic pain with or without nerve root involvement, and for the pain from intra-abdominal infiltration.

Epidural opiates are especially useful if the patient seems to have a morphine responsive pain but the overall amount of oral or subcutaneous opiate is causing excessive drowsiness or confusion or hallucinations. Only about an eighth to a tenth of the total 24-hour oral dose may be needed epidurally.

Intraspinal morphine

Morphine is used in centres where diamorphine is not available (the UK is one of the few countries where diamorphine can be legally administered in routine practice). It is given directly into the CSF (i.e. intrathecally) as well as epidurally.

A number of side-effects can occur with intraspinal opiates, but delayed respiratory depression has to be especially considered when morphine is given. Such an effect can occur hours after the initial administration. This seemingly represents the time taken for the morphine to diffuse upwards within the circulating CSF to be absorbed by the brain tissues, including the respiratory centre. Such delayed respiratory depression is infrequent with epidural diamorphine.

Closed systems

For prolonged epidural or intrathecal administration the epidural catheter may be implanted beneath the skin. Using a tunnelling technique the catheter is 'threaded' subcutaneously around to the anterior chest wall where its' free end is attached to a reservoir also buried beneath the skin. The reservoir can be filled daily by the percutaneous injection of the appropriate amount of opiate. Alternatively the free end can be brought out and attached to some form of pump and the opiate administered continuously. These closed systems are expensive.

Intrathecal block

A possible indication for an intrathecal block is pain in the perineum, usually from cancer of the rectum. A small amount of phenol in glycerine is injected via a needle inserted between the fifth lumbar vertebra and the sacrum. The patient is tilted backwards (at an angle of 30° and maintained like that for half an hour so that the solution drops down to pool around the lower sacral roots). This indication is a good example of the need for careful consideration and careful selection of patients when neurolytic solutions are to be used. With this procedure there is a real risk of bladder and rectal dysfunction, because among the sacral nerve roots affected by the chemical lesion are those which supply the rectal and bladder sphincters.

Intrathecal diamorphine and bupivacaine

A number of units in the UK, disappointed with the results of epidural analgesia in some patients with intractable cancer pain, have commenced using intrathecal diamorphine and bupivacaine. Results have been variable and this approach is still being evaluated.

The sensory fibres carrying visceral pain

These fibres accompany the autonomic nerves and are usually interrupted at the sympathetic ganglia.

Coeliac plexus block

One of the most useful techniques is the coeliac plexus block. This is especially helpful for intractable pain in the upper abdomen and back, associated with, carcinoma of the pancreas or stomach. The plexus also receives pain fibres from the gallbladder, liver, kidney, adrenal and ureter. The block is carried out under local anaesthesia with the patient lying face downwards. The needle is inserted through the skin to either side of the vertebral column just under the 12th rib. Using X-ray image intensification the needles are advanced upwards and inwards to the front of the aorta. If a 'prognostic block' is being carried out, i.e. to observe if the procedure will relieve the pain, local anaesthetic solution is injected through each needle. If destruction of the nerve plexus has been decided upon an equal volume of absolute alcohol and local anaesthetic is injected. A coeliac plexus block requires admission to hospital for about 3 days. Its effect may last for about 6 months and often complete abolition of the pain is achieved.

Lumbar sympathetic block

A block of the lumbar sympathetic ganglia is another very useful procedure for bladder and rectal pain, especially tenesmus. The ganglia also receive pain fibres from the uterus, ovary and testis. The block is carried out in much the same way as the coeliac plexus block but at a slightly lower level. The neurolytic solution usually used is phenol in water. This procedure also will require the patient to be admitted to hospital for about 3 days.

When to refer to the anaesthetist or pain clinic

The possibility of some form of nerve block should be considered for any cancer pain not responding to drug therapy. The anaesthetist will be only too willing to discuss whether or not a nerve block is appropriate for a particular problem.

The possibility of a nerve block should be considered when the following types of pain cannot be controlled with drug measures.

- Pain that is 'anatomically suitable', that is unilateral pain, on one side of chest, upper abdomen or trunk, or in a leg or arm.
- Pain across the upper abdomen or radiating through to the back from cancer affecting the stomach, liver, gall bladder or adrenal.
- Pelvic pain.
- Rectal/bladder tenesmus.
- Lower back pain, alone or with nerve root pain radiating down one or both legs.
- Pain controlled at rest but not on movement.

Other 'special therapeutic pieces'

Expert assistance from a variety of specialities may be needed if the pain remains difficult to control or certain pathological conditions develop. Certain 'special therapeutic pieces' may need to become incorporated into the mosaic of pain management. These include hormone therapy and chemotherapy, general surgery, orthopaedic surgery, neurosurgery.

Hormone therapy and chemotherapy

Modification of the cancer by either of these methods alleviate pain and they may be considered even in an advanced malignancy. Examples of hormone therapy include progestogens for metastatic breast and renal carcinoma and anti-androgen therapy for advanced prostatic carcinoma. Chemotherapy may be used occasionally, for example for pain relief in advanced breast and head and neck cancer, but the benefits need to be weighed very carefully against the side-effects.

General surgery

The general surgeon may be able to help alleviate pain due to advanced cancer in certain circumstances. Surgical intervention may relieve pain by such procedures as laying open painful intestinal–cutaneous fistulae, draining superficial abscesses, relieving intestinal obstruction by a colostomy or a by-pass operation.

Orthopaedic surgery

Orthopaedic management of skeletal metastases may achieve considerable pain relief. Treatment may be required for a pathological fracture, impending fracture or spinal instability.

Pathological fracture. For a pathological fracture some form of internal fixation is commonly carried out, followed by radiotherapy. Local irradiation is an essential part of treatment in order to inhibit further tumour growth.

Impending fracture. There is a high risk of fracture of a long bone if a large bone destroying (lytic) metastasis is present. (Such metastases are not seen on X-ray until at least 50 per cent of the bone has been destroyed.) Some form of internal stabilisation of the weakened bone is then necessary, followed by radiotherapy.

The unstable spine. The spine may become unstable as a result of bone destruction of the vertebrae and any movement is associated with severe pain. X-rays show various degrees of vertebral collapse. Various methods of stabilisation are used and fixing the vertebrae at and around the level of the bone metastases to a rod or rectangle can bring immense relief of pain. Post-operative irradiation is essential.

Neurosurgery

Recourse to neurosurgical techniques to relieve advanced cancer pain varies from centre to centre. In general it is an infrequent approach.

Cordotomy. When pain remains intractable a procedure such as cordotomy may be indicated. This involves sectioning the tracts which convey pain stimuli from the spinal cord to the brain in the antero-lateral quadrant of the spinal cord. Such a procedure is used mainly for pain on one side of the body below the mid-chest.

Percutaneous and surgical cordotomy. Cordotomy is achieved in two ways; percutaneous or surgical. In the former a needle is inserted between the first and second cervical vertebrae under X-ray control. The patient is not anaesthetised, but sedated with premedication. Using an electrode a heat lesion is produced in the antero-lateral quadrant of the spinal cord. Surgical cordotomy is an operative procedure under anaesthesia and is usually carried out in the upper thoracic region. The antero-lateral quadrant of the spinal cord is cut under direct vision.

A decreasing demand. The increasing use of other techniques, especially implanted drug delivery systems for the chronic administration of epidural or intrathecal opiates, has greatly reduced the need for cordotomy. Similarly there is a decreasing demand for other approaches such as the ablation of the pituitary gland, section of dorsal roots of spinal nerves, or the use of stereotactic surgery. In the latter, various nerve tracts or collections of nerve cells are destroyed by means of a probe or energy beam directed through the brain.

Conclusions

The nurse has a unique, privileged position having trusted, close contact with patients. Such a relationship should be used to the full to help relieve the pains of advanced cancer. The nurse should consistently keep in mind the following considerations.

- Cancer pain is not inevitable. It is treatable and controllable.
- The majority of cancer patients have more than one pain.
- Assessment of a patient's 'pain' is essential. Repeated review is equally important – new pains develop, old ones recur.
- It is essential to stand back and look at the person's 'total pain'.
- Analgesics are the mainstay of pain relief. For persistent pain they should be taken 'by mouth', 'by the clock' and 'by the ladder' (World Health Organization, 1986).
- Morphine is the opioid of choice. Addiction, tolerance and respiratory depression are myths.
- Analgesics are only one of a number of measures and each patient should have a personal 'mosaic of therapies'.
- If pain persists ask questions. Is the pain morphine responsive? Has the 'whole person' been addressed? Is the patient frightened, angry, depressed or lonely? Have co-analgesic drugs been considered? Is there any indication for radiotherapy or nerve blocks? Has some basic principle been overlooked?
- Pain is only one of many distressing symptoms of advanced cancer. Pain control should be but one part of a comprehensive approach to the care of the patient and family.

References

ATKINSON, R. E., SCHOFIELD, P. A. and MELLOR, P. (1989). Buprenorphine morphine transfer trial in cancer pain. *Meeting of Intractable Pain Society of Great Britain and Ireland*, Nottingham.

DOYLE, D. (1987). *Domiciliary Terminal Care*. Churchill Livingstone, Edinburgh.
McCAFFERY, M. and BEEB, A. (1989). *Pain. Clinical Manual for Nursing Practice*. Mosby.
MANNIX, K. A. and RAWLINS, M. D. (1987). The management of bone metastases: non-steroidal anti-inflammatory drugs. *Palliative Medicine* 1, 128–31.
NELSON-JONES, R. (1988). *Practical Counselling and Helping Skills*, 2nd edn. Cassell Education, London.
RAIMAN, J. (1988). *Nursing Issues and Research in Terminal Care*. John Wiley, Chichester.
REGNARD, C. F. B. and TEMPEST, S. (1992). *Guide to Symptom Relief in Advanced Cancer*. Haigh & Hochland.
TTS–FENTANYL MULTICENTRE STUDY GROUP (1994). *Journal of drug Development* 6, 93–7.
TWYCROSS, R. G. and LACK, A. (1984). *Symptom Control in Far Advanced Cancer*. Pitman, London.
VENTAFRIDDA, V., SGANZERLA, E. P., FORCHI, C., POZZI, G. and CORDINI, G. (1979). Transcutaneous nerve stimulation in cancer pain. *Advances in Pain Research and Therapy*, Vol. 2. Raven Press, New York.
WALL, P. D. (1987). Foreword in *Pain Control*, Jane Latham. Austen Cornish Publishers with The Lisa Sainsbury Foundation.
WOOD, M. (1989). Pain control and hypnosis. *Nursing Times* 85, 38–40.
WORLD HEALTH ORGANIZATION (1986). *Cancer Pain Relief*.
ZECH, D. J. F., LEHMANN, K. A. and GROND, S. (1994). Transdermal (TTS) Fentanyl in cancer pain managment. *Progress in Palliative Care* 2, 37–42.
ZENZ, M. (1988). Personal communication in R. G. Twycross, Opioid analgesics in cancer pain: current practice and controversies. *Cancer Surveys* 7, 29–53.

Further reading

McCAFFERY, M. and BEEB, A. (1989). *Pain. Clinical Manual for Nursing Practice*. Mosby.
REGNARD, C. F. B. and TEMPEST, S. (1992). *Guide to Symptom Relief in Advanced Cancer*. Haigh & Hochland.
TWYCROSS, R. (1994). *Pain Relief in Advanced Cancer*. Churchill Livingstone, Edinburgh.
TWYCROSS, R. (1994). *Introducing Palliative Care*. Radcliffe Medical Press.
WORLD HEALTH ORGANIZATION (1986). *Cancer Pain Relief*.

4

The management of other frequently encountered symptoms

Ilora Finlay

'I do not want two diseases, one God made and one the doctor made.'

Napoleon Bonaparte

Symptom analysis

The most important first step towards symptom control is to understand why the symptom has occurred. For every symptom that the patient reports, the cause must be determined; knowledge of the cause of the symptom will guide overall management, including appropriate prescribing. Any symptom can be caused by:

- the cancer itself;
- treatments both past and present; and
- other concurrent illnesses.

It is also important to remember that the patient's experience of a symptom will be worsened by fear, worries or depression; the distress caused by symptoms is cumulative, so a patient with several symptoms will rapidly feel worn down by them and increasingly despondent.

Discovering the cause of each symptom depends on the best of medical diagnostic skills and the most accurate nursing observations. Teamwork in which these two perspectives are shared will piece together the clues as to the cause of the symptom. Clinical review is essential as the patient's disease progresses. As one symptom comes under control another one often emerges, to prompt again the diagnostic question 'why' (see Fig. 4.1).

Cancers cause symptoms by the direct pressure the growing tumour causes onto normal structures, e.g. bowel obstruction, spinal cord compression (see below). The tumour mass also causes metabolic effects by this compression, e.g. uraemia from ureteric obstruction. Tumours themselves are sometimes metabolically active, secreting molecules such as parathyroid hormone-like substance which causes hypercalcaemia (see below) or cachexin causing severe weight loss.

Symptoms caused by the treatments may be related to past treatments, for example, post-surgical adhesions, post-chemotherapy neuropathy or neutropenia, post-radiotherapy tiredness. Current treatments such as drug side-effects are extremely common, but some symptoms can be anticipated, e.g. prescribing laxatives as soon as starting a patient on opioids. The symptoms caused by treatments can therefore be considered under past, current and future (preventable) problems.

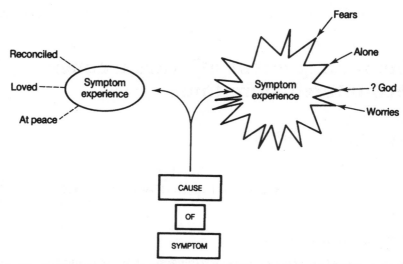

Fig. 4.1 The interplay between the pysche and pain. The same symptom will be perceived as terrible by the frightened patient and less distressingly when the patient is calm.

Patients already immunocompromised by their disease and treatments are more likely to develop intercurrent infections such as herpes zoster. Infections may be masked by the patient's other drugs and therefore more difficult to detect. Coincidental disease such as rheumatoid disease or cardiac disease will continue to be present even when the patient has cancer; treatments may aggravate symptoms related to cancer, e.g. the dose of antihypertensives and anti-angina drugs can often be lowered or stopped in patients on opioids, as opioids can cause postural hypotension and hence dizziness.

Pain has had much publicity and so patients are more willing to complain of pain, with the hope and expectation of analgesia. Other symptoms such as weakness and anorexia are viewed by patients, and often the professionals, with a sense of hopelessness and the feeling nothing can be done. The negative attitude of professionals isolates patients to suffer alone and to keep distress to themselves.

In taking the history, each symptom must be elicited along with associated factors; for example, it is not enough to know that the patient is vomiting – concomitant nausea, the nature, volume and timing of the vomit, abdominal distension, constipation, urinary symptoms, headache on waking and dyspepsia are all important diagnostic pointers to the cause of the vomiting. The clinical picture is always complex in these patients – a patient on opioids will often have a dry mouth, increasing the risk of oral candida with taste distortion which then aggravates anorexia. Nausea caused by opioids may compound nausea caused by liver metastases; in such a complex picture the individual elements must be teased out in order to target treatments for rapid symptom control. Attention to detail is imperative to obtain symptom control.

Patients are often on multiple drug therapies and great care should be taken to make the dosing regime as easy as possible for the patient. Oral therapies should be palatable and timed to coincide with other treatment so that the patient is not muddled by the medication regime itself. Painful intramuscular injections should be avoided, but even the subcutaneous injection of drugs can be irritant and sting, e.g. cyclizine. Intravenous administration is the route of choice when a rapid effect if required. Rectal drugs are useful for the patient at home who cannot tolerate oral medication (example, nausea and vomiting).

In this chapter frequently encountered symptoms will be discussed (see Table 4.1) will be discussed. In addition, the common medical emergencies of hypercalcaemia, spinal cord compression and superior vena caval obstruction will be dealt with briefly.

Nausea and vomiting

About one-third of patients with cancer experience nausea and vomiting. Nausea is often neglected as patients under-report their symptoms and episodes of vomiting are readily noticed by family and professionals. Nausea makes a person withdrawn from their surroundings, pale, sweaty, feel faint, listless and 'off food'; the nauseated patient may simply complain of loss of appetite.

The mechanisms of nausea and vomiting are complex and the causes many (see Fig. 4.2). There are different centres in the brain involved, but can be grouped together into main areas: the chemoreceptor trigger zone (CTZ) where blood-borne toxins and drugs are detected, and the integrated vomiting centre (IVC) in the medulla. The IVC coordinates the whole process of nausea, retching and vomiting,

Table 4.1 Results of the survey of 200 consecutive admissions to Holme Tower Marie Curie Home, Penarth, Wales in 1989. Published on Interactive Video Disc, produced by Marie Curie Education Department

Symptoms on admission	% incidence of symptoms (i.e. % of patients with this symptom)
Pain	62
Weakness	39
Constipation	34
Nausea and vomiting	30
Dypsnoea	26
Fear	20
Confusion	16
Anorexia	14
Depression	8
Incontinence	8
Lymphoedema	7
Skin problems	5
Fungating lesions	5
Sore mouth	4
Ascites	3
Dysphagia	2
Cough	0

with afferent impulses coming from the CTZ and from higher centres in the brain, including memories, from the vestibular apparatus via the eighth nerve and via the vagus from the gut and liver. The sensory cranial nerves (sights and smells) also have an input. The different antiemetics act on different parts of this process, which explains the variability of response to antiemetics when they are prescribed in an irrational and haphazard way; the drug used must be appropriate to the cause of nausea and vomiting (Ferry and Cullen, 1991) (see Fig. 4.3).

Cancer often heightens the sense of smell. Cooking odours and perfumes can provoke nausea. Memory is also important – taste, smells and sights associated with previous episodes of vomiting rapidly reactivate the vomiting process; this is why drugs which have been associated with a patient vomiting will be adamantly refused by the patient who feels sick at the mere sight of the substance. Patients undergoing chemotherapy can experience alteration of taste and develop taste aversions with conditioned nausea.

Nutrition remains an important challenge for the nauseated patient. Low fat, bland foods may be tolerated and savoury foods preferred to sweet (see Chapter 6 on nutrition), but the anxiety generated in patients and carers about food intake must not be underestimated.

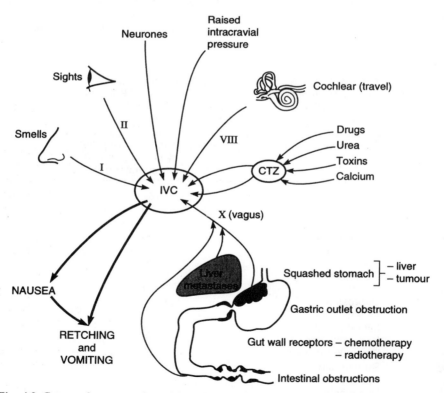

Fig. 4.2 Causes of nausea and vomiting. The cause of the nausea and vomiting must be understood before an appropriate antiemetic (see Fig. 4.3) can be chosen.

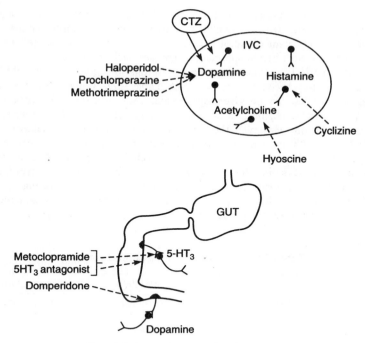

Fig. 4.3 Sites of action of antiemetics.

The symptoms and clinical picture guide diagnosis of the cause (Fig. 4.2) (Twycross and Lack, 1986). A large mass in the epigastrium compressing the stomach will give the patient a sense of fullness on eating or drinking with regurgitation and vomiting. Obstruction at the gastric outlet results in vomiting of undigested food soon after eating. Metoclopramide and domperidone both increase gastric emptying through the pylorus and can be helpful given before food in these patients. Patients with raised intracranial pressure may have large volume projectile vomits with little antecedent nausea; treatment with steroids or radiotherapy to lower the raised intracranial pressure, plus a gastrokinetic agent such as metoclopramide can help.

Patients with multiple small liver metastases have severe nausea, weakness and anorexia and sometimes improve on low-dose oral steroids. About one-third of patients will experience some nausea when starting opioids. This drug toxic effect is mediated via the CTZ, involving a dopamine pathway; haloperidol and methotrimeprazine are potent central antidopaminergic drugs with good effect, but have the disadvantage of extrapyramidal side-effects in some patients (Oliver, 1985).

Radiotherapy to the upper abdomen and chemotherapy frequently evoke severe nausea, by direct effect on gut wall receptors, which is why 5-HT$_3$ antagonists such as odansetron are particularly effective for chemotherapy induced vomiting. They are expensive and their role for other types of vomiting has not been well defined.

The majority of patients with intestinal obstruction present with nausea and vomiting. Treatment will be considered in a separate section below. Hypercalcaemia is an important cause of severe nausea and vomiting, which can now be treated effectively with bisphosphonate drugs (see section below).

When the patient is vomiting, drugs cannot be given orally. Rectal and subcutaneous routes become important (see Table 4.2). When a syringe driver is available, antiemetics can be given by subcutaneous infusion. Methotrimeprazine, and to some extent cyclizine, are both irritant and can cause sterile abscess formation at the needle site. However, they are both potent antiemetics. Haloperidol 5 mg and cyclizine 150–200 mg can be combined in the same syringe with diamorphine if necessary (Dover, 1987; Oliver, 1985). The cyclizine acts on H1 histamine and acetylcholine pathways in the IVC, whilst haloperidol is antidopamine. This combination therefore is extremely useful in severe nausea and vomiting from many causes (Finlay, 1991). Methotrimeprazine is also a potent central antiemetic and quite sedative; the dose range is 25–75 mg in 24 h. Metoclopramide 10 mg

Table 4.2 Antiemetics in nausea and vomiting

Drug	Dose	Timing	Indication	Disadvantages
Cyclizine	50 mg s/c	4 hrly	Good for established vomiting	Painful injection; causes dry mouth
Haloperidol	5 mg s/c oral	once daily	Opiate induced vomiting	Sedative; risk of extrapyramidal side-effects*
Methotromeprazine	25 mg s/c oral	25 mg 8 hrly	Opiate induced vomiting	Very sedative, risk of extrapyramidal side-effects*
Metoclopramide	1–2 mg/kg body per day in divided doses		Chemotherapy; radiotherapy; gut damage	Risk of extrapyramidal side-effects*
Domperidone	30 mg pr	6 hrly	Acts via rectal route	Ineffective in opiate induced and other central causes of vomiiting
Hyoscine	0.4 mg s/c	4 hrly	Weak antiemetic; action centrally	Very dry mouth; slows gut peristalsis
Ondansetron	8 mg i/v	8 hrly	Chemotherapy	Constipation

* Extrapyramidal side-effects
(1) Occulogyric crisis, seen in the young, especially women
(2) Parkinsonian rigidity, usually of gradual onset over a few days

Reversal of the extrapyramidal side-effects is by procyclidine injection. This is a medical emergency.

intravenously can rapidly gain control of the vomiting and can then also be given by subcutaneous infusion at doses of 1–2 mg per kilogram body weight per 24 h. Once control has been gained over vomiting, the dose of antiemetic can often be reduced for maintenance control and oral antiemetics taken.

Intestinal obstruction

Patients with intra-abdominal tumours, particularly ovarian tumours are at risk of bowel obstruction. Foul-smelling vomitus which is sludge-like in appearance (partly digested food) is often the first and only sign of obstruction. Colic and abdominal distension suggest a lower bowel obstruction; many patients continue to have some bowel action despite a subacute obstruction. When obstruction is a single site, particularly of the lower bowel, surgery to by-pass the obstruction can result in many months of good-quality life, but patients with small bowel obstruction often have multiple sites of obstruction, making surgery inappropriate.

Drip and suck regimes have little to offer. A subcutaneous infusion of combined antiemetics (e.g. cyclizine and haloperidol) will often provide good symptom control and antispasmodic agents (e.g. hyoscine butylbromide 60–120 mg, often with diamorphine) will control bowel colic. In a small number of patients, high-dose steroids (dexamethasone 8 mg a day for 4 or 5 days) will help relieve symptoms. Octreotide, which reduces the volume of gastrointestinal secretions, may help those patients whose symptoms persist despite other treatments (Mercadante, 1993)

Constipation

Constipation is often an avoidable complication of therapy. It can mimic bowel obstruction and rigorous steps should be taken to ensure that severe constipation is avoided in all patients. As with other symptoms, the cause determines treatment (Fig. 4.4); poor fluid intake and the many drugs which slow gut peristalsis are often culprits (e.g. group II codeine-type analgesics, group III strong opioids) (Sykes, 1990) (see Table 4.3).

The stool must be kept soft by keeping water in the lumen of the bowel with a small bowel osmotic flushing agent such as magnesium hydroxide or an osmotic agent which prevents fluid resorption in the large bowel, e.g. lactulose, lactitol. Peristalsis can be stimulated with senna, danthron or sodium picosulphate. When stimulant drugs are used a softening agent should be given concurrently, e.g. senna liquid 10 ml bd plus magnesium hydroxide 10 ml bd or lactulose 20 ml bd. Without a stool softener agent the stimulant laxatives will cause severe colic (Regnard, 1988).

Lactulose is very sweet with an oily texture and can cause flatus; some patients prefer powdered lactitol, a flavourless, non-absorbable sugar which can be sprinkled on food or in drinks.

Docusate is a pure stool softener, which in high dose (8–12 tablets a day) can help to keep the stool as soft as toothpaste and prevent constipation precipitating intestinal obstruction in patients with narrow bowel lumen from tumour or adhesions. Patients at risk of intestinal obstruction should also avoid non-digestible foods such as orange pith and grape skins.

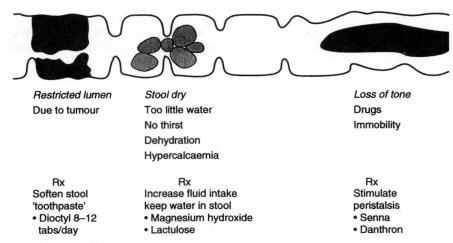

Restricted lumen	Stool dry	Loss of tone
Due to tumour	Too little water	Drugs
	No thirst	Immobility
	Dehydration	
	Hypercalcaemia	
Rx	Rx	Rx
Soften stool	Increase fluid intake	Stimulate
'toothpaste'	keep water in stool	peristalsis
• Dioctyl 8–12	• Magnesium hydroxide	• Senna
tabs/day	• Lactulose	• Danthron

Fig. 4.4 Constipation. The cause of constipation must be sought before deciding which laxative to give.

All too often the patients present with constipation; a confirmatory gentle digital examination of the rectum is essential. Rectal measures only empty the lower few inches of the bowel, so oral laxatives must always be given concurrently to empty the colon. Single dose micro–enemas or glycerine suppositories can help the patient defaecate. An arachis oil retention enema will help lubricate hard stool from the sigmoid colon down into the rectum and through the anus; sometimes a stimulant phosphate enema needs to be given 12–24 h after an arachis oil retention enema. Manual removal of the faeces from the rectum should be a last resort. This is extremely distressing for the patient and should never be performed without adequate analgesia and sedation. Sublingual dextromoramide 10 mg with 1 mg lorazepam is a useful combination for the patient at home, given at least half and hour before commencing manual removal of faeces.

Table 4.3 Constipation and laxatives

Drug	Effect	Dose	Indication
Senna liquid	Bowel stimulation	10 ml bd/tds	On opiates
Senna tabs	Bowel stimulation	2 tabs tds	On opiates
Magnesium hydroxide	Small bowel flusher	10 mls bd/tds	With senna in patients on opiates
Lactulose	Stool softener	up to 60 ml a day	With Senna
Lactitol	Stool softener	1–4 sachets/day	With Senna
Codanthrusate Codalax	Bowel stimulation with stool softener	10 ml bd/qds	On opiates
Dioctyl	Stool softener	4–12 tabs/day	Avoid bowel obstruction

The paraplegic patient with no rectal sensation may tolerate occasional manual removal or regular rectal clearance with powerful stimulant suppositories such as carbalax. Paraplegic patients are the only group who may benefit from a mild degree of constipation when planned rectal emptying can avoid embarrassing incontinence. However, severe constipation with consequent overflow diarrhoea must be avoided.

Diarrhoea

The commonest cause of diarrhoea in cancer patients is constipation with overflow. However, some patients whose common bile duct or pancreatic duct is obstructed by tumour will have malabsorption-type stools which tend to be foul smelling, pale or putty coloured and float in the toilet bowl. Examination of the stool will help identify the cause of the diarrhoea (Table 4.4). Where tumour surface is secreting mucous into the bowel lumen, steroids given as a predsol retention enema to have a direct effect on the tumour surface will help. With fungating tumours into the rectum, radiotherapy or surgical laser-resection may help.

Fistulae into the vagina

In patients with carcinoma of the cervix and other pelvic tumours that have received radiotherapy, there is a risk of a fistulae developing between bowel or bladder into the vagina. This is extremely distressing. The vagina is often exquisitely tender, but gentle douching of the vagina, the use of metronidazole to decrease smell and a urinary catheter in the bladder sometimes helps. A defunctioning colostomy to relieve the distress of faeces coming through the vagina can help, but results are poor when fistulae are multiple. The vulval skin should be protected with thick layers of barrier cream, such as zinc-containing cream. Adherent dressings such as granuflex should be avoided. Emulsifying ointment can be used to wash the area, with analgesic cover from a short-acting opioid (e.g. dextromoramide) or a non-steroidal anti-inflammatory agent.

Table 4.4 Diarrhoea

Stool type		Cause
Grey, floating	= Malabsorption	Blind loop syndrome, pancreatic duct blocked
Watery, undigested food	= Intestinal hurry	Infection, laxative overdose, shortened bowel
Black	= Melaena	GI bleeding
Brown, sticky fluid, occasional pellets	= Overflow	Constipation
Mucoid	= Tumour secretions	Tumour in lumen of bowel

Bladder problems

Cystitis is very common and painful (Regnard and Mannix, 1991). Smelly urine, incontinence or dysuria warrant immediate treatment with an antibiotic such as trimethoprim or ampicillin which will give good symptom relief whilst the result of an MSU is awaited.

Catheterisation should be avoided wherever possible, because catheters can be uncomfortable and risk ascending infection. Both men and women should have lignocaine gel inserted into the urethra before catheterisation which can be exquisitely painful for some patients, especially those with pelvic tumours. Where by-passing of the catheter occurs, a smaller catheter should be inserted (Belfield, 1988). Cloudy urine in the catheter should be treated immediately with daily bladder washouts.

Bladder spasms from tumours in the bladder can be exquisitely painful. When analgesics and anti-spasmodics fail, caudal block or lumbar sympathectomy may help.

Anorexia

Anorexia is very commonly associated with cancer at all stages of disease. It may be the first symptom before frank nausea develops, may be associated with a heightened sense of smell or result from oral candida infection causing altered taste. Corticosteroids have been advocated for many years to increase appetite, but their effect is unpredictable, they cause gastric irritation and predisposed to oral candida, skin fragility and pressure sores. However, corticosteroids can provide a sense of well-being in some patients, but the effect is often short-lived and, whilst useful, they should be used with caution.

The family trying to feed an anorexic patient, need help to understand that there is nutritional value in soups and fluids; small meals or snacks frequently can provide a good balanced diet rather than needing a full meal (see Chapter 6 on nutrition). Food preparation is a way of showing love; the carer can feel rejected and a failure when the anorexic patient is unable to eat food which has been carefully prepared.

Many different diets have been advocated to 'fight the cancer', but objective evidence is lacking. Many of these diets raise false hopes and are expensive and time consuming for the family. Patients and relatives can increase calorific intake with cream and butter; high-fluid intake with soup, gravies and sauces is important. Relatives need help to understand that the patient is not being starved to death and fears over nutrition need understanding (McKillop, 1988).

Artificial feeding

When patients are in the palliative phase of their illness, parenteral feeding usually adds nothing to quality or quantity of life. A small number of patients with swallowing difficulties from head and neck or oesophageal tumours may find a feeding gastrostomy helpful to avoid hunger, maintain a good nutritional status and as an easy route to give drugs. Percutaneous gastrostomy is a simple surgical procedure; the wishes of the patient must be carefully considered and gastrostomy is often favoured by those patients frightened by their inability to eat (Boyd and Keeken, 1994).

Mouth care

Oral candida infections are extremely common (Finlay, 1986), particularly in patients with dentures, with oral mucosa damaged through radiotherapy or surgery or with a dry mouth caused by drugs. Taste disturbance and a dirty furred tongue may be presenting features with the small white plaques typical of oral candida visible around the teeth, gums, palate or inside the cheeks (Aldred, 1991). Candida often extends into the oropharynx and oesophagus causing dysphagia.

Oral hygiene is the single most important factor in care. A soft toothbrush and toothpaste and oral bicarbonate solution will help clean the mouth. Topical treatments such as nystatin or amphotericin are widely used, but tend to only be effective during the course of treatment. The new systemic antifungal agents such as ketoconazole or fluconazole are extremely effective in short courses, although ketoconazole should be avoided in patients with hepatic disease or for a prolonged course of therapy (Meunier *et al.*, 1990).

Ill-fitting dentures need relining or replacing to avoid mouth ulceration from mucosal damage. In the immunocompromised patient, herpes simplex will cause multiple mouth ulcers.

Vitamin deficiencies in patients with a poor diet are common and can cause smooth red tongue and mucosa, particularly vitamin B and C deficiency.

Dysphagia

Candida infection of the oesophagus is common and easily treated with a systemic agent such as fluconazole 50 mg a day for one week. Obstruction of the oesophagus by tumour may need insertion of an Atkinson or similar tube; mediastinal tumours causing extrinsic compression of the oesophagus warrant radiotherapy. High-dose dexamethasone (12–16 mg per day) can temporarily improve swallowing through reducing peritumour oedema. When swallowing of the dexamethasone tablets is difficult they can be dispersed or given as soluble betamethasone or as a subcutaneous injection. Intraluminal radiotherapy of the oesophagus and laser resections of oesophageal tumours are available in some expert units.

Dyspnoea

Dyspnoea is extremely distressing, making the patient feel they are suffocating. Dyspnoea generates tremendous fear and panic. The danger is to mistake the dyspnoea for a panic attack.

The causes of dyspnoea (Fig. 4.5) are various. Baseline observation will provide clues to the cause (Table 4.5). Respiratory rate, pulse rate, blood pressure and any cyanosis are crucial observations. The history of the onset, presence or absence of cough, pleuritic pain and changes in sputum volume and colour must be carefully assessed. Bronchospasm can be caused by cardiac failure (cardiac asthma) or be secondary to retained secretions or tumour in the bronchi. Nebulised bronchodilators will help with wheezing, but the underlying cause must be determined. Cardiac failure requires vigorous treatment with diuretics to avoid the distress of a patient drowning in their own secretions (Allen, 1985). Tumour compressing the trachea or main bronchus or causing haemoptysis requires

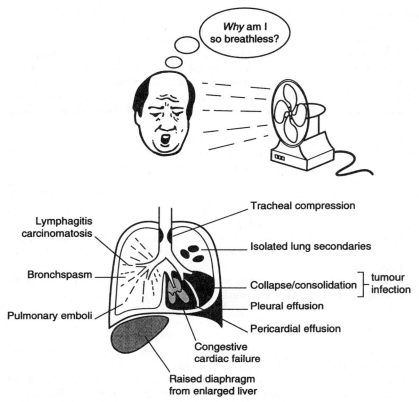

Fig. 4.5 Treat the cause of dyspnoea. facial cooling with a fan will ease the sensation of dyspnoea, but the cause to be treated will lie in the chest.

radiotherapy. Expectorated blood is extremely frightening for patients and relatives and may be the herald sign preceding a massive haemoptysis (Jones and Davies, 1990). When a massive haemoptysis occurs, the patient should be sedated as quickly as possible to decrease their distress and dark red towels used to disguise and soak up the large volumes of blood.

Pleural effusion can be drained through a small plastic cannula (Mansi and Hanks, 1989) almost painlessly – this can be done at home if the patient is too ill or too distressed to be moved. Chest infections causing symptoms warrant treatment with the appropriate oral antibiotics. If the patient deteriorates further and is unable to take oral medication it may become injudicious to resort to burdensome parenteral antibiotics, but the ethics of each case must be considered individually.

Another ethical dilemma occurs over pulmonary emboli. Clotting abnormalities associated with malignancy make patients prone to thrombosis and pulmonary emboli, but their response to anticoagulants can be unpredictable and difficult to control. Multiple small emboli causing recurrent episodes of dyspnoea usually warrant anticoagulation with warfarin. Large single emboli are usually rapidly fatal and symptomatic treatment with sedation and opioids may at times be more appropriate.

Table 4.5 Observations which suggest various causes of dyspnoea

Causes of dyspnoea	Pointer signs/symptoms
Tracheal compression	• Stidor/wheeze audible on inspiration and expiration. NB easily mistaken for wheezing • Inspiratory and expiratory effort
Tumour at epiglottis	• Marked inspiratory stridor sometimes partly relieved by sitting forwards. NB consider tracheostomy
Infection	• Sputum volume increase • Sputum colour change • Pyrexia is not always present early • Tachycardia, sweating
Pulmonary emboli	• Sudden episodes of deterioration (may be multiple and small) • Tachycardia • Apyrexial, no chest signs
Congestive failure	• Tachycardia • Patient prefers sitting up, worse on lying • Frothy white sputum when severe
Lymphangitis Lung secondaries	• Steady deterioration • Dyspnoea on exertion, progresses to dyspnoea at rest
Pleural effusion	• Steady deterioration, may be rapid • No vocal resonance felt when a hand put on the chest wall over the effusion • Stony dull to percussion • Trachea may be deviated towards the unaffected side
Anaemia	• Marked pallor • Marked tachycardia • Wide pulse pressure • Air hunger

Persistent irritant cough caused by lung metastases requires a clinical oncology opinion to consider radiotherapy or chemotherapy. Cough suppressants such as linctus codeine are remarkably ineffective and methadone linctus (2 mg/5 ml once or twice a day) may be more effective. Nebulised opioids can be helpful in a small number of patients. The local anaesthetic effect of nebulised lignocaine means that the patient is at risk of choking when swallowing and it has been shown to be no more effective than nebulised saline (Wilcock *et al.*, 1994).

Even after treating the underlying cause, the patient with an area of poorly ventilated lung will have a shunting of blood through that area and will therefore remain anoxic and dyspnoeic. Oxygen by mask does little to relieve this as the blood is shunted through an unventilated lung. Facial cooling relieves the sensation of dyspnoea, which is why patients feel like 'sitting by an open drafty window'; the breeze from a small electric fan can be very effective.

The patient's central respiratory drive can be damped down by judicious use of opioids (Bruera *et al.*, 1990). Oral morphine should be titrated in small (10 per cent) dose increments above the pain threshold until the sensation of severe dyspnoea is eased. The respiratory rate must be monitored and will fall as the dose of opioid rises. The side-effect of drowsiness may be a price worth paying to relieve the dying patient from the sensation of struggling to breathe and allow the patient to rest with peace and dignity. Low-dose midazolam will relieve panic. In severely dyspnoeic patients eating and talking will always be an effort, but neither patient nor family should have to experience distress.

Itch

Itching of dry scaly skin is easily relieved with simple emollients such as emulsifying ointment. When bath oils are used they can be applied directly to the patient's damp skin after a bath, rather than put in the bath water; they make the bath surface dangerously slippery.

Severe itching due to liver failure is sometimes partly relieved by topical cetomacragol and oral stanozolol. Questran, which decreases the bile salt concentration in the blood is extremely unpalatable to take and often ineffective for itch.

Whenever a skin rash is present a dermatology opinion should be sought. Scabies is a common cause of severe itching in the non–icteric patient.

Ascites

Intra-abdominal tumours and hepatic metastases can be associated with a rapidly accumulating ascites (Morris, 1984). A patient's girth increases, the abdomen feels heavy and uncomfortable and some patients find sitting difficult. Backache is often associated with large volumes of ascitic fluid. In patients with carcinoma of the ovary and intra-abdominal tumours the ascitic fluid may be thick and loculated.

Diuretics such as spironolactone have been recommended for patients with ascites, but often seem poorly effective. The discomfort of large volumes of ascitic fluid can be relieved by draining ascites via a small intravenous cannula inserted through the abdominal wall. The puncture site can be sealed with cyanoacrylate glue (superglue) to the skin to avoid persistent leakage of fluid (Blackwell and Burrow, 1994). The protein depletion that occurs when ascites is drained can result in a rapid deterioration of the patient's general condition so volumes of more than 3 litres should not be drained off in one go. If ascitic fluid is rapidly reaccumulating the surgical insertion of a Le Veen or similar shunt can be extremely beneficial; through this system the ascitic fluid drains directly back into the patient's circulation avoiding protein depletion (Morris, 1984).

Fungating lesions

A tumour beneath the skin or fungating through the skin surface is a visible reminder to the patient of their disease. When the skin is broken, the necrotic tissue at the tumour surface smells, oozes and can be extremely distressing. Sensitive and tactful nursing are required. It is important to remember the patient will be very embarrassed by the smell and soiling caused by exudate at the tumour surface as well as the indignity of having a sensitive part of the body destroyed (*The Lancet*, 1990). All too often the breast, genital area or part of the face become eroded by locally aggressive tumour. The goals in nursing care are different to the goals for surgical wounds, since fungating lesions will not heal and look worse as the tumour grows. The treatment aim is to contain the exudate, eradicate smell and achieve a cosmetically acceptable dressing for the patient. Palliative radiotherapy should always be considered as it can shrink the tumour and decrease the exudate from the tumour surface.

Anaerobic organisms living in the crevices of a tumour surface cause smell. Dead black and grey slough must be debrided with a scalpel blade and forceps. Small amounts remaining may then be digested off using scherisorb gel. Granu-flex dressings may help remove slough but the sticky layer tends to damage adjacent skin. Metronidazole kills the anaerobes on the tumour surface and topical metronidazole as a 0.8 per cent gel is remarkably effective (Newman *et al.*, 1989) (Fig. 4.6). Continued bacterial colonisation can be decreased with topical 0.5 per cent silver nitrate solution or with flamazine cream which contains silver nitrate. In patients with deep fistulation into the tumour surface, systemic metronidazole may be needed, although it does tend to cause gastrointestinal upset.

The quality of a patient's life must be preserved at all times. Dressing changes must not be painful; adequate analgesic cover is often attained with sublingual dextromoramide 10 mg half an hour before starting the dressing. Bleeding points require topically applied adrenalin solution or a seaweed alginate dressing over the bleeding points. The alginate dressings are useful to control bleeding, but tend to increase the amount of oozing and exudate from the surface.

Non-stick dressings should be applied to the tumour surface and can be coated

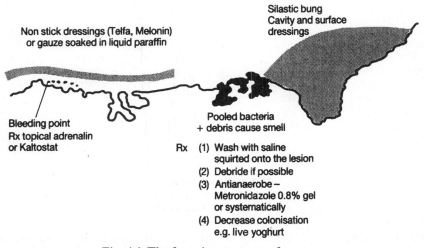

Fig. 4.6 The fungating tumour surface.

with topical metronidazole gel before application. Absorbent gauze and gamgee can then be applied to absorb excessive exudate. Netelast and tubigauze stocking dressings avoid the skin damage caused by adhesive tapes. Silastic foam dressings, which absorb exudate well, can be moulded to fit cavities. They can be rinsed out in chlorhexidine solution and re-used.

Both medical and nursing input are required in planning management of fungating lesions. While doing a dressing great sensitivity is need; facial expression can give away far more than ever intended and the patient's sense of dignity must be maintained.

Weakness

Weakness is one of the commonest symptoms associated with advancing cancer. The assessment of a patient by physiotherapist and occupational therapist can provide diagnostic information, provide the patient with walking aids and home adaptations to maximise mobility and can be extremely psychologically supportive to the patient whose decreasing mobility is a reminder of increasing disease (Fig. 4.7).

Treatable causes of weakness must be excluded (Regnard and Mannix, 1992). These include Parkinsonian side-effects of drugs, metabolic disturbances such as hypercalcaemia or hypokalaemia and the toxic effect of any infection. Parkinsonian patients often have rigidity and poverty of movement rather than a gross tremor. All central dopamine antagonists, which includes most antiemetics, risk these extrapyramidal side-effects. In patients whose immune system is already compromised, infections have few clinical pointers.

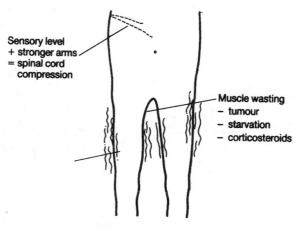

Sensory level
+ stronger arms
= spinal cord
compression

Muscle wasting
– tumour
– starvation
– corticosteroids

Generalised rapid weakness
– Parkinsonian effects of drugs
– Metabolic disturbance Ca^{++}; Na^{+}; K^{+}
– Toxic from infection

Fig. 4.7 Common causes of 'going off his legs'. Leg weakness must not be assumed to be an irreversible or untreatable effect of tumour.

Severe muscle wasting is a side-effect of corticosteroids, although tumours and low nutritional intake also cause muscle wasting *per se*. Lambert–Eaton syndrome associated with carcinoma of the lung is improved by treatment of the primary tumour (Elvington, 1992).

Spinal cord compression is a medical emergency (see below). It is the most important cause of progressive weakness. It is a medical emergency requiring immediate treatment the same day.

Insomnia

Lack of sleep decreases the patient's ability to cope with the difficulties of the disease. The distress caused by symptoms is worsened by fatigue and a vicious circle ensures. No hypnotic will compensate for poor symptom control. Patients must have pain control and feel physically comfortable. In addition, they need to feel warm, loved, secure and at peace within themselves. With attention to all of these details, most patients do not need a hypnotic. However, it may be useful to give drugs with sedative side-effects (e.g. haloperidol or methotrimeprazine) at night rather than during the day. Good physical and psychosocial care of a patient are the most important aids to sleep; a worried or frightened patient will not sleep.

Fear and anxiety

The eyes are said to the window of the mind. The patient's eyes, wide and staring, describe the terror of facing the unknown. As pressures pile in on patients who have to come to terms with the end of their life, often prematurely, they need to be able to voice these fears (Maguire *et al.*, 1993). Often patient's fears can be allayed. Fears are based on previous experiences or situations witnessed in others. Many patients are grateful for the reassurance that they will not 'go out of their mind' or 'stop being themselves' and they will not become used to their pain killers. The patient's confidence in the professionals' commitment to care is essential to relieve the fear of the unknown. Patients must know that their dignity will be maintained to the end and their family will be supported throughout.

Where a young parent is dying, open discussion over what to tell the children and their future care arrangements is important and should be instigated earlier rather than later.

Depression

A depressed mood and sadness are appropriate responses as a patient faces death. It is quite understandable that the patient feels sad, angry, bitter and anticipates the grief of impending loss in leaving loved ones and in losing health and autonomy. It is important to differentiate this 'appropriate sadness' from 'clinical depression' since a clinical depression will improve with treatment, but antidepressants are not happy making drugs. Inappropriate prescribing will make the patient feel sedated and experience drug side-effects which compound their misery and distress.

So how can the depressed patient be differentiated from the sad patient? Feelings of worthlessness, hopelessness and excessive guilt are pointers to a depressive syndrome in the terminally ill patient. Suicidal thoughts occur in depression; it is important to ensure that they are not a desperate cry for help as a result of poor symptom control when the symptoms such as pain need treatment as well as the depression.

Other symptoms commonly associated with depression such as insomnia, weight loss, fatigue are attributable to the cancer and therefore are not useful diagnostic pointers in these patients. Drug side-effects such as corticosteroid-induced psychosis can mimic depression. Early morning wakening in a patient with good pain control is a useful pointer to clinical depression, but must not be confused with the patient who is wakened by breakthrough pain. The depressed patient's mood on wakening is often low whereas the person who is appropriately sad experiences a build-up of emotion as the day goes on as different reminders of the illness become evident during the day.

Depression is often mixed with anxiety state and must not be confused with fear. Fears must be allayed. The patient needs to be able to talk about these fears. In general, benzodiazepines are unhelpful since they do not treat clinical depression, they may result in disinhibition of the patient and an increase in emotional lability, or a feeling of drowsiness and an increase in depression. In addition, after only a short time, a withdrawal anxiety can occur in between doses, making the situation worse.

When treatment is to be instigated with an antidepressant the choice depends on other pharmacological actions that are desired (Goldberg, 1987). Tricyclic antidepressants, particularly amitriptyline are useful for patients who also have some neuropathic pain (see Chapter 3 on pain) and .drugs such as clomipramine have a mild anxiolytic effect. They can be given at night or in divided doses through the day. Tricyclic antidepressants such as desipramine or nortriptylene have relatively low anticholinergic activity and so they are useful when anticholinergic properties should be avoided, such as patients who have had urinary retention, excessively dry mouth or patients on several drugs with anticholinergic properties, when an anticholinergic delirium could be precipitated.

The newer antidepressants appear to have little clinical advantage over the tricyclic group although they are less sedative. Fluoxetine is the most useful of the second generation antidepressants though it can cause mild nausea and a short period of increased anxiety initially. Several drug interactions have been reported.

The antidepressant effect of most drugs takes about 10 days to occur. When depression does not respond rapidly to treatment or if the patient's depression is worsening despite treatment, a psychiatric opinion should be sought.

Lymphoedema

Unfortunately, lymphoedema commonly occurs after mastectomy, particularly with axillary radiotherapy. Gross lymphoedema of the legs is also seen when patients have tumour in the abdomen involving para-aortic nodes and can be difficult to differentiate from venous thrombosis of the internal iliac veins (see Chapter 5).

Arm lymphoedema requires two main strategies. Firstly, the collapsed lymphatics beyond the site of obstruction need encouragement to open again with gentle massage or effleurage (Todd, 1993). A specialised physiotherapist is required to guide therapy. Rhythmic gentle massage should be undertaken working furthest away from the affected site and gradually massaging the area to include zones nearer and nearer the affected site. The second part of treatment requires compression bandaging which must be expertly and carefully applied. Compression bandaging which becomes tight or wrinkled will not provide even pressure and must be reapplied immediately. Badly applied compression bandaging can result in nerve damage. Sequential compression sleeves can assist with the massage process (Flowtron) and can be an adjunct to massage and compression bandaging. Diuretics have no place in the management of lymphoedema as they make the patient dehydrated but do nothing to relieve the obstruction or decrease fluid in the affected limb.

The skin of a lymphoedematous limb requires care to avoid abrasions. Bacterial cellulitis develops rapidly in a lymphoedematous limb and can be extremely difficult to eliminate, even with intravenous antibiotics. Meticulous care to nails and the skin around nails is important, and any evidence of athlete's foot should be treated immediately with topical antifungal agents. At the first sign of inflammation, antibiotics should be started, remembering of course that fungi may have entered percutaneously.

Lymphoedema of the lower limbs can also be treated by compression bandaging and massage. When the lymphoedema extends up to the waist, vigorous compression of the lower limbs will only result in swelling in the genital area and may be extremely uncomfortable for the patient. Male patients will need encouragement to apply gentle external pressure over an oedematous penis and scrotum to decrease the swelling. Obstruction to urinary outflow does not usually occur. In these patients a slow-acting diuretic such as spironolactone at low dose may occasionally help, and steroids may decrease peritumour oedema when there is para-aortic node involvement. A radiotherapy opinion should always be sought since some relief following radiotherapy of affected nodes can occur.

The dilemma of corticosteroids

Corticosteroids are used widely in palliative care for the relief of compression syndromes and of raised intracranial pressure. However, their indiscriminate use can create more problems than they relieve. Apart from the well-known gastric irritant effect, patients' tendency to develop a steroid psychosis cannot be predicted. Only a few exhibit a full-blown psychosis, but many patients experience a degree of emotional lability when on steroids, making them over-react to situations and feel anxious, weepy, frightened and insecure. These psychological alterations are distressing for the patient to experience and for the family to witness.

Steroids cause insomnia and agitation if given at night; no dose of steroids should be given after 6.00 pm for the patient who plans to go to sleep about 11.00 pm. The skin changes induced by steroids increase the risk of pressure sores. Steroids depress the immune response slightly and therefore symptoms of infection tend to be masked, making diagnosis more difficult. Steroids also have a diabetogenic effect.

The cushingoid face and facial hair that are common side-effects of high-dose steroid administration can be extremely distressing. The damage from this altered body image should not be underestimated. Muscle wasting of proximal muscle groups is a specific side-effect of corticosteroids and is slow to reverse after stopping the steroids.

Cerebral tumours and metastases

Cerebral tumours can be particularly distressing. Tumours involving the frontal lobe area can result in personality change, although, fortunately, these are rarely seen. Neurosurgery can sometimes be palliative in debulking tumours and will allow radical radiotherapy. Corticosteroids should be avoided early because of long-term side-effects (Kirkham, 1988). The tumour itself is usually surrounded by an area of oedema and hyperaemia; this is the area affected by high-dose corticosteroids, but the malignancy is unaffected. This decrease in oedema and hyperaemia can give a temporary relief of pressure effects, but, as the tumour grows, the pressure effects will recur and be resistant to corticosteroids. A good response to corticosteroids may suggest the patient will respond to further radiotherapy of the brain tumour.

When neurological function needs to be transiently regained for special events such as a family wedding, high-dose corticosteroids can be used to 'buy back' a little time. However, there are dangers in fluctuating the dose of corticosteroids between high and low dose and the use of steroids in this way needs careful ethical consideration otherwise the patient appears to transiently dramatically improve only to deteriorate again. When patients become less well it may be appropriate to tail down the corticosteroids and allow the patient to slip into coma, rather than lingering through a twilight state of awareness of tremendous disability.

In patients who can no longer swallow their steroids, the dose should be tailed down, but should not be abruptly stopped. The patient who has experienced adrenal suppression and has their steroids withdrawn will feel awful; a small subcutaneous dose daily may be appropriate for a few days until the patient becomes comatose.

Even when patients are extremely ill they have a right to their autonomy and there is no place for paternalism in deciding whether to increase or decrease steroids. Patient and family should be involved in the decision where possible and should feel in agreement with the decision taken. The role of the professional is to advise and suggest and should neither exclude nor override a patient's wishes. The aim must be to obtain the best possible outcome for the each patient at each point in the illness, given the realistic goals available within the limitations of the disease process.

Medical emergencies in palliative care

Spinal cord compression

Spinal cord compression is a disastrous complication of malignancy. Tumour compression of the cord will cause a progression of symptoms, often over several days, that can be halted by immediate radiotherapy or surgery if appropriate. Compression of the cervical, thoracic or upper lumbar spine will result in paraplegia at whatever level the compression occurs (Kramer, 1992). In the lower lumbar spine, compression of the cauda equina will cause specific symptoms and is also a medical emergency. In general, the patient who has rapidly progressing weakness of the legs and central pain in thoracic or cervical spine should raise a high index of suspicion. Sometimes the patient is tender on percussion over the specific vertebrae at the level of the tumour and may have some pain radiating out along the dermatome at that area (radicular pain). There may be paraesthesia and tingling in the limbs with decreased sensation and a feeling of heaviness and difficulty in moving the legs. Often the first sign is that the patient's have difficulty walking upstairs, although compression of the cervical spine also causes arm weakness. Examination of the patient may reveal a level of sensory loss corresponding to the level of the cord compression. There may be a very narrow band of increased sensation at this level with sensory loss below. As motor and sensory loss worsen, the paraplegia develops. This is irreversible and followed by loss of sphincter control. Compression of the cauda equina results in early bladder and bowel disturbance without the limb weakness.

All patients suspected of cord compression must be treated actively immediately – to wait until sphincters are lost is negligent. Paraplegia is terrible enough let alone when compounded by incontinence. Investigation with magnetic resonance imaging (MRI) scanning will show areas of tumour and radiotherapy can be commenced the same day. Patients with a spinal cord compression should be given steroids immediately, even prior to transfer to a radiotherapy unit, to decrease peritumour oedema and help preserve some neurological function during the delay involved in travelling.

Hypercalcaemia

Hypercalcaemia occurs in about 10 per cent of patients with cancer and is not restricted to tumours that metastasise to bone (Heath, 1989). A disturbance of bone metabolism results in the rapid reabsorption of calcium from bones occurring more quickly than the calcium load can be excreted through the kidney (Heller, 1986).

The patient with hypercalcaemia is often drowsy, constipated, nauseated with severe vomiting and dehydrated with a dry mouth. Unfortunately, all these symptoms are commonly seen in cancer patients, so a high index of suspicion of hypercalcaemia should be maintained at all times. A serum calcium and serum albumin should be done together, since the serum calcium must be corrected for a low albumin (Iqbal, 1968). The following SI unit equation is useful:

Corrected serum calcium = measured serum calcium + 0.02 (42-serum albumin)

Levels above 2.6 mmol/l are raised and those above 3.4 mmol/l are life-threatening.

Hypercalcaemia requires immediate admission to an in-patient unit and intravenous rehydration. The bisphosphonate drugs given intravenously can provide an excellent response; the serum calcium falls within 72 h giving dramatic relief in symptoms. Patients should not die prematurely from a condition that is now easily treated. It is important to remember that a few months of life can be very important to a patient, particularly a young parent preparing his or her family for life after bereavement. Patients with hypercalcaemia can look extremely ill before treatment but improve dramatically.

Superior vena caval obstruction

Mediastinal tumour compressing the superior vena cava results in gross swelling distorting the face and neck. Distended veins may be visible over the upper chest wall. Radiotherapy and high-dose steroids can reduce the bulk of the obstruction and give relief.

Conclusion

Perhaps the first rule in treating patients is to believe the patient. The question 'What is the worse thing for you at the moment?' can get the problem list into the patient's order of priorities and often takes the professional carers by surprise. The second rule is to never abandon the patient. When health professionals feel there is nothing more that can be done they, as carers, should review the situation as there is always comfort that can be given by caring and continuing to support.

There is no shame in needing to ask for help and advice from other colleagues and recognising honestly when other input to the clinical problem is required. The primary care team will maintain their principle role in providing care to the patients at home, calling on others when appropriate to do so. No individual professional should believe that they are omnipotent. Good patient care is only achieved by close integration of all specialist services.

The challenge to the professional is to continue to ask the question 'why', to elucidate the cause of each problem. When the cause is known, treatment can be administered scientifically and rapid relief of symptoms attained. There is no place for haphazard cookbook prescribing and each patient must be assessed individually.

References

ALDRED, M., ADDY, M., BAGG, J. and FINLAY, I. (1991). Oral health in the terminally ill. *Special Care in Dentistry* 11, 59–62

ALLEN, S. C. (1985). Respiratory disease: managing residual symptoms. *Geriatric Medicine*, 15–20 June.

BELFIELD, P. W. (1988). Urinary catheters. *British Medical Journal* 296, 836–7.

BLACKWELL, N. and BURROW, M. (1994). A sticky tip (letter). *Palliative Medicine* 8, 269–70.

BOYD, K. J. and KEEKEN, L. (1994). Tube feeding in palliative care: benefits and problems. *Palliative Medicine* 8, 156–8.

BRUERA, E., MACMILLAN, K., PITHER, J. *et al.* (1990). Effects of morphine on the dyspnoea of terminal cancer patients. *Journal of Pain and Symptom Management*, 5(6), 341–4.

DOVER, S. B. (1987). Syringe driver in terminal care. *British Medical Journal* 294, 553–4.

ELVINGTON, G. (1992). The Lambert–Eaton myasthenic syndrome. *Palliative Medicine* 6, 9–17

FERRY, D. R. and CULLEN, M. H. (1991), Nausea and vomiting. *Medical International* 3892–3.

FINLAY, I. G. (1986). Oral symptoms and candida in the terminally ill. *British Medical Journal* 292, 592–3.

FINLAY, I. G. (1991). Rational use of antiemetics in the terminally ill. *Update* 16 September, 2–6.

GOLDBERG, R. J. (1987). Management of depression in the patient with advanced cancer. *Journal of the American Medical Association* 246, 373–6.

HEATH, D. E. (1989). Hypercalcaemia of malignancy. *Palliative Medicine* 3, 1–11.

HELLER, S. R. and HOSKING, D. J. (1986). Renal handling of calcium and sodium in metastatic and non-metastatic malignancy. *British Medical Journal* 29, 583–5.

IQBAL, S. J., GILES, M., LEDGER, S., NANJI, N. and HOWL, T. (1968). Need for albumin adjustments of urgent total serum calcium. *The Lancet* 24/31 December, 1477–8.

JONES, D. K. and DAVIES, R. J. (1990). Massive haemoptysis. *British Medical Journal* 300, 889–90.

KIRKHAM, S. R. (1988). The palliation of cerebral tumours with high-dose dexamethasone: a review. *Palliative Medicine* 2, 27–33.

KRAMER, J. A. (1992). Spinal cord compression in malignancy. *Palliative Medicine* 6, 202–11.

McKILLOP W. J., STEWART, W. E., GINSBURG, A. D. and STEWART, S. S. (1988). Cancer patients conception of their disease and its treatment. *British Journal of Cancer* 58, 355–8.

MAGUIRE, P., FAULKNER, A. and REGNARD, C. (1993). Managing the anxious patient with advancing disease – a flow diagram. *Palliative Medicine* 7, 239–44.

MANSI, J. L. and HANKS, G. W. (1989). Drainage of malignant effusions. *The Lancet*, 1 July, 43.

MEUNIER, S., GERAIN, J. and SNORCK, R. (1990). Oral treatment of oropharyngeal candidiasis with nystatin versus ketoconazole in cancer patients, a randomised study. *Drug Investigation* 2, 71–5.

MERCADANTE, S., SPALDIO, E. and CARACENI, A. (1993). Octreotide in relieving gastrointestinal symptoms due to bowel obstruction. *Palliative Medicine* 7, 295–9.

MORRIS, J. S. (1984). Ascites. *British Medical Journal* 289, 209.

NEWMAN, V., ALWOOD, A. L. and OAKES, R. A. (1989). Use of metronidazole gel to control smell from fungating lesions. *Palliative Medicine* 3, 303–5.

OLIVER, D. J. (1985). The use of methotrimeprazine in terminal care: a review. *Palliative Medicine* 2, 21–6.

REGNARD, C. (1988). Constipation: an algorithm. *Palliative Medicine* 2, 34–5, 54–5.

REGNARD, C. and COMISKEY, M. (1992). Nausea and vomiting in advanced cancer – a flow diagram. *Palliative Medicine* 6, 146–51.

REGNARD, C. and MANNIX, K. (1991). Urinary problems in advanced cancer – a flow diagram. *Palliative Medicine* 5, 344–8.

REGNARD, C. and MANNIX, K. (1992). Weakness and fatigue in advanced cancer – a flow diagram. *Palliative Medicine* 6, 105–10.

SYKES, N. (1990). The management of nausea and vomiting. *The Practitioner*, 234, 286–90.

THE LANCET (1990). Editorial. Management of smelly tumours. *The Lancet* 20 January, 141–2.

TODD, J. (1993). Lymphoedema: a guide to pathogenesis and management. *Oncology Newsletter* 1, 3–5

TWYCROSS, R. and LACK, S. (1986). Constipation. In: *Control of Alimentary Symptoms in Far Advanced Cancer*, pp. 166–207. Churchill Livingstone.

WILCOCK, A., CORCORAN, R. and TATTERSFIELD, A. E. (1994). Safety and efficacy of nebulised lignocaine in patients with cancer and breathlessness. *Palliative Medicine* 8, 35–8.

Further reading

ALDRED, M., ADDY, M., BAGG, J. and FINLAY, I. (1991). Oral health in the terminally ill. *Special Care in Dentistry* 11, 59–62

McKILLOP W. J., STEWART, W. E., GINSBURG, A. D. and STEWART, S. S. (1988). Cancer patients conception of their disease and its treatment. *British Journal of Cancer* 58, 355–8.

MERCADANTE, S., SPALDIO, E. and CARACENI, A. (1993). Octreotide in relieving gastrointestinal symptoms due to bowel obstruction. *Palliative Medicine* 7, 295–9.

REGNARD, C. and COMISKEY, M. (1992). Nausea and vomiting in advanced cancer – a flow diagram. *Palliative Medicine* 6, 146–51.

5

Lymphoedema

Caroline Badger

'The most important requirement of the art of healing is that no mistakes or neglect occur.'

from Huang Ti Nei Ching Su Wen
(The Yellow Emperor's Classic on Internal Medicine)

Introduction

It is likely that in any clinical setting where the patients are weak, debilitated, immobile, elderly or very sick, oedema will manifest as a problem; it follows therefore that cancer patients, particularly those with advanced disease, are a vulnerable group.

A distinction is made here between transient acute oedema, such as that following an injury (which should resolve by itself) and chronic oedema. Chronic oedema is a progressive condition resulting from insufficiency, or failure, of the lymph system, with or without co-existent venous insufficiency and it will not resolve without intervention When oedema results purely from lymphatic insufficiency it is known as lymphoedema, if there is a venous component to the swelling the term lymphovenous oedema is usually used.

The lymph system

One of the main functions of the lymph system is to act as an 'overflow pipe' system, returning excess interstitial fluid to the blood circulation. Only about 10 per cent of the fluid that filters from the blood into the interstitium is drained by lymphatic vessels, the remaining 90 per cent is re-absorbed into the venous end of the capillary loop. Together with interstitial fluid, proteins too large to pass back through blood capillary walls are also removed from the tissues by the lymph system. The propulsion of lymph through the system is not provided by the heart: flow is dependent largely on the action of the muscle pump in limbs and the massaging effects of local tissue movement. The large lymphatic vessels have contractile walls and are valved to ensure that the flow of lymph is unidirectional. Lymph will pass through a series of at least one or more lymph nodes before joining the blood circulation via the thoracic duct; nodes act as filters to substances such as bacteria or malignant cells.

Oedema arises when there is a discrepancy between the amount of fluid that the lymph system has to transport and its actual transport capacity. If drainage routes are reduced (as, for example, when lymph nodes are excised or irradiated) then clearly the remaining routes have to take on an extra load; the result is overloading of the system which eventually fails, leading to an accumulation of fluid in the affected subcutaneous tissues of the body. On the other hand the cause might lie in an increase in the amount of fluid being formed in the interstitium (as, for example, in the case of venous insufficiency); the lymphatics respond initially by increasing lymph flow but if the increased level of tissue fluid persists the lymphatic vessels are once again overloaded and begin to fail, and once again swelling appears.

Oedema and the cancer patient

Cancer patients often develop oedema as the result of a variety of factors; in addition to the underlying mechanisms outlined above they may be suffering from hypoproteinaemia, heart failure, or be taking fluid-retaining drugs. While the principles of treatment remain the same regardless of the cause, the approach to treatment, realistic goals and the use of additional treatments will vary according to the cause and type of oedema. A careful and thorough assessment of the patient is therefore essential in order to select the most appropriate treatment.

Treatment may either be active (Badger and Twycross, 1988) in nature or palliative (Mortimer *et al.*, 1993), the indications for active treatment are detailed in Fig. 5.1. The same four main components of treatment (Fig. 5.2) are used in both active and palliative treatment, the difference being that in palliative treatment the way in which the components are combined and the intensity with which they are used, may vary. Each of the four elements of treatment has a distinct role to play and in order for active treatment to be successful the four components are always used in combination. In palliative treatment each element may be used separately to achieve a specific effect.

Before treatment can be selected a thorough history must be taken and a careful clinical examination performed.

Assessment

Assessment should take into account the extent, as well as the degree, of oedema: if oedema involves the trunk as well a limb or limbs, treatment will have to include the trunk in order to achieve drainage from the limbs. Pinching folds of skin simultaneously on both sides of the body is the most reliable method of

---

- Oedema is chronic.

- The cause of the oedema is reversible.

- The cause of the oedema is irreversible *but* there are sufficient drainage routes for lymph to allow the reduction of oedema.

- The patient's life expectancy is longer than a few weeks.

- The patient wishes to have treatment.

Fig. 5.1 Indications for the active treatment of oedema.

- Care of the skin.

- External compression or support.

- Manual lymph drainage.

- Exercise.

Fig. 5.2 The four main components of treatment.

detecting oedema on the trunk: oedematous tissue is more difficult to pick up and will feel thicker. Marks left by clothing/underwear will also provide clues as to the presence of oedema.

The presence of arterial problems will preclude the use of compression: if the ankle/brachial index is greater than 0.8 then gentle support (less than 10 mmHg at the ankle) may be applied.

Veins that fail to collapse on elevation and/or the appearance of obvious collateral veins suggest venous obstruction of some kind. Oedema as a result of deep vein thrombosis is not of itself an indication for compression treatment, since any accompanying oedema will resolve with treatment of the blood clot. If a thrombus forms in an already oedematous lower limb, or if the oedema fails to resolve, compression treatment with bandages or elastic hosiery is usually postponed until at least eight weeks following the start of anticoagulant therapy, to avoid the risk of emboli; this is not a problem if the thrombus has followed total occlusion of a blood vessel by progressing tumour. Where upper limbs are concerned compression is often used from the onset of anticoagulant treatment, the rationale being that the blood vessels and thrombi are so much smaller that any emboli are unlikely to be large enough to cause trouble.

If cellulitis is present antibiotics must be started (simple penicillin V, or erythromycin if the patient is allergic to penicillin) and treatment of the oedema should be postponed until the infection has resolved. Fungal infections, such as athlete's foot, are common and can easily be treated with antifungal creams or powders.

As always it is essential to determine the type and cause of any pain or discomfort before deciding on treatment.

The extent and site of any tumour will have an impact on any goals set in relation to the oedema as will the tumour's responsiveness to cancer treatment; if the tumour can be influenced by treatment then an active approach to treating the oedema may be possible.

If active treatment is being pursued then accurate measurement of limb volume, at the very least, limb circumferences at set points, are essential in order to determine the effectiveness of treatment. If treatment is palliative then clearly any troublesome symptoms should be reviewed on a regular basis in order to know whether treatment is proving helpful.

Common scenarios

Once the type and cause of oedema and any accompanying complications have been identified, and realistic goals of treatment decided upon with the patient, the most appropriate treatment can be selected. The following examples illustrate three common scenarios frequently encountered in palliative care settings. The underlying mechanisms and characteristic problems associated with each type of oedema are described and suggestions made for treatment in each case.

Lymphoedema resulting from cancer treatment

The surgical treatment of cancer often involves lymphatic drainage routes: lymph nodes may be partially or wholly excised and the lymphatic vessels transected, with a consequent interruption to, or reduction in, potential pathways for the drainage of interstitial fluid. If radiotherapy is added, the resultant progressive scarring can reduce the drainage capacity of the lymph system still further. Under these circumstances the load on the lymphatics (that is the amount of fluid being formed in the interstitium) is not increased, but the capacity of the lymph system to transport this normal load is reduced; as a consequence fluid accumulates in the interstitium eventually giving rise to obvious swelling of the affected part of the body.

Characteristic problems

Lymphoedema is a high-protein oedema: the lymphatics are the only means by which large proteins are removed from the interstitium, so that any reduction in the drainage capacity of the lymph system leads to an increase in the protein concentration of tissue fluid. The presence of static, protein-rich fluid in the interstitium sets up a chronic inflammatory process which causes the skin and subcutaneous tissues to change. The thickened, leathery appearance of the skin resembles elephant hide and is the reason why long-standing lymphoedema is commonly called 'elephantiasis'. While lymphoedema is soft and pitting in its early stages, the progressive fibrosis of the tissues is responsible for the characteristic non-pitting nature of chronic lymphoedema. Skin creases and natural skin folds are enhanced as the tissues thicken and a distortion in the normal shape of the limb is quite common.

Lymphoedema leads to a reduction in local immunity in the affected area, so that recurrent episodes of cellulitis are frequently a problem; occasionally there is an obvious cause for the cellulitis – an insect bite, a cut or abrasion, or even a fungal infection such as athlete's foot – but often there is no visible portal of entry for bacteria and the attack appears more inflammatory in nature than infective. Repeated attacks of infection cause further damage to lymphatic vessels and so treatment is best aimed at prevention.

Treatment

In patients with a life expectancy of more than a few weeks, who do not have localised recurrence of a tumour affecting lymph drainage, it is reasonable to aim for reduction and control of swelling. The main aims of treatment are illustrated in Fig. 5.3.

Treatment is normally carried out in two phases. The initial reduction phase

- To reduce the volume of the limb.

- To restore the limb to a normal shape.

- To soften fibrotic subcutaneous tissues.

- To eliminate recurrent infection.

Fig. 5.3 The aims of active treatment.

usually lasts anywhere between 2 and 4 weeks and involves treatment (see Fig. 5.2) of the patient by a specialist practitioner.

Skin care is an essential part of treatment. In lymphoedema the skin is usually very dry and prone to cracking. An intact and supple skin will reduce the risk of infection. Hyperkeratosis, another common problem, can be treated with salicylic acid ointment.

External compression is applied using a multilayer technique of bandaging (Badger, 1992). Low-stretch bandages are used (Rosidal K – Lohmann; Comprilan – Beiersdorf) in order to achieve a relatively low resting pressure that rises when the limb is active. Compression raises interstitial pressure, limits the formation of tissue fluid and provides a firm outer casing against which the muscles in the limb can pump. Since pressure is applied in a gradient that reduces towards the root of the limb, fluid is encouraged to drain towards the body. The foam padding used under the bandages helps to create a smooth profile on which to bandage, overcoming the problems of distortion in the shape of the limb as well as protecting the joints and flexures of the limb.

As has already been mentioned movement is essential for good lymph flow. Exercises are used to promote the drainage of lymph and discourage pooling of fluid in the limbs.

The manual drainage of lymph involves a specific technique of massage. The aim is to move fluid from oedematous areas of the body to uncongested areas where lymphatics are functioning normally. Fluid is moved by whatever routes are possible (i.e. tissue planes or via lymphatics or veins). Aromatherapy massage or other therapeutic techniques of massage are not a substitute for manual lymph drainage and may, indeed, make swelling worse. A simplified form of manual lymph drainage 'simple massage' (Regnard *et al.*, 1991) can be taught to patients or their carers.

The second phase of treatment is the maintenance of any improvement and relies on the patient following a regime at home, while receiving regular monitoring of progress by a suitably experienced practitioner. The regime consists of continuing the daily programme of skin care, exercises to promote lymph drainage, wearing strong compression hosiery and regular sessions of self-massage.

Oedema resulting from tumour obstruction

A tumour mass can interfere with the drainage of lymph by obstructing lymph nodes or vessels, as may the diffuse spread of tumour cells through small lymphatic vessels. In such cases there is often a venous component to the oedema since, in addition to obstructing lymphatic vessels, tumour may also compress or obstruct blood vessels. Pressure in the obstructed vein rises and there is a consequent increase in the filtration of fluid from the blood into the interstitium. Obstruction to venous outflow may also result in the formation of a thrombus in the vein. Unlike the case of pure lymphoedema described above, the picture here is one of an increased load on the lymphatics (more fluid is formed in the interstitium) as well as a reduction in the lymphatic systems capacity to drain it.

Characteristic problems

The problems of increased size, distortion in the shape of the limb and recurrent infection may all affect this group too. If tumour is extensive, or if there is a cutaneous spread, the affected oedematous tissues tend to be tense, hard and indurated. Elephantiastic changes in the skin are often more pronounced (particularly in the upper limb). Superficial skin lymphatics may become dilated; initially they have the appearance of blisters, but gradually they become more organised and solid. Weeping of lymph through the skin (lymphorrhoea) is frequently a problem and there may also be ulceration in areas of tumour infiltration.

If venous blood flow is compromised there may be signs of venous hypertension: veins that don't collapse when the limb is raised or the appearance of obvious collateral veins.

Oedema will usually extend beyond the root of the limb, i.e. the groin or axilla, onto the adjacent quadrant of the trunk front and back. In the case of recurrence of breast cancer, for example, oedema may extend beyond the arm, up the side of the neck and down as far as the waist. Extensive pelvic tumour may result in bilateral oedema of the lower limbs extending beyond the groins to involve the genitals, and in extreme cases up as far as the nipples.

Movement of affected joints is often severely restricted by oedema, particularly in the upper limb: if movement has been discouraged, for instance if the patient has been advised to rest the limb, stiffness and immobility set in very rapidly.

Pain or discomfort usually arises from an intense feeling of pressure in the affected tissues, a feeling that the limb is about to burst. Neurological symptoms are probably more likely to be due to the tumour than to the oedema, although swelling may exacerbate the symptoms. Feelings of a deep, intense aching are probably the result of venous congestion. If the skin is ulcerated or there is lymphorrhoea there may well be a cellulitis in the limb and this will be another source of discomfort.

Treatment

While local tumour remains uncontrolled reduction of the oedema is an unrealistic aim. This is particularly true when the trunk is congested, since treatment aimed at reducing the volume of limbs will only result in an increase of oedema on the body. Palliative treatment, however, is possible and much can be done to relieve discomfort. A thorough assessment will reveal what the patient considers to be the most troublesome problem.

While diuretics have no useful role in the treatment of pure lymphoedema they may be appropriate if oedema is venous in origin or if it has been exacerbated by fluid retention. A combination of high–dose steroids and a diuretic is worth considering when oedema results from lymphatic/venous obstruction as a result of a tumour mass: steroids may have an effect on reducing peritumour swelling and as a consequence may relieve some degree of obstruction.

Oedematous skin is vulnerable to trauma and slow to heal so that great care must be taken to preserve a supple and intact skin. If the skin is already damaged then scrupulous skin hygiene is necessary to prevent infection. Lymphorrhoea (leakage of lymph through the skin) is treated with bandaging for the first 24–48 h until the leakage has stopped; hosiery is then fitted to prevent a re–occurrence.

Feelings of intense pressure in the limb can be countered by the application of external support. A variety of different products can be used ranging from shaped Tubigrip (single or double layer) to off-the-shelf hosiery to low-stretch bandages; bandages are simply wrapped around the limb to provide support, rather than applied under tension. Factors that will influence the choice of support are illustrated in Fig. 5.4.

Tubular supports and elastic hosiery are best used when the skin is in a reasonable condition since pulling the garment on and off may damage fragile or broken skin. Mobility in the limb will need to be considered since a degree of joint movement will be needed in order to apply the garment. A wide range of sizes is available, but grossly swollen limbs may need to be bandaged. The garment should fit snugly, but should not constrict and should always feel comfortable; remember that the aim is to support swollen tissues not to reduce volume. It may be easier to fit two layers of a bigger size sleeve or stocking than a single layer of a tighter-fitting garment.

Once in place, garments should never be turned down at the top – any excess in the length of the garment should be eased evenly down the length of the limb – nor should the material be allowed to wrinkle or crease: turning the garment down will create a tourniquet effect, while wrinkles and creases will tend to rub the skin and may cause damage and discomfort.

In cases where the limb is gross in size, or where joints are stiff and/or fixed, or where the skin is weeping, damaged or fragile, the limb will need to be bandaged. Any necessary dressings can be applied first and then the multilayer bandaging applied over the top. Be guided by the patient when it comes to the amount of pressure used since this will vary from patient to patient: insufficient pressure will not relieve the bursting feeling while too much will be uncomfortable. Bandaging should never impede movement of affected joints.

- The condition of the skin.

- The mobility of affected joints.

- The size of the limb.

- Availability of resources.

- The patient's preference.

Fig. 5.4 Factors that influence the choice of external support.

When the treatment of oedema is active, rather than palliative, bandages must be replaced once in every 24 h but in the palliative approach, provided the patient has full sensation in the limb and the skin is intact, bandages may be left in place for 2 or 3 days. Hosiery is usually removed at night and put on first thing in the morning.

Exercise of the main muscles that are important for pumping (i.e. the forearm muscles for the upper limb and the calf muscles in the lower limb) will enhance flow and discourage pooling of blood and lymph. In addition, regular gentle exercise of the joints will help to prevent stiffening and/or preserve residual joint movement. Exercises may be passive if the patient is unable to perform active movements.

Manual lymph drainage or simple massage can be used to ease fluid congestion on the trunk and relieve tension in the tissues of the affected limb. The effect tends to be short-lived, so that it is often the case that frequent sessions are needed throughout the day; the help of relatives or friends could be enlisted to carry out the massage.

Dependency oedema

Dependency oedema affects, as the name suggests, limbs that are immobile and dependent for much of the time. The sort of patients that are most at risk are those with paralysed limbs, perhaps due to brachial plexus damage as a result of breast cancer or due to spinal cord compression by tumour, and those who are weak, less mobile and spending a large part of the day sitting in a chair with legs down.

Oedema develops under these circumstances because of a lack of propulsion to blood and lymph in the limb. The movement of lymph through the lymphatic system is largely dependent upon the local massaging action of moving tissues. Muscle pumping, so important in helping venous blood to return to the heart, also plays an important part in propelling lymph. If movement and muscular activity decreases or are absent in a limb, then pooling of blood and lymph occurs, exacerbated by the effects of gravity.

Characteristic problems

This type of oedema is usually soft and pitting unless it has been present for some time, in which case the patient may exhibit signs of the skin and tissue changes associated with lymphatic insufficiency. Characteristically the swelling predominantly affects the distal portion of the limb: in an immobile patient both lower limbs will tend to be affected with most, if not all, of the swelling gathered around the feet and ankles, while in the paralysed upper limb it is usually the hand and forearm that is worst affected, while the shoulder and upper arm are often clear of oedema.

Oedema may be slight to begin with but, unless movement is restored or treatment instituted, the oedema will progressively worsen. Other problems will ensue: oedematous skin is vulnerable to injury, slow to heal, and provides a focus for infection; water is heavy and the increased weight of swollen limbs places an additional burden on a patient who already has problems with mobility and may be weak and debilitated. Heavy swollen legs can make all the difference between a patient preserving what little mobility remains or becoming bed-bound and may, indeed, be the only thing preventing a patient from going home.

Treatment

This type of oedema responds well to pressure and is usually relatively easy to reduce because it is displaced easily. With respect to lower limb oedema, if the oedema is mild, of recent onset and hasn't resulted in gross distortion of the shape of the limb, then it is probably sufficient to fit the patient with below knee compression stockings. Gentle compression (anything from 15 to 25 mmHg at the ankle) should be all that is required, in combination with some gentle regular movement of the limb and elevation to the horizontal when resting. When the limb is paralysed and movement and/or elevation not possible, then higher compression (20–40 mmHg at the ankle) will probably be necessary. If application of the stronger hosiery proves difficult then it is useful to note that the same effect of increased pressure can be obtained by the application of two layers of the lower class of stockings.

When the degree of oedema is more severe, the shape of the limb significantly distorted, or the problem so long-standing that fibrosis of the affected tissues is present, then more intensive measures are required. Provided oedema doesn't extend to the trunk a short course of pneumatic compression therapy (Flowtron, Lymphapress), say 1–2 h, should reduce the swelling and soften the tissues. Stockings should then be fitted immediately to support the drained tissues. Once again class 1 should be sufficient for patients with residual movement in the limbs while stronger compression will be required if paralysis is present and/or elevation of the limb is not possible.

In cases of dependency oedema of the upper limb, many of the same principles apply, with the exception of the use of the pneumatic compression pump. Dependency oedema in the upper limb will almost exclusively be the result of reduced mobility due to neurological damage rather than as a result of weakness or debility. The ensuing stasis is nearly always compounded by compromised lymph drainage in the affected upper quadrant of the body which results from the cancer treatment or from obstruction by tumour. The use of pneumatic compression therapy runs the risk of overloading lymphatics beyond the root of the limb, causing fluid congestion in the tissues of the shoulder, chest or upper back

Since most of the swelling is likely to be concentrated in the hand and fingers these areas may be grossly distorted, in which case multilayer bandages are the first line treatment. If the swelling is not severe and is soft and pitting then a compression glove should successfully reduce and control swelling in the fingers and the addition of a compression sleeve with attached handpiece should reduce and control the hand and arm swelling. Most elastic arm sleeves come in one compression class only, but once again two layers of sleeve will increase the compression. The same indications for exercise and elevation will apply for upper limbs as lower limbs.

Oedema can be a distressing and unpleasant condition for the cancer patient, resulting in considerable physical and psychosocial handicap. If signs of oedema are actively sought treatment can be instituted early on; many of the problems associated with established oedema can then be avoided and much of the distress alleviated.

References

BADGER, C (1992). External compression and support in the management of chronic oedema. In: PRITCHARD, A. P. and MALLETT, J. (eds), *The Royal Marsden Hospital Manual of Clinical Nursing Procedures*, pp. 211–20, 3rd edn. Blackwell Scientific, Oxford.

BADGER, C. and TWYCROSS, R. (1988). *Management of Lymphoedema: Guidelines.* Sobell Study Centre. Oxford.

MORTIMER, P., BADGER, C. and HALL, J. (1993). Lymphoedema. In: DOYLE, D., HANKS, G. and MACDONALD, N. (eds), *Oxford Textbook of Palliative Medicine*, pp. 407–15. Oxford University Press, Oxford.

REGNARD, C., BADGER, C. and MORTIMER, P. (1991). *Lymphoedema: Advice on Treatment*, 2nd edn. Beaconsfield Publishers, Beaconsfield.

Further reading

BADGER, C. and REGNARD, C. (1989). Oedema in advanced disease: a flow diagram. *Palliative Medicine*, 3, 213–15.

BADGER, C., MORTIMER, P., REGNARD, C. and TWYCROSS, R. (1988). Pain in the chronically swollen limb. In: PARTSCH H. (ed.), *Progress in Lymphology – XI*, pp. 243–5. Elsevier Science, Amsterdam.

JEFFS, E. (1993). The effect of acute inflammatory episodes (cellulitis) on the treatment of lymphoedema. *Journal of Tissue Viability* 3(2) 51–5.

MORTIMER, P. (1990). Investigation and management of lymphoedema. *Vascular Medicine Review* 1, 1–20.

THOMAS, S. (1990). Bandages and bandaging: the science behind the art. *CARE Science and Practice*, 8(2) 56–60.

WILLIAMS, A. (1993). *Lymphoedema Services Directory*. Sobell Study Centre, Oxford.

6

Nutritional care

Charlette R. Gallagher-Allred

Caring for the dying patient and family is as important to any health-care professional involved with palliative care as treatment of the symptoms resulting from
the underlying disease. To care means that we accept the patient and family and
deal with the issues and concerns that are important to them. Nutrition is often a
major issue and concern of dying patients and their families.

The meaning of food and nutrition

Food carries biological, emotional and sociological meanings. It means different
things to different people, and, within the same person it has different meanings
depending on whether they are ill or well.

The act of serving food to others, regardless of setting, carries a highly
symbolic value. It characterises the social and community values of 'being thy
brother's keeper' (Callahan, 1983). Food also carries with it religious, cultural and
ethnic values that have meaning to patients, families and health-care professionals.
In order to fully appreciate the meaning food has in the lives of patients, those
involved with palliative care would do well to identify the meaning food has in
their own lives.

The dying process can alter a patient's nutritional needs in three ways.

- The anatomical, physiological, and metabolic changes that occur because of various diseases can decrease gastrointestinal absorption and increase nutrient
  requirements, such as frequently occurs in patients with acquired immune deficiency syndrome (AIDS) who often develop severe diarrhoea and malabsorption.
- The dying process itself slows many body functions, including gastric emptying,
  which results in increased satiety, decreased hunger and frequent food intolerances.
- Medical interventions, such as curative chemotherapy, alter metabolic processes
  and frequently result in increased nutrient requirements. Even palliative medications such as narcotics alter nutrient needs when side-effects occur, such as
  nausea, vomiting and constipation.

Overlaid on these *physical* conditions are changes in the desire for food because
of the *psychological* changes that accompany the grief process. For example, the
dying patient often holds different views of food depending on his or her stage of
death and dying. A patient in the denial stage may demand tube or parenteral
feeding stating, 'I'm not ill'. An angry patient may express anger and guilt
through statements such as, 'I ate a high-fibre diet all my life and I *still* got colon
cancer'. A patient during the bargaining stage of death and dying may ask, 'If I

give up alcohol, will my liver cancer stop spreading?' Depressed patients are often anorectic and do not eat, but the acceptance stage may be signalled by an increase in appetite as the patient is relieved of denial, anger, bargaining and depression.

Goals of nutritional care

Overall goals of palliative care are to maximise enjoyment and minimise pain. When eating and mealtimes can accomplish either of these goals, they should be used to advantage. If eating is not an enjoyable experience, on the other hand, its practice should not be overemphasised. It is at this time that the nurse can be a strong patient advocate and family ally by reassuring both that loving care can be demonstrated in ways other than through feeding.

The goals in the provision of nutritional care to dying patients and their families include the following.

- Relief of troublesome symptoms (diet can be an effective adjunct to medical and nursing interventions).
- Enhancement of pleasurable experiences of living.
- Prevention or treatment of malnutrition, which could be the unavoidable cause of death, if death by starvation or dehydration is unacceptable to the patient, family, and/or health-care team.

The nurse's role in achieving nutritional goals

'The role of the nurse in nutritional care of the terminally ill is first, to come to terms with personal, psychological, and moral and ethical issues surrounding nutrition and hydration on an individual level; and second, to enter into a partnership with the patient and family and guide them through the storm of emotions and questions using a framework based on principles of ethics, crisis intervention, and effective communication.' (Mauer Baack, 1993, p. 1).

Following such self-understanding, the nurse will perform several functions in order to achieve the goals in the provision of nutritional care to dying patients and their families, including the following.

- Assess the patient's physical and psychological condition for the role that curative and palliative treatments, food and mealtimes have on causing symptoms; ascertain if dietary modifications can alleviate these symptoms and improve well-being.
- Identify the patient and family's nutritional concerns and dietary questions.
- Establish goals of treatment and integrate dietary interventions as appropriate into the overall plan of care.
- Counsel the patient and family on specific and practical dietary modifications that can enhance well-being.
- Re-evaluate nutritional goals and intervention periodically, and implement changes when appropriate.

Assess the patient's condition

Assessment is the first component in the provision of nutritional care to dying patients and their families. A plan of care can only be as good as the completeness and accuracy of the data collected and the assessment of the patient's condition and the family's situation.

Figure 6.1 is an assessment instrument that includes important nutrition-related questions that the nurse might ask the patient and family during an initial visit and during on-going visits. Answers to these questions will give clues about the nutritional status and eating behaviour of the patient. In addition, it might alert the nurse to the need for the services of a dietician or nutritionist.

Identify patient and family concerns

Figure 6.1 also includes questions about specific nutrition issues and dietary concerns that patients and their families may wish to express. The nurse will want to be attentive for off-handed concerns that expose hidden fears, such as those given below.

- 'If I don't drink anything, will dehydration be painful?'
- 'I'd like to eat, but I'm afraid I'll choke and be unable to breathe if I eat too much.'
- 'If I had eaten "right" would I have avoided cancer?'
- 'I'm sure people will think I look too thin in the coffin.'

Integrate nutrition into the plan of care

After the information from the nutrition assessment tool is collected and assessed, a nutrition problem list can be delineated. Nutritional goals that are consistent with other medical and nursing goals should then be established. Following the delineation of appropriate palliative nutrition therapies to treat each nutrition problem, the problems, goals, and therapies are written into the plan of care.

When identifying goals and suggesting appropriate therapies, the nurse will want to take the patient and family's ethnic, cultural and religious background into consideration. Despite the well-known adage that it is hazardous to apply stereotypes to individual patients, peoples of various backgrounds do have different views and do respond differently to food, symptoms, pain, health-care delivery systems and dying. The views and responses of others are often greatly different from our own. To be helpful to patients and their families, nurses must not only recognise that individual differences exist but must also be supportive of these differences (Gallagher-Allred, 1989, p. 127).

Counsel on appropriate dietary modifications

Anticipatory guidance is an important aspect of the nutritional care plan. When counselling the patient and family on how to manage the symptoms associated with dying, the nurse anticipates those problems most likely to occur and guides the patient and family in making plans to handle them, thereby alleviating their fears of future problems. Information about diet and nutrition that the patient and family will benefit from counselling by the nurse includes the following (Gallagher-Allred, 1989, p. 223).

- How the disease process and the process of dying can affect the patient's desire for food.

1. Does the patient experience any of the following problems?
   - nausea and /or vomiting   Yes ☐   No ☐
     if so, is it associated with
     — taste of specific foods   Yes ☐   No ☐
     — sight or smell of particular foods   Yes ☐   No ☐
     — temperature of foods   Yes ☐   No ☐
   - diarrhoea   Yes ☐   No ☐
   - constipation or gastrointestinal obstruction   Yes ☐   No ☐
   - mouth sores   Yes ☐   No ☐
   - difficulty swallowing   Yes ☐   No ☐
   - dry mouth   Yes ☐   No ☐
   - poor appetite   Yes ☐   No ☐
     if so, is it caused by:
     — pain or other symptoms   Yes ☐   No ☐
     — depression or anxiety   Yes ☐   No ☐
     — early satiety, fatigue, or weakness   Yes ☐   No ☐
   - pressure sores   Yes ☐   No ☐

2. Does the patient take any vitamin, mineral, other food supplements?   Yes ☐   No ☐

3. Does the patient have a gastrointestinal or intravenous feeding tube in place?   Yes ☐   No ☐

4. Does the patient or family express significant remorse about weight change?   Yes ☐   No ☐
   - If the patient has lost a lot of weight, does the weight change make the patient more dependent on others?   Yes ☐   No ☐
   - Does the patient or family want to try to reverse the weight loss with enteral or parenteral nutritional support?   Yes ☐   No ☐

5. Does the family exhibit any of the following behaviours?   Yes ☐   No ☐
   - inappropriate use of food as a crutch for emotional problems   Yes ☐   No ☐
   - belief that disease is caused by what the patient did or did not eat   Yes ☐   No ☐
   - fear that if the patient doesn't eat, he or she will feel hunger pains   Yes ☐   No ☐
   - fear that if the patient becomes dehydrated, he or she will die soon   Yes ☐   No ☐
   - belief in unorthodox nutritional therapies such as vitamin C, laetrile, the macrobiotic diet, enzymes   Yes ☐   No ☐

Fig. 6.1 Nutrition assessment instrument.

- How changes in a patient's appetite and ability to eat can cause changes in food intake, bodily appearance and bodily function.
- Specific dietary measures for symptom control.
- Relief measures that will be available as the patient's condition deteriorates.
- The availability of community nutrition and food resources.
- How to reach the nurse when questions arise and assistance is needed.

Armed with an individualised and appropriate nutritional care plan, the nurse should experience a great deal of satisfaction in implementing the plan. An effective counsellor will use the following information and skills in carrying out the plan of care, and counselling the patient and family on their nutrition issues and dietary concerns (Gallagher-Allred, 1989, p. 261).

- Knowledge about what losses mean to patients and their families.
- Knowledge of the stage of dying of the patient and the individual members of the patient's family.
- Ability to listen actively.
- Well-honed communication techniques.

Counselling and communication techniques are discussed further in Chapters 18 and 19.

Re-evaluate goals and intervention

Self-evaluation, evaluation of the established plan of care, and evaluation of the ability of the patient and the patient's family to achieve desired goals should be a part of the nurse's standard procedure during and after each visit. It is only with such evaluation that progress can be noted and the care plan be modified as necessary.

Two dietary situations that nurses frequently encounter are (i) the patient who cannot and will not eat (the family often wants to push this patient to eat more than the patient can or is willing); and (ii) the patient who can and wants to eat but needs assistance in knowing what to eat and how to maximise the quality of mealtimes.

Helping the patient who cannot and will not eat

Anorexia and cachexia are hallmark conditions of many end-stage chronic diseases. This is particularly true for patients with incurable cancer, renal disease, pulmonary disease, AIDS and heart failure. Suggested causes include abnormal host metabolism of protein, carbohydrate, fat, hormones, fluids and electrolytes; disease elaboration of cachexia-inducing substances; and debilitating effects of various therapies.

Cancer-related anorexia and cachexia are particularly common phenomena that nurses must address. Tumours cause early satiety (especially with lung, stomach, and pancreatic tumours), specific food aversions (particularly to protein-containing foods such as beef and pork with almost all tumours), nausea and vomiting (especially with liver cancer or metastases to the liver and as a result of narcotics and other therapies), and decreased interest in foods (particularly with an external tumour compression or partial obstruction of any part of the gastrointestinal tract). Although weight loss in the cancer patient is a worrisome sign, treatment unfortunately does not necessarily improve the patient's well-being or survival (DeWys and Kubota, 1981; Nixon *et al.*, 1981).

Although anorexia and cachexia commonly occur with incurable disease, they are not always problems to the patient and family. Indeed, one task of the nurse is to ascertain whether either or both are of significant concern and, if so, whether the problem is the patient's, the family's, or both. Often anorexia and cachexia are more problematic for the family than the patient.

Cachexia may be a problem for patients and families because they do not understand what causes it or how it occurs. Patients and their families should be told that, contrary to the popular misconception, cancer does not cause loss of body weight by eating away body parts like a worm eats a leaf. Hearing this can help alleviate the fear that something ugly is happening inside the body.

In working with an anxious family with a patient who cannot or will not eat, the nurse should attempt to diminish the effects of the no-win situation. Treatment is best directed at ameliorating social consequences such as embarrassment of the patient at his or her gaunt appearance and physical complications. Teaching the family about the effects that the disease and dying process have is also important. The family's anxieties can be diminished and the patient can be freed from the pressure to eat when attention is shifted from maintaining the patient's nutritional status to enhancing patient comfort through providing small appetising meals. Sometimes it is most appropriate to offer the patient no food unless the patient requests it. Although this shift may be difficult at first for the family, it brings considerable relief to both patient and family in the long run (Gallagher-Allred, 1989, p. 220).

Helpful phrases in discouraging the 'he must eat or he will die' syndrome include the following.

- 'The disease controls his appetite; pushing him to eat will cause the tumour to grow and won't do him any good now.'
- 'He's sick and will be sick even if he eats.'
- 'Pushing him to eat will only make him uncomfortable.'
- 'It's important to show him you love him in ways other than through food.'
- 'Let him sit with you and eat what he wants.'
- 'Try not to worry that he eats poorly; it doesn't seem to bother him.'

Dehydration has been called a natural anaesthesia for dying patients because it appears to decrease the patient's perception of suffering by reducing the level of consciousness. The concomitant dry mouth effect associated with dehydration can be relieved through ice chips, lubricants and other simple suggestions (Zerwekh, 1983).

If the patient's life expectancy is measured in weeks or days, dehydration, as a natural course of events, may be preferred to aggressive nutritional support through tube feedings and/or total parenteral nutrition (TPN) if such feedings cause discomfort. By foregoing aggressive therapy, the following conditions may result which will benefit the patient (Cataldi-Betcher *et al.*, 1983; Dresser and Boisaubin, 1985; Hacklor Fetsch and Shandor Miles, 1986; Zerwekh, 1984, 1987; Musgrave 1990).

- Decreased gastrointestinal and venous distension.

- Decreased nausea, vomiting and potential for aspiration.
- Decreased diarrhoea.
- Decreased pulmonary secretions resulting in less coughing, less fear of choking and drowning, and less rattling secretions.
- Decreased urine flow and need to void.

For some patients the procedures required in order to avert malnutrition and dehydration are so onerous that the benefits are inconsequential or meaningless. Is not to intervene acceptable, or is it tantamount to murder? The choice lies in doing what is in the patient's best interests after the goals to be accomplished have been considered and the expected benefits and burdens have been analysed by the patient, the patient's family, and competent health care professionals (President's Commission for the Study of Ethical Problems in Medicine and Biomedical and Behavioral Research, 1983, pp. 1–12).

It has been the experience of this author and others (Lynn and Osterweiss, 1985; Kaye, 1990) that palliative care patients with advanced cancer rarely find any advantage to aggressive nutritional support via tube or parenteral feedings. Instead, patients who are allowed to eat and drink as desired, and who are not pushed to do so if they do not desire or are unable, is a viable alternative. A previously placed tube for enteral feedings or an intravenous line for TPN may not need to be discontinued, however, unless the patient desires. Even though the feeding tube may be in place, there is no moral reason for using the tube for feeding (President's Commission for the Study of Ethical Problems in Medicine and Biomedical and Behavioral Research, 1983, pp. 1–12; Boisaubin, 1984; Lo and Jonsen, 1980; American Dietetic Association, 1992; Young *et al.*, 1992).

Helping the patient who can and wants to eat

For patients who want to eat and who can be helped to eat better, the importance of improving appetite and enabling them to eat as normally as possible cannot be overestimated. The nurse's role is of paramount importance in this patient situation. Medications, such as corticosteroids and megestrol acetate (Mahayni and Minor, 1991; Bruera *et al.*, 1990; Tchekmedyian *et al.*, 1992), alcohol as an aperitif, tricyclic antidepressants, and dronabinol (Conant *et al.*, 1991) can be administered to improve appetite and mood (Grauer, 1993). Improving a poor self-image through suggestions such as clothes that are worn, a hairdresser appointment or a dental appointment, can also improve a patient's appetite.

If anorexia is due to correctable causes and the patient has a predicted life expectancy of several months, the correctable causes should be treated aggressively if desired by the patient. Likewise, treatment should be aggressive if the patient's anorexia appears to be an isolated symptom and the suspected consequence is malnutrition that could compromise both the quality and quantity of the patient's remaining days. Suggestions for improving oral intake of adults and children through use of food have been summarised in Table 6.1.

Commercial medical nutritional supplements also may be warranted for adult patients and children who want a high calorie intake in a small volume. Medical nutritional supplements are often appreciated by weak patients and their families because the patient can drink the highly fortified liquid products with minimal effort and the family members feel that they are providing 'something special'.

Table 6.1 Suggestions for improving oral intake. (Adapted from Gallagher-Allred, 1989, pp. 221 and 269, with permission of Aspen Publishers, Inc.)

- Feed the patient when hungry, changing mealtimes if needed. Note the patient's best meals and make these the largest meals.
- Serve a small serving of the patient's favourite foods on a small plate.
- Gently encourage, but do not nag, the patient to eat; remove uneaten food without undue comment.
- Cold foods are generally preferred to hot foods. Reassure parents of a dying child that they do not have to serve a hot, nutritious meal daily for the child; encourage them not to feel guilty if the child wants nothing or only wants a fast-food hamburger or fries.
- Set an attractive table and plate, using a plate garnish or table flower if enjoyed by the patient. In an institutional setting, serve the patient's food on trays set with embroidered tray cloths and pretty china or stoneware, rather than on traditional paper underliners and dishes. Allow the patient's personal china and utensils from home to be used if feasible.
- Make mealtimes sociable and enjoyable, vary the place of eating and remove bedpans from the room.
- Children can be encouraged to drink by playing games; it is fun for a child to drink fluids in out-of-the-ordinary ways, such as through a syringe, in small medicine cups, and by eating juice bars or ice lollies. Remove toys from the bed, turn off the television, bring in friends for a meal. Children will enjoy a packed lunch on occasion, and they enjoy eating foods that have been cut into interesting shapes or look like favourite characters.
- Suggest the patient rest before eating; most children and adults feel more like eating when they are relaxed.
- Encourage high-calorie foods day or night, including eggnog, milkshake, custard, pudding, peanut butter, cream soups, cheese, fizzy drinks, pie, sherbet, and cheesecake. In an institutional setting, consider serving foods from a hot trolley instead of or in addition to allowing patients to choose their meals in advance. Consider soup and soft sandwiches for midday meals. Try to supply as much variety in food selection as possible, including regional favourites.
- Provide lipped dishes for those patients who have arm and hand weakness; use rubber grips on ordinary cutlery for those with a weak grip.
- In an institutional setting, have a dining room available, with a home-like atmosphere, where patients can eat and patients and families can eat together. Allow the family to eat with the patient in the patient's room if desired. Have staff available to feed patients who are unable to feed themselves. Do not hurry patients to eat.
- Liberalise diets as much as possible; rarely are diabetic or low-sodium diets essential, but if they are, consider low simple sugar foods and no regular salt packets instead of more restricted diets.

Enteral tube feedings, in addition to oral intake or as the sole source of nutrition, may also be appropriate in feeding the patient who can and wants to eat. Liquid commercial nutritional products are usually administered from a small-bore, flexible catheter that in most patients is passed through the nose into the stomach or upper small intestine. The tube may also be passed directly into the stomach through the abdominal wall.

If tube feedings are desired, the nurse will need to make decisions concerning the osmolality of the solution, whether the solution will be administered by continuous drip, or by intermittent feeding, and the rate the solution is to be delivered (McCamish and Crocker, 1993). In general, the formulas to be administered should be isotonic solutions. Depending on the patient's ability to tolerate the solution, feedings should be started with a continuous drip at full strength if isotonic solutions are used, or at half strength if hypertonic solutions are used. An appropriate beginning rate is usually 50 ml/h (up to a final rate of 100–125 ml/h), or the concentration can be increased (half to three-quarter to full strength), depending on patient tolerance and nutritional goals. Many patients and families prefer intermittent tube feedings to continuous drip because that method seems more like a meal than drip delivery via pump.

In theory, a continuous drip administration of 100–125 ml/h of full-strength (1 kcal/ml) solution is the maximum amount needed if weight maintenance is the goal (2400–3000 kcal) for most patients. In practice, however, only 1000–1800 kcal/day (continuous drip for 10–15 h) is generally needed to achieve satiety and comfort. Greater amounts frequently cause complications, including fluid overload, cramps, diarrhoea, reflux and aspiration; enhanced tumour growth may also occur (Shika and Brennan, 1989; Torosian and Daly, 1986).

A case can be made for limited use of TPN in palliative care. When patients are in the early stages of their disease, they are often able to lead full and active lives. TPN may be appropriate if patients are unable to ingest enough calories orally or via enteral tube feeding to sustain their activity level due to a poorly functioning or non-functioning gastrointestinal tract (Fainsinger *et al.*, 1992). An inoperable bowel obstruction or short bowel syndrome are two examples of such medical situations.

On the other hand, TPN is generally not well tolerated by terminally ill patients, and rarely does parenteral feeding reduce the distress of anorexia and cachexia when the terminal stage is reached. Instead, TPN often subjects the patient to new problems that are more distressing and to prolong suffering that would not have been faced had parenteral feeding been foregone (Billings, 1985). If TPN is desired, it is best begun in the hospital setting before the patient is returned to the home or long-term care facility. Home and long-term care facility administration should be under close monitoring of a specially trained care team.

Dietary therapy for common nutritional problems

Although dying often brings many less-than-desirable side-effects, it would be wrong to view dying as a 'disease' hungry for medical 'remedies'. However, the nurse can give the patient and family many helpful dietary suggestions for symptom control, so that they can maximise comfort during the dying patient's remaining days.

Table 6.2 provides suggestions for appropriate dietary therapy for common

Table 6.2. Dietary therapy for common symptoms in palliative care. Note that not all of the identified treatments may be appropriate for all diseases or conditions. (Adapted from Gallagher-Allred, 1989, pp. 221 and 269, with permission of Aspen Publishers, Inc.)

Belching
- Allow the patient to make the final choice of foods to eat and avoid, but consider testing the patient's tolerance to gas-producing foods, such as the following: beer, carbonated beverages, alcohol, dairy products if lactose intolerant, nuts, beans, onions, peas, corn, cucumbers, radishes, cabbage, broccoli, Brussels sprouts, spinach, cauliflower, high-fat foods, yeast and mushrooms.
- Encourage the patient to eat solids at mealtimes and drink liquids between meals instead of with solid foods.
- Advise the patient to avoid eating quickly and reclining immediately after eating; encourage the patient to relax before, during, and after meals.
- Advise the patient to avoid overeating, avoid sucking through straws, avoid chewing gum, and to keep the mouth closed when chewing and swallowing.

Constipation
- Encourage the patient to eat foods high in fibre (bran; whole grains; fruits, especially pineapple, prunes and raisins; vegetables; nuts; and legumes) if adequate fluid intake can be maintained. Avoid high-fibre foods if dehydration, severe constipation, or obstruction are anticipated.
- Increase fluid intake as tolerated; encourage fruit juices, prune juice, and cider. If liked by the patient, a recipe (1–2 ounces with the evening meal of a mixture of 2 cups apple-sauce, 2 cups unprocessed bran, and 1 cup 100 per cent prune juice) is effective and may reduce laxative use.
- Discontinue calcium and iron supplementation if used; limit cheese, rich desserts, and other foods if constipating.

Diarrhoea
- Let the patient make the final choice of foods to eat and avoid, but suggest omission of the following foods if they cause diarrhoea: milk, ice cream, whole-grain breads and cereals, nuts, beans, peas, greens, fruits with seeds and skins, fresh pineapple, raisins, cider, prune juice, raw vegetables, gas-forming vegetables, alcohol and caffeine-containing beverages.
- Encourage the patient to eat bananas, apple-sauce, peeled apple, tapioca, rice, peanut butter, refined grains, crackers, pasta, cream of wheat, oatmeal and cooked vegetables.
- Encourage the patient to avoid liquids with a meal and instead to drink liquids an hour after a meal.
- Encourage the patient to relax before, during, and after a meal.
- Enteral and/or parenteral nutritional support in the AIDS patient may be appropriate if the patient has a lengthy life expectancy and the cause of the diarrhoea is known and treatable; if tube feedings or oral diet is appropriate, they should be high in calories and protein and low in fibre, lactose and fat.
- If dehydration is a problem, encourage high-potassium foods.

Hypercalcaemia
- Allow the hypercalcaemic patient to eat foods high in calcium such as dairy products if desired, but encourage the patient to avoid calcium and vitamin D supplementation; restriction of high-calcium foods is rarely helpful.
- Encourage the patient to drink lots of fluids, particularly carbonated beverages containing phosphoric acid if the patient enjoys them.

Mental disorders
- Encourage the patient to avoid alcohol and caffeine-containing foods, such as coffee, tea and chocolate, if they contribute to anxiety, sleep deprivation or depression.

- If the patient is drowsy or apathetic, suggest that the family may need to feed the patient. Encourage them to prepare the patient's favourite foods, usually in soft form to be served with a spoon or bite-size so the patient might self-feed. Help the family protect the patient and others from the patient by shutting off or removing knobs from stoves, removing matches and locking doors to cabinets or closets that contain poisons, alcohol or medications. Put away electrical appliances, such as mixers, food processors, can openers and waffle irons; unplug microwave ovens.
- If the patient is agitated or confused, caution the family about the dangers of hand-feeding the patient. Suggest feeding with a spoon and not allowing the patient to handle feeding utensils, plates, glass, etc. Encourage the family to tell the patient what time of day it is, what meal is served, and what foods are served. Remind the patient that the foods served are favourites. Make mealtimes enjoyable by reminiscing about pleasant events in the patient's life. Consider the pros and cons of waking the patient if asleep at mealtimes.
- If the patient is stuporous or comatose, counsel the family that semi-starvation and dehydration are not painful to the patient; explore with them the pros and cons of enteral and parenteral nutritional support if they request information.

Mouth problems
- If the patient says that foods taste bitter, encourage poultry, fish, dairy products, eggs, milk and cheese; bitter-tasting foods usually include red meat, sour juices, coffee, tea, tomatoes and chocolate. Suggest cooking foods in glass or porcelain instead of in metal containers, and avoid serving foods on metal or with metallic utensils. Encourage sweet fruit drinks, carbonated beverages, ice lollies and seasonings, herbs and spices to enhance flavours.
- If the patient says that foods taste 'old', try adding sugar; sour and salty tastes often taste 'old'.
- If the patient says that foods taste too sweet, suggest drinking sour juices, and cooking with lemon juice, vinegar, spices, herbs and mint; add pickles to appropriate foods.
- If the patient says that foods have no taste, suggest marinating appropriate foods, serving highly seasoned foods, adding sugar and eating foods at room temperature.
- If the patient has difficulty swallowing, suggest small frequent meals of soft foods (pureed if needed), advise against foods that might irritate the mouth and oesophagus, such as acidic juices or fruits, spicy foods, very hot or cold foods, alcohol and carbonated beverages.
- If the patient has mouth sores, suggest blenderised and cold foods; gravies, cream soups, eggnog, milkshakes, cream pies, cheesecake, macaroni and cheese, and casseroles are well-liked. Suggest the patient avoid alcohol and acidic, spicy, rough, hot and highly salted foods.
- If the patient has a dry mouth, suggest frequent sips of water, juice, ice chips, ice lollies, ice cream, fruitades, or slushy frozen baby foods mixed with fruit juice. Sucking on hard sweets may stimulate saliva. Solid foods should be moist, pureed as needed, and not too tart or too hot or cold if mouth sores are present.

Nausea and vomiting
- Encourage the patient to avoid eating if nauseated or if nausea is anticipated.
- Suggest small meals of cool non-odorous foods. Many patients find it helpful to avoid fatty, greasy or fried foods; avoid mixing hot and cold foods at the same meal; avoid high-bulk meals; and avoid nausea-precipitating foods, such as overly sweet foods, alcohol, spicy foods and tobacco with meals.
- Encourage the patient to eat slowly and avoid overeating. Relaxing before and after meals and avoiding physical activity and lying flat for two hours after eating may also help.
- Suggest that the patient not prepare own food.

Obstruction (gastrointestinal)
- If oral intake is not contraindicated, encourage the patient to eat small meals that are low in fibre, low in residue, and blenderised or strained. Many patients will prefer to eat their favourite foods, enjoy large meals, and then vomit frequently. A gastric tube, open to straight or intermittent drain, may alleviate the need for regular vomiting.
- With 'squashed stomach syndrome', encourage the patient to eat small frequent meals, avoid nausea-producing foods, odorous foods, gas-producing foods, and high-fat or fried foods. Limit fluid with meals, taking fluids an hour before and after meals.

symptoms in palliative care. Because the majority of palliative care patients are diagnosed with incurable cancer, the suggestions are primarily based on responses from treating cancer patients. As the world's population ages and chronic degenerative diseases, including renal disease, cardiovascular failure, pulmonary failure and organic brain syndrome, have more time to exert their ravishing effects, we may be caring more for these patients in the future. In Table 6.2, reference is made to specific diseases, but the diarrhoea associated with post-surgical dumping and AIDS, and the nausea and vomiting associated with gastrointestinal obstruction and narcotic use, are included under the symptoms of diarrhoea and nausea and vomiting, respectively. The reader is cautioned that not all of the identified treatments may be appropriate for all diseases or conditions.

Food service suggestions

Food service in an in-patient palliative care setting must reflect the philosophy of maximising patient comfort and enhancing quality of life (Drew Kidd and Lane, 1993). Menu development should reflect the ethnic, cultural and regional food preferences of the population. Regardless of meal pattern selected (e.g. three or four meals, lighter meals or heavier meals, etc.), there must be flexibility for reheating menu items or preparing a quick meal when a patient desires. Allowing patients to select menus as close to serving time as possible may help to allay anorexia. Small portions attractively garnished and plated in a dining atmosphere conducive to patient and family socialisation also contribute to better patient meal acceptance. Family members' assistance with feeding further enhances the dining experience.

In the palliative care setting, some patients and families may express a desire for additional fibre, others for low-fat foods, still others for meals that reflect personal nutritional beliefs. Specific dietary modifications, such as low sodium, low fat and diabetic requirements also may be needed. In most cases, however, these restrictions are liberalised to allow the patient maximum pleasure, variety and choice. Fluctuations in patients' mental alertness, level of responsiveness, dental status, and swallowing difficulties may indicate the need for consistency modifications as soft, mechanical soft, pureed or blenderised foods. Simple, easy-to-prepare foods served in smaller portions are more acceptable to patients than complicated, labour-intensive recipes. Comfort or familiar foods also are enjoyed and better tolerated. Some examples of universally selected comfort foods are macaroni and cheese, grilled cheese sandwiches, peanut butter and jelly sandwiches, toast, crackers, soups, fresh fruits and soft salads.

Several considerations for planning menus that will maximise success of a food service operation have been identified (Drew Kidd and Lane, 1993).

- What is the equipment available for food preparation?
- What is the budget allowance for food, labour and supplies?
- What are the availability and skills of food service production personnel?
- What type of production system (e.g. cook/serve, cook/chill, etc.) will be used?
- What type of tray delivery system will be used? Will communal dining be offered?
- What distance must the food be transported for service to the patient?
- How much space is available for food storage, preparation and service?

- In what form will food be purchased – fresh, frozen, convenience, etc.?
- What type of menu will be used – selective, non-selective, cyclic, restaurant-style?
- Can the menu be adapted to seasonal and market conditions where popular menu items can be incorporated with cost-effectiveness?
- Does the menu balance production work-load from day-to-day?

In-patient palliative care facilities often provide a family kitchen, including personal china, flatware and crystal storage, refrigerated storage, and re-heating system, to handle foods brought from home. A family kitchen allows flexibility for meal service and supports family and friends in their caring efforts to nourish. Public health rules for labelling and dating food items and safe storage time limits should be enforced. The importance of food sanitation and safety cannot be over-emphasised in a setting where many patients are immune-compromised.

By serving nutritious, attractively prepared food for visual and physical pleasure, the palliative care facility's food service staff has the opportunity to enrich patients' lives at a time when the smallest pleasure is truly treasured (Drew Kidd and Lane, 1993).

Ethical and legal considerations in nutritional support

The ethical and legal considerations in nutritional support of palliative care patients are increasingly being debated, which is due in part to recent technological advances in nutrition support that enable us to keep people alive longer than meaningful life can be maintained.

'To feed or not to feed', as with other methods of treatment, requires that those involved with palliative care ask the underlying questions, 'What good will it accomplish for the patient?' and 'Do the benefits of nutrition support outweigh the burdens?'.

To answer these questions, it is important to first establish the clinical facts regarding each patient's situation and effectively communicate these to the patient and family. The benefits and burdens the patient may experience by the provision of or the withholding/withdrawal of nutrition support also should be delineated for the patient and family. The patient's and family's educated perspective, based on their personal value system, then should be the cornerstone of the decision-making process.

In the United States, enteral and parenteral nutrition support are provided often to palliative care patients. Following are examples of patients for whom enteral or parenteral feedings are appropriate (McCamish and Crocker, 1993, p. 109).

- Those who have a feeding tube or line in place and want it used [e.g. patients with amyotrophic lateral sclerosis (ALS) or head and neck cancer].
- Those for whom an untimely and uncomfortable death may occur without enteral or parenteral nutrition.
- Those for whom it is important to prolong life so that an important event can occur before the patient dies (e.g. to attend a grandchild's graduation or wedding or to get business affairs in order).
- Those for whom there is a threat of legal action if the tube/line is not placed or used when the patient's wishes are not known.

- Those for whom the tube/line is a source of control or denial.

When dealing with the ethical issue of withholding or withdrawing nutrition support, the following three questions should be addressed (Young *et al.*, 1992).

- Is artificial nutrition/hydration considered medical therapy?
- Can competent patients refuse artificial nutrition/hydration?
- Can an incompetent patient have artificial nutrition/hydration withdrawn based on a surrogate's request?

Case law in the United States at this time does not supply definitive answers to these questions, despite the most recent, lengthy and tangled court decision concerning the Nancy Cruzan case (Supreme Court Opinions, 1991). Three relevant opinions are often expressed, however, which appear to transcend national boundaries (McCamish and Crocker, 1993).

- Withholding and withdrawing nutrition support have the same ethical significance.
- Artificial nutrition and hydration is considered medical therapy and can be refused by competent patients and surrogates of incompetent patients under certain circumstances.
- Patient autonomy is a guiding ethical principle.

An additional question concerns how one decides if or how to feed a permanently unconscious child. Nutrition and hydration are rarely withheld in permanently unconscious children in the United States. This may be due partly to difficulties in diagnosis (Ashwal *et al.*, 1992). Mostly, however, it is probably due to attitudes toward children generally and a particularly strong desire to nurture them (Miller-Thiel *et al.*, 1993). Such attitudes are changing, especially as we struggle to give children the same consideration we give to adults.

When addressing appropriate versus inappropriate use of any medical technology including artificial nutrition and hydration, one should consider when the therapy is futile (McCamish and Crocker, 1993). If provision of nutritional support imposes a severe burden on the patient, or if the patient will not actually benefit from such treatment, the efforts can be determined futile. The concept of futility should be applied cautiously, however, since a possibly helpful medical therapy may not be offered and might even be withheld if it is deemed not beneficial. The way in which futility is defined, therefore, is important. It is essential to establish not only the probability that the nutritional intervention will be successful, but also the goals by which success will be measured (Singer and Siegler, 1991).

Three conditions when nutritional support might result in disproportionate burden to the patient include (i) when nutritional support would be a futile treatment, (ii) when no possibility of benefit could occur with nutritional support, and (iii) when the burden outweighs the benefit (Lynn and Childress, 1983).

It is necessary to emphasise that, in circumstances where the patient expires when artificial nutrition and hydration is withdrawn, the cause of death is the underlying disease or condition, not the withdrawal of the nutrition support (McCamish and Crocker, 1993). Many clinicians and ethicists maintain that withdrawing nutrition and hydration falls into the 'allowing to die' category, instead of 'killing.' In the past, prior to the availability of artificial nutrition and hydration support technology, similar patients would have died of their disease. Advances in nutrition and hydration technology have not changed this and, therefore, absence of nutrition support is not the specific cause of death. This concept is very important to emphasise with patients and their families. Families already carry a sufficiently heavy burden without adding to it the burden of guilt due to a decision to withdraw artificial nutrition and hydration.

Within the same context, 'withholding' and 'withdrawing' artificial nutrition and hydration are considered to have the same ethical significance, even though the removal of artificial nutrition and hydration may be psychologically and emotionally much more difficult. This should not, however, lead to withholding this therapy in an attempt to avoid a difficult decision regarding withdrawing support in the future (McCamish and Crocker, 1993).

In working with patients and families who may consider the use of or the withholding/withdrawal of nutrition support, the nurse's role is to be with the patient and family and guide them through the following steps (Gallagher-Allred, 1989, p. 240).

- Listen carefully to the patient's and family's concerns.
- Clarify options.
- Provide pros and cons of each option.
- Support the patient–family choice.
- Encourage deliberative palliative care team decisions that are consistent with patient and family wishes.

These steps will help the nurse in other situations, such as how to deal with questions about unorthodox nutritional therapies or claims that have not been scientifically validated. For several reasons – including ignorance, hope and fear of abandonment – many people cling to nutritional claims that have no proven basis or may have been disproved. The first goals of the nurse are to understand the patient's point of view and then to acknowledge the patient's concern as real. After identifying the patient's concerns, it will be necessary to deal with the patient's ignorance or feelings in a caring manner. Discuss the treatment fully and outline the pros and cons dispassionately and in a non-judgemental way (Gallagher-Allred, 1989, pp. 226–7).

Although it may be appropriate to do so, there is no obligation on the part of the nurse to dispel the hopes that an unorthodox nutritional therapy or claim may bring a patient, unless what is being practised is harmful or unless the costs outweigh the benefits. Try to identify whether the unorthodox practice is producing a positive psychological effect. If so, then the cost-to-benefit ratio can be determined and a decision whether to discuss the practice with the patient can be made somewhat objectively (Gallagher-Allred, 1989, p. 227).

In closing, the nurse should discuss with dying patients and their families any guilt feelings they may have that they caused the patient's incurable illness by foods that were or were not eaten. Not to dispel these feelings is to leave in place an inhumane weight of guilt. The goal of palliative care nurses is to comfort patients and their families. Relieving them of this possible guilt is consistent with this goal (Cassileth *et al.*, 1985).

Acknowledgement

Acknowledgement is due to Aspen Publishers, Inc., Maryland, for permission to include material based on, and Fig. 6.1, Table 6.1 and Table 6.2, from Gallagher-Allred (1989).

References

AMERICAN DIETETIC ASSOCIATION (1992). Position of The American Dietetic Association: issues in feeding the terminally ill adult. *Journal of the American Dietetic Association* **92**, 996–1002.

ASHWAL, S., BALE, J. F., COULTER D. L. *et al.* (1992). The persistent vegetative state in children: report of the Child Neurology Society Ethics Committee. *Annals of Neurology* **32**(40), 570–6.

BILLINGS, J. A. (1985). *Outpatient Management of Advanced Cancer: Symptom Control. Support and Hospice-in-the-Home.* J. B. Lippincott, Philadelphia, Pennsylvania.

BOISAUBIN, E. V. (1984). Ethical issues in the nutritional support of the terminal patient. *Journal of the American Dietetic Association* **84**, 529–31.

BRUERA, E., MACMILLAN, K., KUEHN, N., HANSON, J. and MACDONALD, R. N. (1990). A controlled trial of megestrol acetate on appetite, caloric intake, nutritional status, and other symptoms in patients with advanced cancer. *Cancer* **66**, 1279–82.

CALLAHAN, D. (1983). In feeding the dying. *Hastings Center Report* **13**, 20–2.

CASSILETH, B., LUSK, E. J., MILLER, D. S., BROWN, L. L. and MILLER, C. (1985). Psychosocial correlates for survival in advanced malignant disease. *New England Journal of Medicine* **312**(24), 1551–5.

CATALDI-BETCHER, E. L., SELTZER, M. H., SLOCUM, B. A. *et al.* (1983). Complications occurring during enteral nutrition support: a prospective study. *Journal of Parenteral and Enteral Nutrition* **7**, 546–52.

CONANT, M., ROY, D., SHEPARD, K. V. and PLASSE, T. F. (1991). Dronabinol enhances appetite and controls weight loss in HIV patients. *Proceedings of ASCO* **10**, 34.

DEWYS, W. D. and KUBOTA, T. T. (1981). Enteral and parenteral nutrition in the care of the cancer patient. *Journal of the American Medical Association* **246**(15), 1725–7.

DRESSER, R. S. and BOISAUBIN, E. V. (1985). Ethics, law and nutritional support. *Archives of Internal Medicine* **145**, 122–4.

DREW KIDD, K and LANE, M. P. (1993). Maximising food service in an inpatient hospice setting. *The Hospice Journal* **9**(2/3), 85–106.

FAINSINGER, R. L., CHAN, K. and BRUERA, E. (1992). Total parenteral nutrition for a terminally ill patient? *Journal of Palliative Care* **8**(2), 30–2.

GALLAGHER-ALLRED, C. R. (1989). *Nutritional Care of the Terminally Ill.* Aspen Publishers, Rockville, Maryland.

GRAUER, P. A. (1993). Appetite stimulants in terminal care: treatment of anorexia. *The Hospice Journal* **9**(2/3), 73–83.

HACKLOR FETSCH, S. and SHANDOR MILES, M. (1986). Children and death. In: O'RAWE AMENTA, M. and BOHNET, N. L. (eds), *Nursing Care of the Terminally Ill*, pp. 215–16. Little, Brown & Co., Boston, Massachusetts.

KAYE, P. (1990). *Symptom Control in Hospice and Palliative Care*. Hospice Education Institute, Essex, Connecticut.

LO, B. and JONSEN, A. R. (1980). Ethical decisions in the care of the patient terminally ill with metastatic cancer. *Annals of Internal Medicine* 92, 107–11.

LYNN, J. and CHILDRESS, J. F. (1983). Must patients always be given food and water? *Hastings Center Report* 13, 17–21.

LYNN, J. and OSTERWEISS, M. (1985). Ethical issues arising in hospice care. In: TORRENS, P. (ed.), *Hospice Programs and Public Policy*, p. 205. American Hospital Association, Chicago, Illinois.

MAHAYNI, H. and MINOR, J. (1991). Megestrol acetate in AIDS-related cachexia. *American Journal of Hospital Pharmacy* 48(1), 2479–80.

MAUER BAACK, C. M. (1993). Nursing's role in the nutritional care of the terminally ill: weathering the storm. *The Hospice Journal* 9(2/3), 1–13.

MCCAMISH, M. A. and CROCKER, N. J. (1993). Enteral and parenteral nutrition support of terminally ill patients: practical and ethical perspectives. *The Hospice Journal* 9(2/3), 107–29.

MILLER-THIEL, J., GLOVER, J. J. and BELIVEAU, E. (1993). Caring for the dying child. *The Hospice Journal* 9(2/3), 55–72.

MUSGRAVE, C. F. (1990). Terminal dehydration: to give or not to give intravenous fluids? *Cancer Nursing* 13(1), 62–6.

NIXON, D. W., LAWSON, D. H., KUTNER, M. *et al.* (1981). Hyperalimentation of the cancer patient with protein-calorie undernutrition. *Cancer Research* 41, 2038–45.

PRESIDENT'S COMMISSION FOR THE STUDY OF ETHICAL PROBLEMS IN MEDICINE AND BIOMEDICAL AND BEHAVIORAL RESEARCH (1983). *Deciding to Forego Life-sustaining Treatment*. United States Government Printing Office, Washington, D.C.

SHIKA, M. and BRENNAN, M. F. (1989). Supportive care of the cancer patient. In: DEVITA, V., HELLMAN, S. and ROSENBERG S. (eds), *Cancer: Principles and Practice of Oncology*, 3rd edn. J. B. Lippincott, Philadelphia, Pennsylvania.

SINGER, P. A. and SIEGLER, M. (1991). Elective use of life-sustaining treatment in internal medicine. *Archives of Internal Medicine* 36, 57–79.

SUPREME COURT OPINIONS (1991). Nancy Beth Cruzan, Petitioners v. Director, Missouri Department of Health *et al. United States Law Week* 58, 4916–41.

TCHEKMEDYIAN, N. S., HICKMAN, M., SIAU, J., GRECO, F. A., KELLER, J., BROWDER, H. and AISNER, J. (1992). Megestrol acetate in cancer anorexia and weight loss. *Cancer* 69(5), 1268–74.

TOROSIAN, M. and DALY, J. (1986). Nutritional support in the cancer-bearing host. *Cancer* 58, 1915–29.

YOUNG, E. A., PERKINS, H. S. and MCCAMISH, M. A. (1992). Ethical dimensions and clinical decisions for parenteral nutrition: in dying as in living. In: ROMBEAU, J. L. and CALDWELL M. D. (eds), *Clinical Nutrition: Parenteral Nutrition*, 2nd edn. W. B. Saunders, Orlando, Florida.

ZERWEKH, J. V. (1983). The dehydration question. *Nursing '83* 13, 47–51.

ZERWEKH, J. V. (1984). The last few days. In: *Hospice and Palliative Nursing Care*, BLUES, A. G. and ZERWEKH, J. V. (eds), p. 180. Grune & Stratton, Orlando, Florida.

ZERWEKH, J. V. (1987). Should fluid and nutritional support be withheld from terminally ill patients? Another opinion. *American Journal of Hospice Care* 4(4), 37–8.

7

Awareness of psychological needs

Morna C. Rutherford and W. Dawn Foxley

'Understanding human needs is half the job of meeting them.'
Adlais Stevenson

Psychological needs are many and varied, reflecting the uniqueness of the individual. As a consequence it would be a formidable task to describe those idiosyncratic needs within the confines of one chapter. A more appropriate approach is to describe the similar reactions people can have in particular circumstances. It is the aim of this chapter to explore the circumstances and psychological reactions of people with cancer and their families during the palliative phase of care.

Basic human needs

Heron's (1977) model provides a useful starting point for understanding the outcome of people's reaction to psychological disruption. He suggests three areas of human need

- the need to love and be loved;
- the need to understand and be understood; and
- the need to choose and be chosen.

An individual who has all personal needs met suffuses characteristics such as enthusiasm, confidence and creativity. Alternatively, neglect of personal needs may cause personal distress (Fig. 7.1). It is possible to consider the distress of people with cancer and their families within the context of this model.

The need to love and to be loved

Heron (1977, p. 2) notes that 'the need is satisfied in mutual loving – a shared celebration of individual strengths and differences'. This sharing enables freedom to fulfil other needs and release creative capacity. Where the need to love and to be loved exists for both patient and family, the chance of *fulfilment* can be eroded by the effect of both cancer and treatment.

Essentially, the experience of cancer is disruptive and multidimensional. The effects on an individual are far reaching, ranging from physical symptoms and functional change to emotional disturbance and existential searching. Invariably, any treatment will involve the introduction of health–care professionals and regimes which underline further the disintegrating power of the cancer process on personal and family cohesion. Clearly, the changes involved affect internal, external and

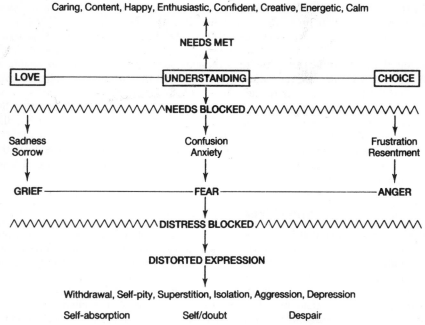

Fig. 7.1 Dynamics of personal needs [modified from Heron (1977)].

relational dimensions, with the danger of separation through illness, hospitalisation or death existing as a threat to the fulfilment of the need for love and security.

For the patient, the need to give and receive love may be marred by changes in self-concept. This affects the ability to relate to self which in turn disrupts the ability to relate to others. Perception of self involves awareness of the whole self and will change as self-awareness alters. For example, following diagnosis, the patient may immediately see him or herself in a different way. After being told her diagnosis, one patient said, 'I feel really strange – like I'm not myself anymore. I know I'm the same person I was yesterday, but I feel all jumbled up inside now.' This example shows how difficult it is to relate to a new self-awareness.

Visible physical changes can impinge upon self-concept in a more direct way providing tangible evidence of change: for example, the surgical removal of a limb. Even body changes which are not outwardly evident can affect self-concept. Another patient described her cancer as a 'Medusa'. Her fear and horror was expressed by this image.

Change in self-concept and body image can lead a patient to lose self-confidence and subsequently withdraw from others. Obvious examples of change are malodorous or disfiguring cancers, change in body function through stoma formation, weight loss or gain, and hair loss. However, uncontrolled symptoms such as pain or sickness can also cause distancing, both physical and psychological, when the need to give and receive love is greatest. The opportunity or ability to love or even be intimate is blocked, resulting in sadness, sorrow and grief (see Fig. 7.1).

Just as changes in self-concept affect the way a person relates to him or herself these changes can in turn affect relationships with others. Griffiths (1989, p. 36) describes how a disfigured person will 'test out' his or her changed appearance. Self-concept often relies on the opinions of people who matter, and a disfigured person will inevitably scrutinise the reactions of family or friends to enable readjustment. Families are then doubly saddled with the vulnerability of their loved one and their own reactions to the changes which affect them.

For families, intimacy with the patient is affected by difficulty in knowing how to relate under changed circumstances. For example, families may avoid handling the person with cancer for fear of causing harm, and if the person with cancer is confused, agitated or drowsy, families may be unable to receive the love they need. It is important, therefore, to make sense of these changes and to find a way of living with them.

The need to understand and be understood

The need for understanding occurs at a practical level and also at a personal level for both patient and family. The practical level includes clear communication if functional problems exist with speech, hearing or language. For example, the use of language and its interpretation may be different for both nurse and patient. At a personal level, it is possible that the patient may not know how to ask for information. The patient may have a need to understand the changes which are occurring and, in order to grasp personal meaning, must firstly be understood by the people from whom assumptions are made too often about the ability of the patient to understand. Even if in full command of the facts, the question 'Why me?' is only too familiar. The resulting cycle of confusion and anxiety may give way to insurmountable fear. Rapid or unpredictable changes can be difficult for both patients and their families to comprehend.

Family members also need to understand and be understood: care may revolve solely around the patient, and family members can feel that nobody is listening to or understanding them. Anxiety within the family is common, especially when considering future implications of the disease process. Lugton (1989a, p. 50) describes anticipatory anxiety in families coping with dying. She states that it is not so much the prospect of death that makes people afraid, but anxiety about the imagined effects of cancer. Experiencing fear, anxiety and confusion can be overwhelming and further remove people from having control over their circumstances. Exercising choice may help regain some sense of this control.

The need to choose and be chosen

The person with cancer can find him or herself 'forced' into a position of dependency and professionals often appear to be in control of the whole process of care, producing resentment and anger. Porter (1988) describes how doctors decide who is eligible for the sick role: they label the sickness, decide on treatment, decide on how the sick person should act and they decide on what will happen after treatment. The patient has no real choice about his or her cancer and its effects, and treatments determined by the type of cancer are usually inflexible. In addition, patients may find that they are no longer able to partake in their usual role in life through limitations such as fatigue and decreased mobility which are imposed on the patient by the disease and/or treatment. Other people may no longer seek the patient's participation in normal daily activities for fear of putting a burden on the patient's failing strength, and so the person with cancer finds he or she is no longer chosen to share in normal life events, resulting in a feeling of 'uselessness'.

Family members are affected also by the inability to make choices. In addition they may not be chosen to give any care to the person they love. Nurses may presume to 'know better', take over the practical side of caring, and families can feel totally inadequate and helpless in offering any vestige of caring left to them.

Clearly, the changes involved in the palliative stage of care can disrupt all three personal needs, profoundly affecting both patient and family. Implications for nurses lie in the awareness of the need to enable the giving and receiving of love, understanding and choice so empowering patients and their families with the ability to be more in control.

Further awareness of the reactions of patients and families can be achieved through conceptualising the process involved when change occurs. Change involves transition from the known to the unknown, resulting in a discontinuation of a certain aspect of that person's life. This is particularly relevant to the diagnosis of cancer a many changes occur and are implied. For example, change in self-concept, role and status may be insidious but nevertheless dramatic, and thoughts of premature death are often inevitable following knowledge of cancer.

Responses to transition

Becoming aware of a potentially life-threatening illness initiates particular responses which are individual, but may also form a pattern. There is a cycle of reactions which form a framework for understanding the dynamics of transition. It is important, however, to note that some people stick at one stage or do not progress through the whole process systematically. Hopson and Adams (1976, pp. 9–15) and Hopson (1982, pp. 124–6) describe a map of self-esteem changes during transition (Fig. 7.2).

Immobilisation

The first stage of immobilisation reflects the shock involved in response to inevitable disruption of life style. Weisman (1979) describes this as 'existential plight' resulting from an abrupt confrontation with indisputable evidence of personal mortality. The person may feel 'paralysed' or 'numb' and be unable to think, understand or manage his or her life. When the person with cancer is told the diagnosis, the degree of shock will depend on how much he or she has already suspected. Some people will state that they knew there was 'something far wrong'. Nevertheless, having this knowledge verbally confirmed will invariable result in shock reaction. The degree of shock will depend also on how the information is conveyed. One patient asked how bad her cancer was, and was told, 'Bad! – don't you know it's terminal?'. Utterly devastated, this patient withdrew from the world for several weeks, refusing to communicate with anyone. The family also can suffer shock which is related to being confronted with the eventual obliteration of a joint future with their loved one. Shock takes time to

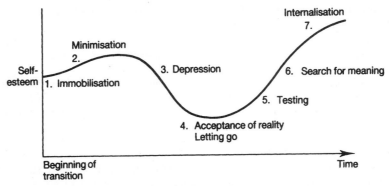

Fig. 7.2 Self-esteem during transitions [from Hopson and Adams (1976, p. 13)].

'settle' and movement into the second stage depends on coping strategies and available support.

Minimisation

One way of moving out of immobilisation is to deny that change has occurred. Some people might say 'It's not possible', 'It can't be happening', 'I don't believe it'. Denial is a coping defence which protects the person from awareness of fear and anxiety. O'Connor (1984, p. 118) states that 'denial of the reality of one's death protects the psyche from the harshness and pain of giving up life'. Denial allows time for meaning to penetrate and for potential strengths to amass, and some people never move beyond this phase. They may take tentative steps onward, but the perceived reality of their situation may be so frightening that denial of reality is in effect preventing their emotional disintegration. Nonetheless, continuing changes can erode this defence. The patient may refuse to change his or her life-style, yet there may be little option when the ability to function becomes increasingly limited. The family also may refuse to change, yet awareness of the patient's struggle with life may be impossible to ignore. A deep inner tension results and profound anxiety is often evident.

Anxiety may proceed to confusion, fear and anger. Confusion can be heard when a person says, 'I just don't know how this could have happened'. Fear can be fragmented into fear of the implications of illness and loss, including worry about distressing symptoms and loss of control.

The injustice of loss may be responded to by anger. This anger can be displaced on to symbols of power, such as the medical profession: the person with cancer may feel that this institution has let him or her down and rage is often an expression of this powerful experience. Outrage can be extremely frightening for both the person and for those close at hand. It is dangerous, however, to suppress this anger, as distorted expression may result in malice, aggression or despair (see Fig. 7.1). Expressing anger can release tensions, engender creativity and increase insight, but it does not change the situation *per se*. Realisation of this may give rise to 'bargaining' (Kubler-Ross, 1969, pp. 72–4), which is a belief that there will be a chance of reward for 'good behaviour'. For example, a person may bargain that giving up smoking will extend life, and if the person believes fully in this bargain, then hope is possible.

Depression

Through time the person experiencing transition may be unable to avoid the realities of change and a spiral of depression can ensue. Lamb and Woods (1981, p. 137) state that the disease process and treatment sometimes causes patients to 'doubt their humanness and the value of living'.

Depression is a difficult concept to define as it can range from sadness to a tangible, heavy blackness which is overwhelming. Some people may express the way they are feeling in terms of regret at missed opportunities, or in terms of hopelessness or powerlessness to change things. Symptoms of depression, such as chronic fatigue, lack of concentration and sleep disturbances, compound the sense of loss of control over circumstances. Transitional depression is linked inevitably to loss.

Figure 7.3 lists some losses and changes for a dying person and the family. Mourning of these losses is expressed through grief which can connect with other emotions such as anger, fear and guilt.

As this stage moves towards the bottom of the transition curve (see Fig. 7.2), the depression will reach its lowest point. A feeling of impasse may develop

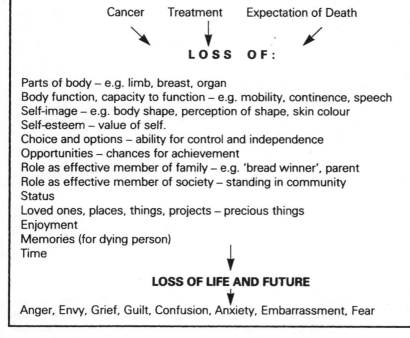

Fig. 7.3 Areas of loss and change.

where, at one and the same time, there is a pervasive sense that life may continue to feel this bad, and increasing awareness that there is no going back. A fear of going on may be tied to a suspicion that life may indeed become even worse.

Acceptance of reality

There is movement into this fourth stage as the person begins to look at what comes ahead and gradually unhook from the past and 'how things used to be'. Kubler-Ross (1969, p. 100) describes this phase of acceptance as being 'almost void of feelings'. This is a deep point in the person's life where he or she realises that life has changed and, in order to come to terms with the change, the person must 'let go' of the past.

Testing

Now there is the opportunity to 'test out' this new way of being in life. Even if a person is dying and is, for example, adjusting to paraplegia, that person may still want to see what can be achieved within the imposed limitations. Personal energy becomes available as the trap of depression is 'discarded'. This is a new reality which is being examined and many 'ups and downs' can be encountered at this stage, releasing emotions such as irritation and agitation. There may even be a sense of 'slipping back' towards depression if plans are frustrated.

Search for meaning

Nevertheless, a shift towards trying to understand the whole process helps to increase self-esteem. When a person is facing death, it may seem that everything is lost. However, if this sixth stage in transition is reached, future goals and impending death converge, and finding meaning becomes a significant step towards self-fulfilment. One patient said, 'It's OK to die. I feel a whole new world is opening up to me.' O'Connor *et al.* (1990) discovered six major themes identified by patients in their search for meaning:

- Seeking an understanding of the personal significance of the cancer diagnosis.
- Looking at the consequences of the cancer diagnosis.
- Review of life.
- Change in outlook toward self, life and others.
- Living with the cancer.
- Hope.

There is a feeling here of placing self in relation to past, present and future life such that existence makes sense. The discovery of hope offers the opportunity to rediscover life.

Internalisation

When meaning is incorporated into life, then growth is possible. Hopson and Adams (1976, p. 5) describe this potential as 'opportunity value' which offers the possibility of increased self-esteem. An example of this can be found in another patient who became severely limited by depression which followed the diagnosis of his cancer. With counselling (see Chapter 18) and the support of his family, he worked through this depressive phase and eventually decided he would 'make the most' of his remaining life. He discovered enough energy to work in his garden hut and use his planning abilities to design kitchen implements for his wife. He described this energy as the freedom to be creative.

Few people move through the transition process in a systematic manner. The progress of cancer and treatment involves many uncertainties and personal variables. Shneidman's (1980) view of the dying process underlines personal uniqueness, observing that an individual's death will reflect their life, and their response to dying will be related to their emotional style. Although people have the potential for growth, not every person will achieve their full potential. The transition map (see Fig. 7.2), offers insight into the importance of completing and moving through each stage in order to achieve increased self-esteem. It is this insight into the process involved throughout transition which can enable nurses to clarify their concepts in relation to care.

Relationships

So far, this chapter has explored disruption of personal needs and sequential reactions to transition. It is important to consider the effect of cancer and treatment on the individual. However, the palliative care will miss an essential dimension of care if professionals involved do not consider the implications and effect of cancer and treatment upon *relationships* within the family. Clearly, if each person within the family is at a different stage in their own transition process, they will have different needs, and may not have the capacity to help each other, yet the *need* to help usually exists. Hospitalisation, treatment, or the disease process itself, may mean separation of family members for the first time in their lives. Distressing symptoms such as pain or confusion can disrupt the close family bonds built in times of health. Within a family there is a need to continue sharing, yet this need may be confronted with the need to protect each other. Protection often takes the form of withholding information which may cause pain. A conspiracy ensues which is difficult to maintain and the family may repress their own grief in order to present a controlled front. This causes severe tension which drives people who love each other further apart.

Family members who have not been close to each other for many years may experience complex emotions including guilt, desperation and relief, resulting in arguments and further disruption. This can be confusing to the nurse who may find it hard to appreciate the family background of turmoil and trouble.

The nurse also is forming a relationship with the patient and family, becoming an integral part of the family unit, and as such may be caught up in the tangled web of inter-family affairs. The needs of the nurse become important here, and are explored at the end of this chapter.

There is the additional dilemma of changing interdependency. Margalith (1987, p. 51) states that 'illness in one member of the family imposes demands on everyone else'. A daughter may find herself nursing her mother in a very intimate way. Inherent in this caring is the painful knowledge and meaning of loss, as this is the mother to whom *she* has always looked for support and nurturing. A struggling young father needs to consider child care, cooking and home management as well as maintaining an essential job when caring for his ill wife. The fight to maintain equilibrium can result in family conflict and breakdown. It is possible, however, for transformation of roles to empower hitherto unknown strengths. Patients have the potential to support their own family: this may be their last gift. It has been found that for some people the diagnosis of cancer may have a positive effect, enabling 'a couple to reassess the value of their relationship' (Lamb and Woods, 1981, p. 140).

Sexuality

The multidimensional effect of cancer and treatment implies an effect on the sexual perception of the individual. Poorman (1983, p. 663) states that 'sexuality is an integral part of every human being and is lived every day of one's life. It is evident in the way one looks. believes, behaves and relates to other human beings'. Sexuality is more than a physical expression; it is all about self-concept, self-esteem and social role, which combine to form the identity of the person. If true holistic care is to be offered to patients and families then considering sexuality must be an integral part of that care.

The sexual urge can be very powerful. It can suppress pain and help people forget their troubles, if only for a short while. It allows a feeling of 'normality' (Buckman 1988, p. 125), a time to be valued again. However, physical effects of cancer may produce difficulties in sexual activity. Pain, fatigue and range of movement difficulties are described by Lamb and Woods (1981, p. 143) as the commonest problems. Nausea, vomiting, halitosis, bowel disturbance and discharging wounds can be added to this list. Radiotherapy, cytotoxic chemotherapy and medication affect patients externally, internally or systematically so affecting sexuality and ways of being with self or another. Surgery involving genitalia, giving vascular impairment or nerve damage is a more obvious cause of lack of sexual response. Hailey and Hardin (1988) found that patients with sex-specific cancer, for example breast or prostate, are more likely than other patients to experience sexual adjustment problems, and males are more likely than females to experience sexual problems after their illness.

Psychological needs are often associated with physical problems. If physical difficulties arise, the patient may feel unattractive or rejected. This in turn can bring feelings of guilt, anger or frustration. Some patients try to avoid the whole issue. The resulting isolation and possible depression becomes another burden at a time when support is most needed.

Symptoms or changed appearance which make sexual contact unattractive, bring problems for the patient's partner. Alternatively, the partner may wish sexual contact, but fear causing pain or trauma.

Some patients have neither the ability nor the urge for full sexual intercourse, yet intimacy and human contact are desired. This is confirmed by Leiber *et al.* (1976) who found that patients with advanced cancer and their spouses experienced simultaneously an increased desire for physical closeness and decreased desire for sexual intercourse. Issues surrounding sexuality should not be deemed to be of concern only to young patients as many more older patients are treated now for cancer (Kaiser, 1992). The importance of touch has long been recognised as essential to human development and this need continues throughout life. The value of holding hands or giving or receiving a cuddle should never be underestimated. Sims (1988, p. 59) states that 'purposeful touch can communicate security, warmth and caring and positively affect emotional self-esteem through conveying acceptance'. Sexual health problems presented by patients and partners sometimes go unheard. It would appear that nurses do not have enough confidence to deal with these problems (Webb, 1987; Smith, 1989; Foxley, 1989). Nurse education can play an important role here. Sexual difficulties must be clearly presented in relation to biological, psychological and social aspects. If feelings in relation to sexuality can be openly discussed, then barriers, such as embarrassment and conservatism, may be dissolved. Equally important is the nurse's own self-concept in relation to personal sexuality. If this is explored in some depth, then freedom to discuss sexuality and sexual matters with patients and their partners may be enhanced. Facilitating the expression of sexuality can only add to the quality of life (Webb and O'Neill, 1988, p. 136).

Meeting needs

Needs are defined as 'circumstances requiring some course of action' (*Concise Oxford Dictionary*). Enhancing awareness of needs will also encompass ways of meeting those needs. When considering the needs of the individual facing death, Orem (1980, p. 145) describes the aims of health care as follows. To enable individuals to:

• Live as themselves.
• Understand their illness and how to participate in their care.
• Be with family, friends and health-care workers in an environment of security and trust.

These aims focus on empowering the patient with control over life, understanding, care, the environment and death. This calls for sensitive care rooted in acceptance, empathy and genuineness. These three conditions are the essential characteristics of a helping relationship and are explored in Chapter 18. It is important for nurses not to make assumptions about patients and their needs, but to make a real attempt to listen to and understand these needs. Facilitating choice marks the respect engendered by total patient care.

When considering how to meet the needs of the family, Hampe's (1975) classic study of the needs of grieving spouses in a hospital setting offers important implications to the care of *all* family members. She found their priorities as follows:

• To be with the dying person.
• To be assured of the comfort of the dying person.
• To be kept informed of the dying person's condition, medical plan and daily progress.
• To be informed of the impending death.
• To ventilate emotions.
• To receive comfort and support from family members.
• To receive acceptance, support and comfort from health professionals.

Lewandowski and Jones (1988, p. 320) support these findings, noting that having *time alone* with the dying person was rated and ranked highest for family members. There is a need to continue sharing life with the patient and this may require permission to be included in the care-giving. Nurses can take the initiative here and plan care *with* the patient and family. It is important to remember that within the relationship of patient and family, it is the nurse who is the newcomer. Gilley (1988, p. 122) states that 'professionals must have a great sensitivity to avoid taking over and being "better" carers than the real carer'.

Respect for the long-standing intimacy of the family's relationship will promote the natural caring capacity of patient and family. Intimacy can be facilitated by privacy, offering the patient freedom to spend time with people who are close. Even when difficult to obtain, ways of being private can be considered with the family. Once included in care, families still need support and comfort, so that they do not feel abandoned.

Reassurance of the comfort of the dying person is only possible if great care is taken to control symptoms and explain progression. Attention to detail, such as the environment and the appearance of the patient, is vital. Hampe (1975, p. 117) states that spouses associated the cleanliness of hospital rooms with the comfort of their mates. Lewandowski and Jones (1988) emphasise that nursing interventions directed toward the *patient* are claimed as most helpful by family members.

Lugton (1989b, p. 29) looked at the support of relatives in a hospice setting. She found that despite welcomed support, one-third of families still found difficulty initiating contact with staff and obtaining the information needed. It is important to create the opportunity for families to ask their questions. Certain disturbing symptoms such as personality change, agitation and breathing difficulties need to be explained clearly. Too much detail, however, can be overwhelming, and the importance of responding with sensitivity to the questions asked becomes fundamental. Preparation for the future is reflected in the need for concise and timely information. Bond (1982, p. 965) observed that it is not always 'what' is said but 'how' it is said that influences satisfaction.

The process of realisation is filled with many emotions which, if contained, results in distorted expression (see Fig. 7.1). Hampe (1975) found that spouses recognised their need to *express* the emotions evoked by increased understanding of circumstances. This finding is consistent with Lewandowski and Jones' (1988) study who found that family members experienced an increasing need to ventilate emotions as they progressed through the phase of living with cancer. The nurse can fulfil a valuable role in providing support, privacy and space for those needing to cry, show anger or express fear. In a secure environment and with support, it may be possible for families to start 'letting go' of the person who is near death.

Children

The needs of children and adolescents in the family may be overlooked. It is just as important for a child or teenager to participate in care, to be assured of the comfort of the dying person and to be allowed the opportunity to prepare for change. Unfortunately, well-meaning protection can separate a child from understanding. A vivid imagination will fill gaps and may produce disproportionate anxiety and fear. Margalith (1987, p. 51) notes that the child's resultant behaviour will exacerbate an already stressful situation. Stedeford's study (1984, p. 32) suggests that the most important factors are the parents' attitude to death, their openness with the children and the amount of support they receive from the extended family. Henley (1986, p. 17) offers guidelines for good practice in caring for dying patients. She states that, '. . . It is most important that children should not be cut off from their dying parent.' Encouraging mutual support within the family will facilitate the involvement of children in the care. Clearly including children in the care-giving and offering the opportunity to ask questions is absolutely vital.

The nurse

Care is a multidimensional process which involves the feelings of the nurse as well as those for whom she or he cares. The person for whom the nurse is caring is usually a stranger, yet the nurse is involved in a very intimate way. Care-giving can unsuspectingly take a nurse closest to her or his own vulnerability. Davies and Oberle (1990) found preserving personal integrity to be a core concept necessary to nursing in palliative care. The ability to maintain self-worth, self-esteem and energy levels is central to the nurses' effective functioning.

Elkind (1982) examined female hospital nurses' views about cancer. Her study suggests that nurses share the fear of cancer felt by women generally. Corner (1988, p. 641) reviewed studies on nurses' attitudes towards cancer. These studies indicate that 'health carers have negative attitudes towards cancer and that behaviour towards the cancer sufferer may be affected as a result'. Maguire (1985) discusses how psychological care can be blocked by nurses' own attitudes, vulnerabilities and fears. This results in distancing tactics and avoidance. Alternatively, Reisetter and Thomas (1986) conclude the possibility that a professional nurse provides nursing care independent of attitudes held. Interestingly, Martocchio (1987) notes that professional competence is necessary but not *sufficient*. A nurse who withholds her full self is unlikely to enable the whole person of the patient.

Individualised care demands a willingness to respect a person's evident needs and to be aware of unseen needs, involving care of the *whole* person. In order to respond *fully* to the wide variety of needs present, the nurse must be aware of the factors which impede his or her ability to care. These factors exist within the client, within the nurse, within their relationship and within the environment. Figure 7.4 illustrates some of these difficulties within the caring process.

The diagnoses of cancer, treatment of the illness and course of the disease create a process of change which requires continual re-examination and readjustment for all involved, including the nurse. Clearly, meeting psychological needs is extremely difficult to achieve. Assessment of needs is thwarted by the danger of stigma, interpretation and poor communication, and planning and management of care is hampered by rigid practices and mismatched priorities. Reviewing the structure of care demands imagination, innovation and team work which includes patients and families. Introducing a flexibility which reflects needs may be risky for a nurse who needs to exercise control, but it is through *sharing* control that balanced care can begin. Support in nursing is essential here to enhance the value of the nurse. Support is discussed further in Chapters 18 and 19. Respecting the choices and the humanity of all people involved is the key. If nurses and patients can discard their assigned roles and find ways of relating to each other as *people*. then a true depth of caring will emerge.

Client	Nurse	Relationship/ Communication	Environment
Physical distress	Expectations	Conspiracy	Lack of privacy
Fear	Assumptions	Ambiguity	Distractions
Guilt	Stereotyping	Dishonesty	Interruptions
Denial	Need for power	Inability to hear	Lack of time
Anger	Need for recognition	Inappropriate language	Lack of opportunity
Embarrassment	Need to be liked	Inappropriate speed of information	Noise
Anxiety	Need to be helpful		Unattractive setting
Depression	Professional role	Inappropriate amount of information	
Withdrawal	Pride		
Pride	Prejudice	Lack of clarity	
Expectations	Personal limitations	Beliefs	
Assumptions	Identification	Culture	
Self-doubt	Disguised reactions		
	Fear		
	Embarrassment		
	Self-doubt		
	Pity		
	Distaste		

DISTANCING-AVOIDANCE
DEFENSIVENESS
INABILITY TO COMPREHEND
MISINTERPRETATION

Fig. 7.4. Barriers to psychological care.

Before she died, a student nurse reflected on the nursing care she was receiving: 'I know, you feel insecure, don't know what to say, don't know what to do. But please believe me, if you care, you can't go wrong. Just admit that you care . . . I have lots I wish we could talk about. It really would not take much more of your time because you are in here quite a bit anyway. If only we could be honest, both admit of our fears, touch one another. If you really care, would you lose so much of your valuable professionalism if you even cried with me? Just person to person? Then, it might not be so hard to die . . . in a hospital . . . with friends close by.'
Anon. (1970). Reproduced with permission of the *American Journal of Nursing*.

Acknowledgements

Thanks go to Professor Stuart Aitken, Department of Geography, San Diego State University; Diana Guthrie, Student Advisory and Counselling Service, University of Edinburgh; Elke Lambers and Dave Mearns, Co-Directors, Person-Centred Therapy (Britain); Alison Shoemark, colleague and friend; and members of the

Scottish PCT Supervision Group. The support and insight gained from all was invaluable. Special thanks also go to Mrs Arlene Ogston for typing, and to Sam for his unfailing patience and respect.

References

ANON (1970). Death in the first person. *American Journal of Nursing* 70(2), 336.

BOND, S. (1982). Communicating with families of cancer patients: the relatives and doctors. *Nursing Times* 9 June, 962–5.

BUCKMAN, R. (1988). *I Don't Know What to Say*. Macmillan, London.

CORNER, J. L. (1988). Assessment of nurses' attitudes towards cancer: critical review of research methods. *Journal of Advanced Nursing* 13, 640–8.

ELKIND, A. K. (1982). Nurses' views about cancer. *Journal of Advanced Nursing* 7(1), 43–50.

DAVIES, B. and OBERLE, K. (1990). Dimensions of the supportive role of the nurse in palliative care. *Oncology Nursing Forum* 17(1), 87–94.

FOXLEY, W. D. (1989). *Sexuality, Nurses and Cancer Patients*. Unpublished paper.

GILLEY, J. (1988). Intimacy and terminal care. *Journal of the Royal College of General Practitioners* 38, 121–2.

GRIFFITHS, E. (1989). More than skin deep. *Nursing Times* 85(40), 34–6.

HAILEY, B. J. and HARDIN, K. N. (1988). Perceptions of seriously ill patients: does diagnosis make a difference? *Patient Education and Counselling* 12, 259–65.

HAMPE, S. O. (1975). Needs of the grieving spouse in a hospital setting. *Nursing Research* 24(2), 113–20.

HENLEY, A. (1986). *Good Practice in Hospital Care for Dying Patients*. Kings Fund, London.

HERON, J. (1977). *Catharsis in Human Development*. Human Potential Research Project, University of Surrey.

HOPSON, B. and ADAMS, J. (1976). Towards an understanding of transition: defining some boundaries of transition dynamics. In: ADAMS, J., HAYES, J. and HOPKINS, B. (eds), *Transition – Understanding and Managing Personal Change*, pp. 3–25. Martin Robertson, London.

Hopson, B. (1982). Transition: understanding and managing personal change. In: CHAPMAN, A. J. and GALE, A. (eds), *Psychology and People*, pp. 120–45. Macmillan, London.

KAISER, F. E. (1992) Sexual function and the older cancer patient. *Oncology* 6(2 Suppl), 112–18.

KUBLER-ROSS, E. (1969). *On Death and Dying*. Souvenir Press, London.

LAMB, M. A. and WOODS, N. F. (1981). Sexuality and the cancer patient. *Cancer Nursing* 4(2), 137–44.

LEIBER, L. *et al.* (1976). The communication of affection between cancer patients and their spouses. *Psychosomatic Medicine* 38(6), 379–89.

LEWANDOWSKI, W. and JONES, S. L. (1988). The family with cancer. *Cancer Nursing* 11(6), 313–21.

LUGTON, J. (1989a). Identifying anxieties. *Nursing Times* 85(17), 50–1.

LUGTON, J. (1989b). Communicating in the hospice. *Nursing Times* 85(16), 28–30.

MAGUIRE, P. (1985). Barriers to psychological care of the dying. *British Medical Journal* 291, 1711–13.

MARGALITH, I. (1987). Holding the family together. *Nursing Times* 83(39), 51–3.

MARTOCCHIO, B. C. (1987) Authenticity, belonging, emotional closeness and self-representation. *Oncology Nursing Forum* **14**(4), 23–7.

O'CONNOR, A. P. *et al.* (1990). Understanding the cancer patient's search for meaning. *Cancer Nursing* **13**(3), 167–75.

O'CONNOR, N. (1984). *Letting Go with Love: The Grieving Process.* La Mariposa Press, Arizona.

OREM, D. E. (1980). *Nursing; Concepts of Practice,* 2nd edn. McGraw-Hill, New York.

POORMAN, S. (1983). Human sexuality and nursing practice. In: STUART, G. W. and SUNDEEN, S. J. (eds), *Principles and Practice and Psychiatric Nursing,* 2nd edn, pp. 661–86. Mosby, Missouri.

PORTER, S. (1988). Siding with the system. *Nursing Times* **84**(41), 30–1.

REISETTER, H. A. and THOMAS, B. (1986). Nursing care of the dying: its relationship to selected nurse characteristics. *International Journal of Nursing Studies* **23**(1), 39–50.

SHNEIDMAN, E. S. (1980) *Voices of Death.* Harper & Row, New York.

SIMS, S. (1988). The significance of touch in palliative care. *Palliative Medicine* 58–61.

SMITH, D. B. (1989). Sexual rehabilitation of the cancer patient. *Cancer Nursing* **12**(1), 10–15.

STEDEFORD, A. (1984). *Facing Death.* Heinemann Medical, London.

WEBB, C. (1987). Nurses knowledge and attitudes about sexuality: report of a study. *Nurse Education Today* **7**(5), 209–14.

WEISMAN, A. D. (1979). *Coping with Cancer.* McGraw-Hill, New York.

WELLS, R. (1986). The great conspiracy. *Nursing Times* 21 May, 22–5.

Further reading

CHAPMAN, A. J. and GALE, A. (Eds) (1982). *Psychology and People.* Macmillan, London.

CHARLES-EDWARDS, A. (1983). *The Nursing Care of the Dying Patient.* Beaconsfield.

KUBLER-ROSS, E. (1975). *Death: The Final Stage of Growth.* Simon & Schuster, New York.

LUGTON, J. (1987). *Communicating with Dying People and their Relatives.* Austen Cornish, London.

PARKES, C. M. (1978). Psychological aspects. In: SAUNDERS, C. M. (ed.), *The Management of Terminal Disease,* pp. 44–64. Edward Arnold, London.

STEDEFORD, A. (1984). *Facing Death.* Heinemann Medical, London.

8

Confusional states

Kathryn A. Mannix

'All the physicians and authors in the world could not give a clear account of his madness. He is mad in patches, full of lucid intervals.'
From Don Quixote, *by Miguel Cervantes (1547–1616)*

What is confusion?

'Confusion' is used to describe many different symptoms, such as incoherent speech, disorientation in time or place, difficulty with concentration, hallucinations or misinterpretations. Use of the word confusion can lead to confusion amongst the carers, because the word may mean something slightly different to different carers. However, all carers understand that it refers to something fundamental and constant about any patient: the thoughts this patient is expressing are different from usual. When visiting a patient who is confused we expect to find muddled thought.

Feeling muddled and being unable to make proper sense of the surroundings can be very frightening. To help a patient who is confused the professional carer must start to calm the patient's fear, try to find the threads of reality in the jumble and help him or her to keep hold of reality as much as possible. At the same time, a cause for the confusion must be found. Confusion is not a diagnosis, it is only a symptom of illness, and we can only hope to reverse the confusion fully by identifying and treating the underlying physical illness.

Some definitions

When an illness is due to physical damage in the body it is an *organic* illness. Confusion is a psychological symptom of an organic illness. Psychiatrists call this an *organic brain syndrome*. There are two recognised organic brain syndromes, acute (sudden and usually reversible) and chronic (slow and continuing). The *chronic organic brain syndrome* is due to death of nerve cells within the brain; it is of gradual onset and gets steadily worse. It is recognised as *dementia*, and it is almost always irreversible. The *acute organic brain syndrome* or *delirium* is due to physical illness in the body which prevents normal brain functioning. It is usually of fairly sudden onset, and instead of getting steadily worse it tends to fluctuate. It is always worth trying to find the physical cause of delirium because treating the cause will usually restore normal brain function.

Table 8.1 shows the main characteristics of these two brain syndromes. Many patients with cancer are elderly and hence some may also have dementia. The important point about delirium is that the person is different from a short time previously. Thus, a demented patient may also become delirious: treatment of the cause of delirium should restore cerebral functioning to its previous (demented) norm.

Table 8.1 Differences between delirium and dementia

Delirium	Dementia
Usually reversible	Irreversible
Clouding of consciousness	Clear consciousness
Misinterpretations	
Hallucinations, especially visual	Hallucinations rare
Release of emotion	Affect may be released or reduced
Fluctuating, often worse at night	Unchanging hour to hour, but slow deterioration over months/years
Sleep disturbances (not enough or too much)	Normal amount of sleep but may sleep at the wrong time
Activity change (retarded or hyperactive)	No activity change
Global cognitive impairment	Often memory change before other changes

Observing and listening to delirious patients shows that their mental processing of information ('cognitive function') is affected in all is aspects; this is called global impairment of cognitive function. The major aspects of psychological function are:

- consciousness
- attention
- mood
- perception
- thinking
- memory
- behaviour.

It will help to explain the changes seen in confused patients if each of these aspects is considered in turn.

Consciousness

This refers to how awake and alert a person is. 'Clouding of consciousness' is the first, almost imperceptible step on a slope from normal alertness down towards coma and death. It is different from sleep, which is a normal, healthy brain function.

Attention

This is the ability to select and concentrate on a particular stimulus, for example to listen to a conversation and ignore distracting noises. Confused patients often appear to be paying less attention than usual, although they may in fact be paying more attention, but they cannot select a particular stimulus and their attention flits between your conversation, noises in the room, thoughts in their head and the colour of the carpet.

Mood (affect)

Most people have a recognisable mood or affect which is 'normal' for them (e.g. anxious, carefree, suspicious) and this is recognised as their personality. People with dementia often display less personality than they used to, becoming rather bland. In delirious patients the opposite is seen: the personality is 'released' and they are unable to damp down some parts of their affect. In this way, anxious individuals may become terrified, carefree people may become euphoric and suspicious people become paranoid. This may occur in dementia but it is less florid.

Perception

This is the process of becoming aware of the information being presented by the sensory nerves, such as a hard bed, the smell of burning toast, the sound of visitors' voices, feeling sick, or having pain. Perception can be altered by the circumstances in which the brain receives messages, and this can lead to misinterpretations. Misinterpretations are more likely to arise in the following instances:

 (i) *When the level of consciousness is reduced,* e.g. during sleep a person may dream about alarm bells ringing when they hear the alarm clock sounding.
 (ii) *While attention is not focused on that sensory pathway,* e.g. while concentrating on typing (visual pathway) the sound of the radio (auditory pathway) may be misinterpreted as the telephone ringing. Darkness reduces a person's ability to attend to visual stimuli and so visual misinterpretations are more common at night.
 (iii) *If a strong emotional state is present,* e.g. after reading ghost stories a person may be frightened by a rustle of the curtains.

By 'turning up the volume' of attention and emotion people can alert themselves to perceive particular stimuli, for example a mother may sleep through the noise of traffic but will awaken instantly if her baby cries.

Emily had a long history of agitated depression, so she surprised herself and her family by how well she coped with the diagnosis of breast cancer at the age of 60 years. She did very well for 8 years, but when she was admitted to the Hospice with bone pain her family asked us not to tell her that her disease was advancing.

Emily did not settle well. She was shouting and fighting with the night nurses, although she remained withdrawn during the day. The night sister noticed Emily kept referring to matches and accusing the night staff of trying to kill her. When she asked Emily if she felt hot, Emily replied that anyone would feel hot if they had been set on fire! Her family told us that Emily had once been in hospital with depression when a schizophrenic patient set fire to the ward, and she had always been very afraid of fires at home after that.

She was found to have a high temperature. Investigations revealed a urinary tract infection, which was treated with antibiotics. One of Emily's daughters came to sleep with her at the hospice for a few days. We explored her fear of burning to death, while her daughter was with her. Emily told us she could feel she was weaker and less well, and she thought that she might be dying. She was very afraid of losing control of herself if she got frightened during dying because she had experienced panic attacks in the past. She was told that when the time came she was likely to lapse into a coma very gently, and found this so comforting that she told this story to all of the patients who had become her friends at the hospice, too!

She went home for a further six months, and came back to the Hospice when she was dying 'because you understand me here . . . '

Thinking

A person's thought content can be recognised by their speech and behaviour. Usually thoughts are connected like links in a chain. When a person thinks, the links into 'what is happening now', 'what happened in the past', 'how I feel inside', 'how my friend seems to be feeling', can be separated out and the person can make sense of a situation.

In delirium the cross-linking becomes less easy to separate and to follow, and the person has difficulty separating internal and external worlds. They may misinterpret memories for present reality, and they speak more slowly, with long pauses as they try to focus their thoughts. Later they lose ability to reason thoughts out, their ability to form abstract thoughts is impaired and they display concrete thinking. Usually they lose insight at the same time, i.e. they do not realise that their thinking has changed in the way that it has, although patients often have a vague feeling that all is not well and many express a fear of madness.

Memory

The decreased ability to receive and process information accurately causes disruption of memory. New information cannot be stored and patients may require the same information to be repeated frequently, although their memory for past events remains intact. When the episode of delirium is past, patients frequently have no memory of it at all, or may only remember meaningless fragments.

Behaviour

As the control of normal behaviour is lost in the muddled mind, people may display signs of their illness by becoming noisy, hyperactive and irritable. More commonly, though, people become slower. Their speech and spontaneous activity are reduced, and repetitive, purposeless movements are common. This preservation of movements or speech seems to be due to an inability to turn off attention from a particular, fragmented thought. This can be very distressing for the patient and for his or her family.

Looking for a cause for confusion

Vulnerability to delirium is known to be increased by increasing age, by serious physical illness, by dehydration, by poor eyesight or hearing, and by dependence on alcohol or sedative drugs. Many of these factors may affect cancer patients, increasing the likeliness of delirium if a further physical stress is added.

In cancer patients it is important to see if there is a treatable cause as quickly as possible, because the last period of a patient's life will be so much more comfortable, and comforting for his or her family, if the patient is lucid and peaceful. Table 8.2 lists some of the causes of delirium which are worth looking for in cancer patients. Of course, there are other causes, but these are the most common or, for rare causes, those which can be treated easily and effectively.

Once the physical cause of delirium is treated it may take several days for the confusion to subside. During that time it is important to continue to reassure the patient and family, and to keep assessing for signs of improvement. Because delirium is a fluctuating condition there may be periods of complete normality

Table 8.2 Causes of delirium in patients with advanced cancer

---

Drugs
  Any drugs acting on the CNS, particularly:
    antidepressants
    anticonvulsants
    sedative drugs
  corticosteroids
  opioids
  anticholinergics
  β-blockers
  diuretics
  digitalis
Remember drug withdrawal, especially
  alcohol
  opioids
  benzodiazepines

Infection
(The patient may not be pyrexial, and very ill patients or those on corticosteroids
may even be hypothermic)
  Chest   ⎫   most common
  Urinary tract ⎬   in the elderly
  Diverticulitis
  Ears   ⎫   most common
  Throat   ⎬   in children
  Pressure sores
  Necrotic tumours

Trauma
  Head injury
  Subdural haematoma

Tumour
  Cerebral primary, cerebral metastases
  'Paraneoplastic' (malignant disease elsewhere)
  Anaemia due to bleeding or bone marrow infiltration

Cardiovascular/respiratory disease (cerebral hypoxia)
  Stroke(s)
  Myocardial infarction (classical symptoms and signs may be absent)
  Heart failure/hypotension/arrhythmias
  Deep venous thrombosis alone or with pulmonary embolism
  Respiratory failure

Biochemical/metabolic
  Electrolyte disturbance (most commonly hyponatraemia, hypokalaemia,
    dehydration, hypercalcaemia)
  Uraemia
  Liver failure
  Hypoglycaemia/ketoacidosis

---

followed by confusion again, which can reduce families to a state of emotional exhaustion as they celebrate 'recovery' only to be plunged back into despair once more. They need support and reassurance to cope with a beloved person who fails to recognise them or even blames them and accuses them of ill-treatment.

George visited his mother Hilda at the hospice every day. She was dying with bladder cancer, but she 'held court' and was queen of the four-bedded bay which she shared with two other patients.

Then George stopped visiting. No-one saw him for days. One of the nurses met him in town, and he angrily told her that his mother had accused him of spending all her money on parties and disreputable women. We asked Hilda directly about this, and she assured us that it was quite true, and George was only waiting for her to die to convert her house into a brothel.

Hilda's husband had left her when George was a little boy. She was afraid that his father's traits were becoming evident in George, and that he would go off the rails when she died. In fact, George had a girlfriend, but he had not told his mother, in case she worried that he would leave home while she was ill.

We attributed Hilda's muddled thoughts to the corticosteroids she was taking for painful pressure on her pelvic nerves, and explained this to George. We tried to stop the corticosteroids, but her pain came back. Gently probing her fears for George she wept to think of him living alone after her death. George was able to ask her how she would feel if he were to marry in the future, and she was overjoyed. He did not risk bringing his girlfriend to meet her, in case this was misconstrued. She continued to ask disinhibited questions about his 'love life' from time to time, but George was able to understand that the origin of this thought was real concern for his future, and he continued to visit regularly until his mother died.

Understanding the confused patient

Definitions and some understanding of what is happening to confused patients' bodies and brains may feel reassuring to the professional carer, but it is not a great deal of help when in the room of a frightened, confused patient whose relatives are looking to the professional carers for help. It is necessary to try to understand what is happening for the patient.

Start by looking at the mind of a normal healthy person – like yourself, perhaps. The thoughts which are reaching your consciousness at this moment are arising from three main areas: from the environment (how warm the room is, how interesting your book is, whether there is a cup of coffee being poured for you); from your body (hunger, gritty eyes, need to sneeze, respiratory movements, posture); and from your subconscious (memories of last weekend, hopes for next holiday, remember to buy some milk today, wonder if your child has got to school safely). If you pay attention to all those thoughts you will get no work done, remember nothing of what you are reading and be too busy getting your coffee to reach for a tissue to catch your sneeze. The mind therefore has a selective filter, which allows a person to concentrate on the job in hand and only allows other thoughts into consciousness if they are important. Figure 8.1 shows how the conscious mind is divided.

Figure 8.2 shows an awake, well person reading a book. The filter to the body

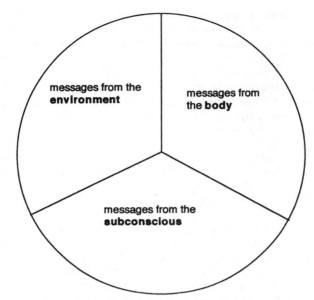

Fig. 8.1 The areas of consciousness.

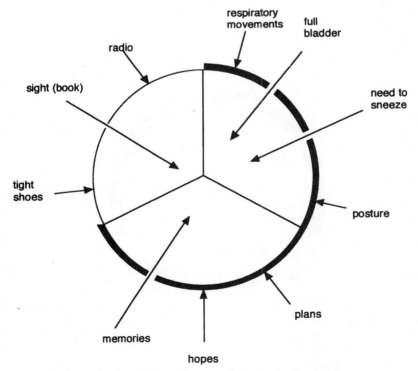

Fig. 8.2 Thoughts reaching consciousness: awake, reacting.

and the subconscious is thick, but it allows relevant thoughts into consciousness (remembering a patient who illustrates the problem you are studying; getting a tissue in time for the sneeze). Note that the boundaries between the different areas of the mind are clear, you can easily separate which messages came from your memory, from your book and from your nose.

Figure 8.3 shows another healthy person, but asleep this time. The boundaries of the three areas of the mind are less clearly demarcated. The environment is being filtered out; although some stimuli from the environment reach consciousness, they may be misinterpreted as part of a dream (telephone ringing becomes a dream about fire-bells). Similarly the body is also being filtered out, but some stimuli still get through (pain, full bladder) and may be misinterpreted because the boundaries are unclear. Thus a person may dream of being attacked because they have pain during sleep. The 'volume control' discussed earlier can be set to alert a person to particular stimuli, such as a full bladder, baby crying or the post arriving.

From this model it can be seen that all the thoughts in a person's consciousness have come from somewhere. They are all rooted in reality – real physical stimuli, real memories, hopes or fears, real feelings within a person's body. It is the same for the confused person, but it seems that the boundaries have broken down and it is difficult for the person to work out where a thought came from. Their filter to the environment is thick so that it is difficult for another person to reach them. This is illustrated in Fig. 8.4.

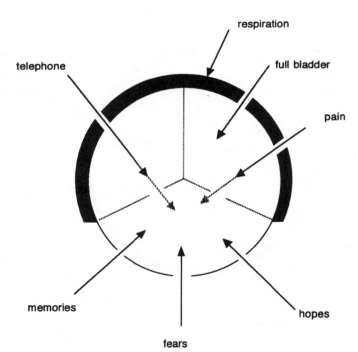

Fig. 8.3 Thoughts reaching consciousness: sleep.

With this model in mind, it becomes easier to understand why confused people have such bizarre experiences. Their 'volume control' is reset by their fear and anxiety, so stimuli they particularly fear or desire are perceived more readily. They may have difficulty in getting a grip on reality, or interpret reality as a dream. By trying to trace their (confused) thought back to its origin in reality, the carer may be able to help to reduce the anxiety and so to turn down the 'volume control' of their fears.

Treatment of confused patients

Recipe
Ingredients:
   1 confused patient
   5 distressed family members
   1 hospital room, with light switch
   3 morning nurses, 2 afternoon nurses, 2 night nurses
   1 ward doctor, 1 on-call doctor
   2 large hospital porters
   1 syringeful of chlorpromazine
   1 green hypodermic needle
   1 wardful of assorted sick patients

Method: Remove the confused patient from his or her familiar bedroom at home, and place in cold hard bed in unfamiliar hospital room. Ask family to leave. Ward doctor should examine patient. Change nurses regularly.
   After 8 hours switch off lights. Leave patient in dark room, and disturb regularly to check that he or she is asleep. When he or she protests, send for on-call doctor.
   Wait until patient becomes frightened. When he or she begins to rise over the edge of the bed, apply one large hospital porter to each arm. On-call doctor should give injection of chlorpromazine into patient's bottom whilst repeating the incantation 'this won't hurt' or 'this is for your own good'.
   Agitate the whole ward for 4 hours and await ward round. Repeat chlorpromazine if patient shows any sign of waking up. Garnish with diazepam suppositories.

It is easy to see why 'confusion' is such a common cause of admission to hospital. Sometimes the patient's behaviour is too violent for him or her to remain at home, sometimes the family is too distressed to cope. It is also easy to see where our management went wrong in retrospect. It is getting it right as we go along that is the challenge.

Refer again to Fig. 8.4. The aim of the health professional is to get the frightened, confused patient back in contact with reality. The carer is in the patient's environment, approaching the patient through his or her sight, hearing and touch. The patient's filter is blocking out the professional carer. How can the carer reach the patient? If sedative drugs are given the thickness of the filter to the environment is increased and the internal divisions of consciousness are broken down even further. Sedating a patient will never improve his or her delirium, although it may seem to improve the plight of the carers. Sometimes sedation really is necessary, for example if, because of fear, the patient becomes a danger to self or others, or if the patient is becoming exhausted. Useful sedative drugs are discussed later in this chapter.

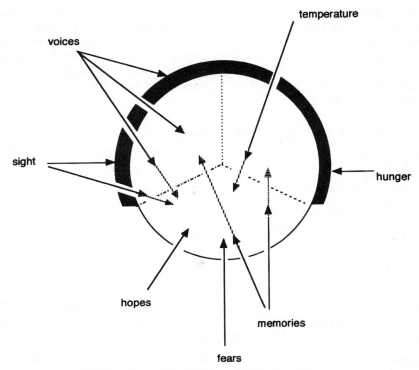

Fig. 8.4 Thoughts reaching consciousness: delirious.

Can a patient be reached via his or her body or subconscious? A gentle touch, holding the patient's hand, smiling, all these are messages of friendship and care which may get through the filter when spoken language is not helping. There is usually comfort from the presence of a trusted friend or relative.

The priorities for management from the patient's point of view are:

1. Stop or reduce the fear.
2. Rationalise the underlying anxieties.
3. Find and treat the cause of delirium.
4. Orientate to reality.

Stop or reduce the fear

There is fear of the situation in which the patient finds him or herself. The carer must help the patient to restore reality. Explain to the patient that if they find they are muddled it is because they are not well. Keep reassuring and smiling. Keep assuming that they will understand at least some of what you say to them.

There is also a fear of madness. This is very common but patients are often unable to express their fear. Patients and families need to be reassured that this muddledness is temporary and is due to the physical illness. We do not think they will go mad. We do not think they are becoming senile.

Hallucinations may occasionally occur and they are often visual. Colluding with the patient is rarely helpful because their mental state is fluctuating; if you agree that you can see the little pink frogs now, then when the patient becomes more lucid later on they may remember you 'went along with them' and stop trusting you – or even believe that you are mad for seeing those things! It is often helpful to acknowledge that the hallucination is real for the patient. 'Yes, I know you can see them and that they are very frightening. I can't see them, but you can. You want them to go away and I want to help you to make them go away'.

Misinterpretations are far more common, but may be mistaken for hallucinations unless a very careful history is taken. With misinterpretations, it is useful to explore the underlying thoughts: 'Did you wish I was your mother when I came in then? Tell me about her. Tell me what she would have done for you?' This should always be accompanied by re-orientating that patient and explaining why they have become muddled ('Your temperature is high, so you are delirious like small children sometimes are'. 'You have a chest infection, so there is less oxygen than usual getting to your brain').

Paula was 33 with two young sons and a husband who worked shifts, so when she was dying of carcinoma of ovary she was admitted to the hospice to try to keep the home 'normal' for the boys. She had a single room and the whole family moved in at weekends. She slept well when they were with her, but during the week she slept badly and got increasingly tired and cross.

One afternoon she asked her Macmillan nurse who was visiting, whether all the patients were discussed like this, because it was stopping her from taking naps. Exploring this strange comment we found that she could overhear voices in the patients' kitchen during the day. Although it was impossible to hear what was being said Paula misinterpreted the voices as a discussion about her illness, as the onset of renal failure made her muddled and unable to separate her own thoughts and fears about her illness from the voices she was hearing. When the family was with her, she was too busy listening to her boys to perceive the sound of voices in the kitchen.

She told us that the voices simply commented on her appearance and state of health. She has been a very attractive woman before her weight loss, and she grieved for her lost looks. Her Macmillan nurse collected her make up and some clothes from home. The ward nurses explained that although the voices were real, the words she heard came from inside Paula's head, and she was able to understand this. Once she knew she was not going mad, she decided to make friends with the voices. When she was dressed with her make up on the voices told her how nice she looked!

The message to the patient must be
- you are safe here;
- this is not your fault;
- you are not going mad.

Rationalise the underlying anxieties

Nightmares and misinterpretations are often clues to the fears in the patient's mind. If the carer can share the fear and help the patient to express it, often the fear can be reduced to more manageable proportions. During nightmares, the patient should be gently woken, re–orientated and the dream explored there and then.

Steve was a diver who worked for an oil company. He had a very rare cancer which progressed slowly and had initially responded to surgery and chemo-therapy. But now he had lung deposits and damage to his pelvic nerves. Having spent long periods working away from home, he was unsure how to talk to his 9- and 12-year-old sons about his disease. He became angry if his doctor tried to discuss the future, saying he had fought his cancer so far and he would not allow it to beat him now.

The doctor noticed that Steve's wife was looking increasingly tired. She told the doctor that Steve was shouting in his sleep and waking everybody up, but the next morning he could not remember any of this. The doctor asked her to wake Steve up next time it happened, and ask him about his dream.

When she did this Steve woke up terrified and gasping. He was dreaming about diving. In his dream he was on a very deep dive, repairing an oil pipe. Then he became aware of difficulty breathing and realised that his air supply was about to run out. He could not attract the attention of his diving buddy. He should not surface and leave the buddy alone, but he would suffocate if he did not surface. While he was deciding what to do his air ran out.

Bravely, his wife asked him why he might have this dream. He told her that he thought it was about dying, and that time was running out. He could not stay with her to bring up their children, and he felt guilty for leaving her.

The next day they told the children about how ill Steve was. Steve said he thought he might die, but that he would never stop loving them. They all cried together. The dream never came back, and Steve died peacefully at home 2 months later.

Find and treat the cause

The list in Table 8.2 shows some of the more common causes of delirium in cancer patients. In patients who are physically very ill unnecessary investigations may cause distress and it is important to assess the patient with care, decide on the most likely causes of confusion, and look for these quickly if they are treatable. If the cause is not treatable this must be explained very carefully to the family, and to the patient if possible, and care must be directed at managing the patient's distress.

Orientation to reality

Throughout the patient's confusion it should be assumed that he or she under-stands what is being said. It will be easier for the patient to be orientated in time if his or her daily schedule is regular, with meals at predictable times, few changes of faces (nursed by family and a few, familiar nurses if possible) and lots of other cues, for example wearing a watch, having today's newspaper near the bed. Remind patients where they are; ask them to try to remember where they are and how they came there. Keep the lights on. Remind them of the date, world news, family news. It is helpful to reinforce reality by asking questions which lead the patient to the correct conclusions, for example:

'What sort of place is this?'

'I'm not sure . . . Queer sort of place if you ask me . . .'.

'Do you see all those beds there? And all these people in pyjamas? So what sort of a place do you think this is?'

'It looks like a hospital to me.'

'Yes, you're right, it is a hospital. We are at the Royal Infirmary. Do you remember coming here?'

'I don't know who sent me here . . .'.

'You came with your son. What is your son's name?'

'Kevin.'

'Yes, Kevin brought you here. You had been staying at Kevin's house. Do you remember?'

'So this a hospital, eh? And Kevin knows I'm here? How long am I staying?'

'You are welcome to stay until you are stronger. You have been very ill and things got muddled in your mind. You are improving. You will be home soon.'

Above all, the confused person needs constant reassurance by calm, sympathetic and familiar people that he or she is safe, is sane and is understood.

Drug treatment for confused patients

Occasionally it becomes necessary to use drugs to manage patients with delirium. There are two particular reasons why drugs may be necessary.

- Uncontrollable terror, sometimes leading to dangerous behaviour.
- Unreachable distress caused by muddled thinking.

With terror or dangerous behaviour it may be necessary to sedate the patient. This means using a drug which is rapidly active and is unlikely to cause serious side-effects. The best drugs in this category are the benzodiazepines, which are sedative, but do not cause hypotension. Diazepam and midazolam are the drugs of choice. Many people use the phenothiazine chlorpromazine, but it can cause hypotension and this is turn can cause myocardial infarction or stroke in at-risk patients. Also, phenothiazines lower the epileptic threshold and so may increase tendency to fitting in patients who are more vulnerable to seizures because of their illness.

With predominantly jumbled thinking an antipsychotic drug is needed. This will help to re-build the divisions within consciousness which are broken down in confusion. The problem is that these drugs all cause some sedation, which increases the barrier through which the carer is trying to reach the patient. The least sedative antipsychotic drugs are the butyrophenones, and haloperidol is the drug of choice.

Occasionally the drug of first choice does not give the desired effect. If this happens, first check compliance; check that the prescribed drug was given at the right dose for the right number of times (see Table 8.3). If the drug of first choice is failing, there should be a drug 'in reserve'. Chlorpromazine, with all its side effects, is probably still the reserve drug of choice; it is sedative (indication 1) and antipsychotic (indication 2). Further details of the use of drugs are given in Table 8.3.

Use of drugs should be confined to the smallest effective dose for the shortest

Table 8.3 Drug treatment for patients with delirium

Problem	Aim	Drug	
		First choice	Second choice
(a) Fear due to muddled thoughts or hallucinations (b) Paranoid behaviour	Rationalise thoughts with minimal sedation, so that patient can discuss fears	Haloperidol 5–10 mg po/sc. Repeat hourly until settled or until 50 mg have been given.* **Watch for changes in muscle tone**	Chlorpromazine 20–25 mg po/im. Repeat hourly until settled. **Watch blood pressure**
(a) Irreversible terror or distress (b) Urgent behaviour control	Sedation	Diazepam 10 mg po/pr. Repeat hourly until settled, or until 60 mg have been given, then observe and only repeat if necessary. Or Midazolam 2.5–5 mg sc or **slowly** iv, repeat sc as necessary to maintain sedation† **Watch respiratory rate**	Chlorpromazine as above

*Maintenance dosage of haloperidol: add up the dose required in the first 24 h, and give this subsequently as a single daily dose. Reduce this daily dose as soon as possible by 5–10 mg daily, and continue to reduce every day until the drug is discontinued or the symptoms reappear.

†Maintenance dose of midazolam varies widely between patients, with an approximate daily dose range of 30–100 mg. This may be administered by syringe driver.

possible time. Where possible, treatment for the cause of delirium should be carried out at the same time. Drugs should be given with the patient's permission, and by mouth, although this is not always possible. If a patient is suspicious about medication it is important to have the drug ready, then negotiate and give the tablets/elixir as soon as the patient agrees to take it. By the time you have gone to the drug cupboard the patient may have forgotten or changed his or her mind.

The correct dose of the drug should be established by starting with small doses, assessing the response and repeating as necessary. If the oral route is not possible, diazepam works quickly by rectum (diazepam injection *per rectum* via 2 ml syringe can be used if no rectal solution or suppositories are available, but remember to take the needle off!) and both midazolam and haloperidol can be given by relatively pain-free subcutaneous injection.

Summary

Confusion is frightening for the patient and for their family. In previously lucid cancer patients it is usually due to an acute organic brain syndrome (delirium) and so a treatable physical cause must be sought.

It is usually possible to understand where the muddled thoughts are arising from, and to comfort the patient's fears even though their thoughts may remain confused.

The priorities for treatment are to stop the patient's fear, rationalise the underlying anxieties, find and treat the physical cause for the confusion and help to reorientate the patient to reality. This means enlisting the help of his or her family to maintain a calm, reassuring environment either at home or in hospital. The patient may need drug treatment, which should preferably be voluntary and by mouth.

Above all, it must always be assumed that a patient understands what is being said. The patient must be reassured that he or she is safe, is not insane, and that the people caring for him or her are trying to understand.

Confusion is often reversible, but even when it cannot be completely resolved it can be understood and made manageable.

Acknowledgements

Dr Andrew Brittlebank and Sister Jeanne Donaghy for their helpful criticisms and suggestions. Dr Averil Stedeford, for diagrams upon which the figures are based, and Heinemann Medical Books Ltd for permission to use these. Mrs Jennifer Trosky, for typing the manuscript.

References

ANDERSON, F. and WILLIAMS, B. (1989). *Practical Management of the Elderly*, pp. 231–4. Basil Blackwell, Oxford.

BREITBART, W. and PASSIK, S. D. (1993). Psychiatric aspects of palliative care: organic mental disorders in the terminally ill. In: DOYLE, D., HANKS, G. W. C. and MACDONALD, N. (eds), *The Oxford Textbook of Palliative Medicine*, pp. 618–21. Oxford University Press, Oxford.

INOUYE, S. K., VAN DYCK, C. H., ALESSI, C. A. *et al.* (1990). Clarifying confusion: the confusion assessment method – a new method for detection of delirium. *Annals of Internal Medicine* 113, 941–8.

INOUYE, S. K., VISCOLI, C. M., HOROWITZ, R. I. *et al.* (1993). A predictive model for delirium in hospitalised elderly medical patients based on admission characteristics. *Annals of Internal Medicine* 119, 474–81

LIPOWSKI, Z. J. (1992). Delirium and impaired consciousness. In: GRIMLEY EVANS, J. and FRANKLIN WILLIAMS, T. (eds), *The Oxford Textbook of Geriatric Medicine*, pp. 490–6. Oxford University Press, Oxford.

REGNARD, C. F. B. and TEMPEST, S. (1992). *A Guide to Symptom Relief in Advanced Cancer*, p. 46. Haigh & Hochland, Manchester.

STEDEFORD, A. (1984). *Facing Death. Patients, Families and Professionals*. Heinemann, Oxford.

STEDEFORD, A. and REGNARD, C. (1991). Confusional states in advanced cancer. *Palliative Medicine* 5, 256–61.

9

Issues of sexuality and intimacy in palliative care

Elizabeth Grigg

'Sexuality involves the totality or being a person and therefore nurses and patients are only given their full respect as people when nursing care has firm foundations in a truly holistic approach incorporating sexuality as a vital aspect of humanity.'

Webb (1985, p. 147)

Introduction

The concept of sexuality and sexual health has become one which over the past decade has taken on a greater emphasis for health–care workers. The advent of the human immunodeficiency virus (HIV) and acquired immune deficiency syndrome (AIDS) has placed sexuality and sexual health–care onto the professional agenda (Faugier, 1993). HIV and AIDS has highlighted the ignorance and prejudice of many care givers and the serious deficiencies in their ability to meet the psycho-social and sexuality needs of their patients. The sexualities of patients, whatever their condition, are almost always overlooked.

According to Gilley (1988) attention to sexuality concerns is singularly lacking in relation to palliative care, a time when people often long for intimate closeness with loved ones. As Webb (1987, p. 75) argues 'communication and love between different people depends upon the integration or somatic, emotional, intellectual and social components comprising the sexuality of each individual'. She continues that 'human beings are sexual in every way all the time; human sexuality is an integral factor in the uniqueness of every person' (Stuart and Sundeen, 1979 cited in Webb, 1987, p. 75). People remain sexual beings until they die.

If nurses are knowledgeable about sexuality in its totality and have learned to accept their own and other people's feelings and beliefs about sexuality, they will be more comfortable in dealing both with professional situations having sexual connotations, such as washing patients of the opposite sex, and with broader issues of sexuality like working with abortion patients (Webb, 1985). According to Webb these nurses will also be able to integrate the concept of sexuality into nursing care. In the process of assessing, planning, implementing and evaluating care, they will be perceptive to signs which draw attention to people's concerns in relation to sexuality and to use nursing judgements about the kind of approaches needed.

Nursing has its own techniques and skills, which are evident in its area of expertise – the sensitivity that most nurses show to the experiences of their patients. Lawler (1991) suggests that this is the 'how' things are done not the 'what' things are done. This makes nursing more of a social entity than merely a science or an art or a mixture of both. Expert nursing practice results not only from knowledge but from the experiences of the social world of nursing.

An historical and societal perspective of sexuality

Henslin and Sagarin (1971), Pocs (1989) and Sardi (1992), state that people of a variety of different civilisations in different historical periods have engaged in a variety of different modes of sexual expression and behaviour. Despite this cultural and historical diversity one important principle should be kept in mind: sexual awareness, attitudes and behaviours are learned within sociocultural contexts that define appropriate sexuality for society's members.

For several centuries, western civilisation has been characterised by an anti-sex ethic, which has normatively limited sexual behaviour to the confines of monogamous pair bonds for the sole purpose of procreation (Pocs, 1989). Changes in the social environment such as the *'liberation of women from the home'* (Pocs, 1989, p. 4), are strengthening the concept of people as sexual beings and posing a challenge to the 'anti-sex ethic' that has traditionally served to orient sexuality.

Western society is now witnessing a gradual convalescence from a disease which Brecher (1988 cited in 'Sardi', 1988) called 'Victorianism', which reinforced the 'moral teachings' of Christianity and was characterised by the belief that all sexualities were wicked, loathsome and would lead to disaster. Sexual repression, on the other hand, would lead people into being frugal and hard working.

In pre-Christian times sexuality was open and accepted as being part of the normal expression of cultures. For example, according to 'Sardi' (1992), G. Rattray Taylor's work *Sex in History*, showed that nudity, in pre-Christian Ireland, was no cause for shame.

By contrast women in Victorian England covered their bodies from neck to below ankle with layers of clothes and according to 'Sardi' (1992) Richard Lewinsohn's research *A History of Sexual Customs*, indicated that their bodies were neither seen nor spoken about. In fact women were often so prude that they would not let themselves be examined by physicians, but indicated on dummies especially set up for the purpose, the spots where they felt pain.

Social change is not easily accomplished. Sociologists generally acknowledge that changes in the social environment are accompanied by the presence of interest groups that offer competing versions of what 'is' or 'should be' appropriate social behaviour (Denisoff and Wahrman, 1979). The contemporary sociocultural changes surrounding sexuality are highly illustrative of such social dynamics (Henslin and Sagarin, 1978).

There are tensions and conflicts arising in the nursing profession as to the definitions, and what 'is' or 'should be' a social policy regarding sexuality 'care' for clients and patients. Literature regarding sexuality in both nursing and wider society remain conflicting and conservative. Moreover, articles on sexuality attitudes within nursing remain scarce compared to articles on, for example, attitudes towards HIV and AIDS.

I have cited some of the articles relating to HIV and AIDS because of the dearth of articles on sexuality in contexts other than in HIV and AIDS. Issues of sexuality and intimacy in palliative care are the same for all people whatever their diagnosis. Many people who are diagnosed with HIV die of an AIDS-related cancer. It is not just because of HIV and AIDS that nurses need to address their attitudes towards sexuality. An holistic approach to nursing care should include all aspects of the person and sexuality is one of these aspects.

Research over the past two decades has led to the conclusion that nurses do not have the necessary theoretical knowledge to be able to teach, counsel or otherwise care for their patients in this area. Nor are they sufficiently aware of and comfortable with their own sexuality to be able to act non-judgementally. Webb (1987) suggests that nurses' rigid and conservative attitudes are likely to influence Both the quality and quantity of their relationships with patients and amongst themselves.

However, given the nature of sexuality and sexual behaviour in western culture, it is not surprising that by far the most problematic areas of nursing are those associated with sexuality (Lawler, 1991). Sexuality comes with a great deal of cultural 'baggage' so that when nurses are confronted with patients, cultural meanings which attend being either a nurse or a patient and the context of care all require management. Much of that management concerns meanings attached to:

> 'The *definition* that patients and nurses place upon the relationship between the physical body and sexual expression' (Lawler, 1991, p. 85).

The definition of sexuality

It is important to expand upon a definition of sexuality because it enhances an understanding of the relevance of sexuality to nursing, both to nurses themselves and to the care that they give to their patients and clients.

Webb (1987, p. 75) states that the term sexuality 'can mean as many different things to as many different people, and a single understanding cannot be reached.' She argues that not only does it reflect the norms and beliefs of a society it also reflects a person's individuality. Gilley (1988) describes sexuality as 'the capacity of the individual to link emotional needs with physical intimacy.'

Similarly Rosemary Hogan defines sexuality in her book *Human Sexuality: A Nursing Perspective* as:

> '. . . considering that sexuality is more than the sex act, it is all that we are as men and women, it encompasses the most intimate feelings and deepest longings of the heart to find meaningful relationships' (Hogan, 1980, cited in Webb, 1985, p. 3).

Lion (1982, cited in Webb, 1985, p. 3) expands upon this definition and explains sexuality as:

> '. . . being much more than the biological side of sex acts, it is the all encompassing emotional aspects of human relationships. It involves the totality of being human and includes all those aspects of the human being that relate to being boy or girl, man or woman, and is an entity subject to lifelong dynamic change. Sexuality reflects a person's character as well as their genital nature.'

According to Webb (1987) this perspective emphasises the changing nature and expression of sexuality throughout the life cycle.

Sexuality has been historically conceptualised as a biological construct in which social processes play a secondary part. Nurses need to understand the definition of sexuality in its totality if they are to provide holistic care (Lawler, 1991). Sexual behaviour and sexual health-care were never mentioned in nurse training. When they began to appear on the curriculum, what was taught was restricted to anatomy, physiology and altered body function, biological aspects only. Although this information is obviously important and necessary, so to is the opportunity to explore personal feelings and attitudes, and their relevance to providing care for others. Thomas (1989) contends that even now, despite some literature on the subject of sexuality, the 'real' matter of sexuality is not even mentioned in nurse training. The rich social meanings which accompany sexuality are ignored.

Sexuality and nursing care

Thomas (1989, p. 49) claims that despite the number of definitions of sexuality which 'encompass the totality of being', it still remains misunderstood as a solely biological sex act, which makes it difficult, not only for nurses to consider their patients' sexual needs, but to actually help them express these needs.

According to Lawler's (1991) research the complex 'social construction or the sexualised body' (p. 113) make it impossible for some nurses to even mention body parts, especially those in the genital area.

Savage (1989), Salvage (1990) and Lawler (1991) propose that one reason many nurses have difficulty is because sexuality has shaped the structure of nursing itself. Society dictates that men and women behave differently and nowhere has the gender role been acted out more faithfully than in nursing.

Male and female nurses are stereotyped, men because they cross their gender role and women because they do not! Because they have taken on a role of person-ifying womanhood, female nurses are most commonly portrayed as 'golden-hearted sex objects' (Savage, 1989, p. 26), while male nurses are emasculated by taking on work involving caring and gentleness – supposedly women's qualities only!

Webb (1985), Savage (1989), Salvage (1990) and Lawler (1991) suggest that sexual stereotyping, which has been reinforced by the media's portrayal of female nurses as 'pornographic sex-symbols' (Salvage, 1990, pp. 22–3), helps shape the relationship that nurses have with their patients. They stress that sexuality is integral to the nurse–patient relationship because of the very nature of nursing and the physical and emotional intimacy it involves. However, the nurse has to make it clear that these acts are non-sexual. How nurses cope depends on their attitudes towards their own sexuality, and the knowledge they have about what sexuality really is.

According to research by Waterhouse and Metcalfe (1991) the majority of patients wish nurses to initiate addressing the issues of sexuality with them. It may be that the influence of medical treatment is directly affecting their biological sexual functioning, or that they have a poor self-concept because of the perception of a changed body image due to illness, and no longer feel sexual or attractive. Whatever the concerns may be they should be identified and discussed. Bor and Watts (1993) argue that some patients are willing to answer the most intimate questions about their sexual behaviour as long as they are not judged or ridiculed.

This ignoring of the sexual side of patients may be attributed to nurses being too embarrassed to address these needs but it could also be because nurses fail to recognise or acknowledge that they exist. This lack of communication about sexuality matters ends up in a conspiracy of silence (Savage, 1989) and nurses use evasive tactics when dealing with sexuality matters (Lawler, 1991).

Currently nurse training does not even address the fact that nurses may feel discomfort when they provide care. For example, Thompson (1990) refers to the need for privacy for adolescent patients on oncology units in order for them to develop their sexual and social relationships. Savage (1990a) argues that nurses feel uneasy about allowing their patients privacy. She continues that it would be simple for nurses to create partial privacy by just pulling the curtains around the bed allowing even the seriously ill physical closeness with partners or friends, but many nurses are reluctant to do this. According to Savage the suggestion of private rooms being provided for patients if they need sexual intimacy causes more unease amongst nurses than the use of screens!

Thompson (1990) believes that the quality of sexual health-care young cancer patients receive is determined by the interest, attitudes and skills of those health professionals who have educated themselves.

Savage (1990b) asserts that if sexuality is to be more centrally incorporated into nursing care, the support available for nurses must be improved.

Sexuality education for nurses

Bell (1989) refers to the three objectives in educating nurses in sexual health, these are: attitudes, knowledge and skills – all of which involve an examination of the sexual self, an awareness of ones own sexuality and an awareness of the possible diversity of other people's sexuality. This, she argues, will create tolerance and acceptance, and enhance attitudes. She presupposes that a knowledge of sexual issues, such as the effects of illness on body image, the consequences of ethnic and religious beliefs relating to sexuality, as well as a knowledge of sexual functioning, response and anatomy, will create a more positive attitude. This should help nurses become more comfortable and competent when interacting with their patients.

Bell (1989), Thomas (1989) and Savage (1990a) stress that skills both in verbal and non-verbal communication are vital in facilitating interaction between the patient and nurse in the area of sexuality.

> 'Nurses need support and encouragement to cope with the presence of sexuality in their work and to incorporate sexual health-care into their nursing practice. But at the same time the difficult nature of sexuality has to be acknowledged and the expectations we have of nurses must be realistic' (Savage, 1989, p. 28).

Sexuality and palliative care for people with cancer

As Bor and Watts (1993, p. 657) argue:

> 'Conversations about death, dying, relationships and sexual matters are among the most challenging and difficult that nurses and other health care providers have with their patients. Cultural taboos, the fear of upsetting patients and underdeveloped counselling and interpersonal skills may present obstacles to more open and effective communication.'

However, as stated above, the majority of patients wish nurses to initiate addressing the issues of sexuality with them and some patients are willing to answer the most intimate questions about their sexual behaviour as long as they are not judged or ridiculed.

The key elements of sexual health as defined by the World Health Organization

(WHO) are relevant and helpful as they recognise that sexuality is related to sexual activity in health, disability or illness. They are:

'1. A capacity to enjoy and control sexual and reproductive behaviour with a social and personal ethic.
2. Freedom from fear, shame, guilt, false beliefs and other psychological factors inhibiting sexual relationships.
3. Freedom from organic disorders, diseases and deficiencies that interfere with sexual and reproductive functions' (Weller, 1993, p. 1).

Chronic disease and disabling illness can have serious effects upon a person's sexuality, sexual expression and identity and upon their sexual health. It may be because of agents influencing physiological functioning or due to the consequences or psychological or social factors. Whatever the reason the nurse's ability to be aware or the concerns a patient or their loved ones may have can have a profound impact on the quality or care given.

Thompson (1990) looks at issues such as body image and self-concept in relation to adolescents with cancer. She discusses the potential effects or cancer treatment that may influence sexual adequacy in adolescents. She argues that adolescents are more sensitive about their bodies than adults:

'Any deformity or imperfection, obvious or hidden, can be so unacceptable to the adolescent that disgust and shame result. Acceptance of personal sexuality also presents problems' (Thompson, 1990, p. 27).

However, I have found that adults can be as sensitive about their bodies as younger people. As 62-year-old Mackenzie stated during her illness:

'Not being able to rely on my own body made me feel sexually insecure, and I withdrew from my relationship because of this . . . I'm really worried that men will stop looking at me now. I'm scared that I've suddenly got no sex appeal I don't feel any less sexy, but it worries me that people will start treating me as though I am sexless' (Mackenzie, 1984, p. 67).

Thompson (1990) provides a useful table, which is reproduced here as Table 9.1, of the potential effects or cancer treatment upon adolescents, which may be injurious to their sexuality and to their sexual expression and identity. A similar table could be applied to people or every age.

Table 9.1 Potential effects of cancer treatment that may influence sexual adequacy in adolescents

Surgery	Radiotherapy	Chemotherapy
Testicular biopsy – fear of mutilation	Testicular radiotherapy – skin changes – sterility	Hair loss Sterility Weight gain/loss
All surgery – residual scarring	Spinal radiotherapy may result	Skin changes Nausea Vomiting
Amputation or affected affected limb/body part – leads to poor body-image	in asymmetry	Use of steroids Facial hair Vaginitis

The person with advanced cancer has probably gone through the traumas or one or many or the listed consequences or treatment. The processes or advanced cancer will result in further significant physiological changes to the body which may have a profound effect upon sexual image and upon sexual feelings. Further changed body shape due to weight loss, or weight gain caused by oedema, can cause deep depression for some people. It is vital that nurses are sensitive to this and are able to provide the appropriate care. If changed body shape is concerning the patient all that may be necessary is the provision or clothes that feel as though they fit. New clothes can increase a person's self worth and help them feel that they are still valued by loved ones.

The body and sexuality are intimately interrelated (Lawler, 1991). According to Lawler's research nurses who have the least difficulty in addressing total body care are those with a relaxed and open attitude towards the body and touching. The British are culturally 'non-touching' and some nurses have to overcome their own sociocultural backgrounds and adjust to a particular professional subculture and its established methods that permits handling other people's bodies. Lawler continues that:

> 'They must also confront the symbolism of certain parts of the body, in particular, parts which have sexual significance, and they must find ways to manage social interaction during those times when they break taken-for-granted rules about the body' (Lawler, 1991, p. 117).

I remember one beautiful elderly lady of about 70 years who was admitted for terminal care. During her dying she struggled to bath every day, to apply make up, perfume and powder and insisted that she had her hair 'done' once a week. She seemed very peaceful when she felt that she looked beautiful. The nurses were aware of her needs and when she could no longer continue with this care herself the nurses were comfortable about doing it for her. It was an important part or her total care. She was happy when her hair was washed and when she was wearing make up and when she knew that she smelt nice. She needed this gentle touching and pampering or her body. She needed to be able to express her sexuality. Towards the end or her illness all she needed was help to do so. It seemed to matter to her as much as being without pain.

According to Lawler (1991) female nurses have more difficulty addressing the sexuality of male patients than vice versa. However it is just as important for men to feel pampered and loved and therefore nurses must be able to:

> 'Negotiate not only normal social boundaries when they touch patients, but, because the body is heavily inscribed with meaning – much of it sexual – nurses' work is socially fragile, and they must learn ways to make their work manageable' (Lawler, 1991, p. 113).

How they cope depends upon, not only expert nursing practice resulting from knowledge and empathy, but from the experiences or the social world or nursing.

According to Lawler there is a point in the male patient's illness when sensuality is not an issue that is considered by female nurses. If a patient is very ill, experiences of a sexual nature are overtaken by the seriousness of the patient's condition. It appears easier for nurses to manage body care for men when they are dying because the care that they give cannot be perceived as sexual.

However, some men do not want care from females. I have known many homosexual men who have requested intimate care only be given to them by male nurses. It may be because they fear they are being judged or ridiculed by heterosexuals because of their sexual orientation. As Hancock states:

'Anything which has sexual overtones stimulates an unholy trinity of inhibition, hypocrisy and prejudice, all of which can and do have a detrimental effect on and care . . . this combined with ignorance produces a seemingly impenetrable barrier' (Hancock, 1991, p. 50).

It is possible that this is what some nurses subscribe to. For example, in 1991 Dennis was requested to run some compulsory HIV/AIDS awareness sessions for all or the staff within his particular health authority. Staff had to attend whether they 'wanted to or not' (Dennis, 1991, p. 55) Nurses formed the largest single occupational group. His observations drew attention to some participants, including nurses, being overtly prejudiced to HIV and AIDS patients because they were perceived as being 'different' or 'not like us' and 'they shouldn't do such things', that is 'take drugs' or 'have relationships with partners of the same sex' (Dennis, 1991, p. 55). Dennis' courses did nothing to change the negative attitudes or some or the participants. These negative attitudes have worrying implications for good patient care.

Sim (1992) does not agree with the toleration or any negative attitudes in nurses, whether it be towards homophobia, drug abuse or risks associated with caring for HIV- or AIDS-infected people. He quotes from a document published by the Royal College of Nursing (RCN):

'Discrimination against particular individuals for whatever reason, should never be tolerated . . . the adoption or a professional attitude requires that all those who need nursing care should receive it without discrimination' (RCN, 1976, cited in Sim, 1992, p. 571).

I worked for a year as a nurse tutor on a palliative care ward for AIDS patients, many or whom were diagnosed with cancer. The atmosphere on the ward was warm and loving. I remember that there were red hearts hanging over some of the beds. There were flowers and plants everywhere. The nurses, mostly male, were very tactile with their patients and with one another. The patients, also mostly male, seemed content. Most or them had partners or loved ones with them for most or the time; sitting on their beds or leaning on their beds, holding hands or stroking each other. Sometimes the curtains were drawn around a bed. If curtains were closed the nurses would never assume access and always asked before going in. Savage (1990a) suggests that once patients have rights over personal space nurses do hesitate and think twice before disturbing someone who has sought seclusion. There was also a bedroom available with a double bed for patients who wished to sleep with their partners.

The care given to the patients, by both the nurses and by the partners, was conducted almost with a reverence. Death seemed to be accepted as a natural progression. Some patients requested some sort or celebration after the event and parties were often held on the ward for staff, friends, other patients and their loved ones. These parties were an expression or the intimacy between everybody involved in the care of people with AIDS in this loving environment.

The nurses cared as much for the loved ones or the patients as they did for the patients. Partners and relatives were encouraged to provide intimate care – if that was what they wanted. I believe it helped the partners and relatives to feel as though they were 'doing something' during a time when there is a strong belief that when someone is dying 'there is nothing else anyone can do'. Lawler (1991) describes the time when someone is dying as a time when they are totally dependent on others for body care. However nurses suggest that they are 'doing nothing' for the patient during this time. Yet as Lawler argues this is possibly the most difficult time for carers in terms or emotional and practical implications.

However, some patients do not wish to be dependent upon partners or relatives for intimate care. For whatever reason they may feel uncomfortable with body care being provided by those closest to them. Nurses need to be responsive to this also.

There was a male patient I knew who wished to be perceived by his wife as being strong and totally independent, even though his illness gradually made him totally dependent upon the care of others. He was nursed at home and initially the district nurses carried out all his care. When he deteriorated and needed almost constant care his wife began to intervene. This caused him great distress and he requested hospitalisation. He eventually died peacefully in hospital. I believe he wished his wife to remember him as an independent figure who was strong enough not to rely upon her for the sort or care a mother gives to a child. He once said to me: 'I want her [his wife] to remember me as a man not as a baby'. He never spoke to her about the care he was receiving and even during the time she stayed at the hospital, when he was dying, she always left his bedside while the nurses provided intimate care. She appeared to love him so much that even though he was probably unaware of her presence, at times, she understood and accepted why he would not have wished her to witness his vulnerability. She was never made to feel guilty by the other carers for not joining in with his care.

Gilley (1988) provides an example or intimacy that is in complete contrast to the one cited above.

> 'There was a couple in their seventies . . . Mrs E became very ill with metastic carcinoma. Mr E nursed her supported by the district nursing team. . . . There was an intimacy in the flat, the curtains were usually closed even by day, the warm lights on in the bedroom, the nursing dressings and paraphernalia kept hidden.
> The outside world seemed far away. Help was accepted from doctors and nurses who were then dispatched kindly on their way, but the real business continued within those four walls.
> I was called in the early hours one cold night. She was near to dying and had been incontinent in their shared bed. Exhausted, he asked me to help change the sheets. As we sorted linen, I shared with him the likelihood that she would die during the night. He knew. 'We've slept together for 50 years. I want one last night with her'. Together we made up the bed with fresh sheets. It was impossible not to think of a bridal bed being prepared. I helped him clean and tidy her. She died in the night' (Gilley, 1988, p. 122).

Kitzinger (1983) describes the sexual relationship or a couple after the woman has had a hysterectomy for cancer. She believes that often the man will start to think more about lovemaking from the woman's perspective and a more sensitive understanding or her needs evolves:

> 'Appalled by the idea that she has had surgery, he slows down, gives more body stimulation and is more gentle.'

Some couples need this type or intimacy even though the partner is very ill. Continuing to have intercourse is a symbol or youth and it may be important for them to have orgasm with intercourse in order to prove to themselves and their partners that they are still sexual beings. When intercourse becomes too difficult to manage couples can still pleasure each other by touching and caressing. Nurses may have to reassure patients that sexual intimacy can be expressed by touching.

Some hospices provide rooms with double beds so that people can have the freedom to lie together for comfort. Some people want to die in their partner's arms. Others wish for isolation. Nurses and care givers must be aware or and respect the diversity or intimate expression. They should accept, empathise and respond to all peoples' differing sexual needs during a time when total care is of paramount importance.

> 'In the same way that a good sexual relationship is the private pleasure of a couple, so must the relationship in terminal care be respected as unique to that couple and part of their intimacy' (Gilley, 1988, p. 122).

Conclusion and discussion

Sexuality, disease, loss and death are some or the most vulnerable aspects or our lives, they often arouse strong feelings and challenge deeply held values.

Nurses, as part or society, reflect the same tolerance (or intolerance) to things that have 'sexual' connotations that others in society do.

If nurses are provided with knowledge about sexuality and are facilitated in becoming more comfortable with their own sexuality and accepting or other people's feelings and beliefs about sexuality, they will be more likely to implement sexuality care to their patients (Bell, 1989; Thomas, 1989; Savage, 1990a, b). However, knowledge alone is not sufficient to enhance nursing care and lower apprehensions about unresolved sexual anxieties (Dennis, 1991; Robbins, 1992) – 'sexuality' care needs support in implementation.

> 'Expert nursing practice results not only from knowledge and empathy but from the experiences of the social world of nursing.'

It is the responsibility or nurse educators to assist learners with holistic and humanistic practice. By providing a safe learning environment, educators specialising in sexuality education should be able to facilitate learners in developing the skills and solutions they will need in implementing sexuality care for patients. In the clinical setting it should be the responsibility or peers and/or supervisors to offer further support. Changes that have taken place in the classroom can be reinforced by observing practice. This reinforcement does not always take place, however, and therefore what is learned in the classroom is not always backed up by observation at the bedside (Birchenall, 1991)

As stated by the Department of Health and the English National Board (1993), the outcomes or sexuality education will only be adequate if all professionals (clinical and educational) have access to it.

Clinical specialists must be comfortable with sexuality issues so that they are able to act as role models for learners, but the learner also has to be equipped to critically examine and reflect upon his/her practice. Sexuality is continual therefore sexuality education should be an on-going process.

Webb (1987) argues that the biological, psychological, social, philosophical and social policy aspects or sexuality in its widest definition need to form part or the curriculum for all nurses, together with work on communication skills including assessment, teaching and counselling skills.

Webb's study places a responsibility on specialist nurse educators to prepare nurses or the future to meet the full range or their professional obligations. Sexuality is one area in which nurse educators must pay full attention as part or the process or accountability for the quality or care which nurses give and which patients receive.

References

BELL, N. (1989). Promoting fulfilment. *Nursing Times* 85, 35–7.

BIRCHENALL, P. D. (1991). Preparing nurse teachers for their future role. *Nurse Education Today* 11, 100–3.

BOR, R. and WATTS, M. (1993). Talking to patients about sexual matters. *British Journal of Nursing* 2, 657–60.

DENNIS, H. (1991) Getting the message. *Nursing Standard* 5, 55–6.

DENNISOFF, R. S. and WAHRMAM, R. (1979). *An Introduction to Sociology.* Macmillan, New York.

FAUGIER, J. (1993). Sexual health education: breaking down the barriers. *A Report of the National Conference for Health and Social Care Professionals.* English National Board and Department of Health.

GILLEY, J. (1988). Intimacy and terminal care. *Journal of the Royal College of General Practitioners* 38, 121–2.

GLOVER, J. (1985). *Human Sexuality in Nursing Care.* Croom Helm.

HANCOCK, C. (1991). The challenge for nurses. *Nursing Standard* 5, No. 17.

HENSLIN, J. M. and SAGARIN, E. (1978). *The Sociology of Sex.* Schocken Books.

KITZINGER, S. (1983). *Women's Experience of Sex.* Penguin.

LAWLER, J. (1991). *Behind The Screens.* Churchill Livingstone.

MACKENZIE, R. (1984). *Menopause.* Reed Books.

POCS, O. (ed.) (1989). *Human Sexuality 88/89.* Illinois State University, IL.

ROBBINS, I. COOPER, A. and BENDER, M. P. (1992). The relationship between knowledge, attitudes and degree of contact with AIDS and HIV. *Journal of Advanced Nursing* 17, 198–203.

SALVAGE, J. (1990). *The Politics of Nursing.* Butterworth–Heinemann.

'SARDI' (1992). *Erotic Love.* Dorset Press.

SAVAGE, J. (1987). *Nurses, Gender and Sexuality.* Heinemann Nursing.

SAVAGE, J. (1989). An uninvited guest. *Nursing Times* 85, 25–8.

SAVAGE, J. (1990a). Sexuality, privacy and nursing care. *Nursing Standard* 4, 37–9.

SAVAGE, J. (1990b). Sexuality and nursing care: setting the scene. *Nursing Standard* 4, 24–5.

SIM, J. (1992). AIDS, nursing and occupational risk: an ethical analysis. *Journal of Advanced Nursing* 17, 569–75.

THOMAS, B. (1989). Asexual patients. *Nursing Times* 86, 49–51.

THOMAS, B. (1990). The human side. *Nursing Times* 86, 28–30.

THOMPSON, J. (1990). Sexuality: the adolescent and cancer. *Nursing Standard* 4, 26–49.

WATERHOUSE, J. and METCALFE, M. (1991). Attitudes toward nurses discussing sexual concerns with patients. *Journal of Advanced Nursing* 16, 1048–54.
WEBB, C. (1985). *Sexuality, Nursing and Health.* John Wiley, Chichester.
WEBB, C. (1987). Nurses' knowledge and attitudes about sexuality in health care – a review of the literature. *Nurse Education Today* 7, 75–87.
WELLER, B. F. (1993). Education for sexual health and sexuality. *Report of York and Guildford Workshops.* November/December 1992. Department of Health and English National Board.

Suggested further reading

BELL, N. (1989). Promoting fulfilment. *Nursing Times* 85, 35–7.
GILLEY, J. (1988). Intimacy and terminal care. *Journal of the Royal College of General Practitioners* 38, 121–2.
GLOVER, J. (1985). *Human Sexuality in Nursing Care.* Croom Helm.
LAWLER, J. (1991). *Behind The Screens.* Churchill Livingstone.
SALVAGE, J. (1990). *The Politics of Nursing.* Butterworth–Heinemann.
'SARDI' (1992). *Erotic Love.* Dorset Press.
SAVAGE, J. (1987). *Nurses, Gender and Sexuality.* Heinemann Nursing.
SAVAGE, J. (1989). An uninvited guest. *Nursing Times* 85, 25–8.
SAVAGE, J. (1990a). Sexuality and nursing care: setting the scene. *Nursing Standard* 4, 24–5.
SAVAGE, J. (1990b). Sexuality, privacy and nursing care. *Nursing Standard* 4, 37–9.
THOMAS, B. (1989). Asexual patients. *Nursing Times* 86, 49–51.
THOMAS, B. (1990). The human side. *Nursing Times* 86, 28–30.
THOMPSON, J. (1990). Sexuality: the adolescent and cancer. *Nursing Standard* 4, 26–49.
WATERHOUSE, J. and METCALFE, M. (1991). Attitudes toward nurses discussing sexual concerns with patients. *Journal of Advanced Nursing* 16, 1048–54.
WEBB, C. (1985). *Sexuality, Nursing and Health.* John Wiley, Chichester.
WEBB, C. (1987). Nurses' knowledge and attitudes about sexuality in health care – a review of the literature. *Nurse Education Today* 7, 75–87.
WELLER, B. F. (1993). Education for sexual health and sexuality. *Report of York and Guildford Workshops.* November/December 1992. Department of Health and English National Board.

10
Day care

Pearl McDaid

'Cogito ergo sum' – I think, therefore I am.

René Descartes (1596–1650)

This statement by Descartes, the French mathematician and philosopher, may be a question that does not require an answer. However, Maslow (1954, 1971), Rogers (1951, 1983), and other humanistic behavioural theorists, suggest that humans seeks reassurance from others in order to be content and secure within themselves.

Since time began, humans have sought the company of others to relieve isolation, to seek peer group support and companionship, to compete, and to enable self-assessment.

Day care centres, in a variety of settings, have evolved over the past five decades in order to provide a forum for identified client groups with unmet social needs. In such centres, therapeutic services are specifically designed to fulfil the requirements of these groups.

Fifty years ago, services for cancer patients were primitive by comparison with those of today. The diagnosis of cancer was often established during an exploratory surgical procedure, when the disease would be found to be widespread and incurable. The use of radiotherapy was limited. Many patients did not survive the post-operative period, and they succumbed with untreatable infections, unrelieved pain and were heavily sedated.

In these more enlightened times, health education and early diagnosis of cancer are the norm, treatment options readily available, and research within the speciality has revolutionised the management and treatment of malignant disease. Many patients are diagnosed and treated whilst continuing to live at home, and are supported by their general practitioner (GP), as well as the hospital specialist. When cure is not an option, referral may be made to hospice or palliative services for support, advice and treatment.

Hospice/palliative day care was piloted during the mid-1970s and is now established as an important component of care for those people suffering from malignant, life-threatening illnesses. There are at present over 200 day care centres listed in the *1994 Directory of Hospice Services in the UK and Republic of Ireland*, compiled by the Hospice Information Service at St Christopher's Hospice, London.

Hospice/palliative day care is complementary to all other cancer services and provides support and surveillance for the patients and their families which could not otherwise be achieved either in hospital or in the community. The primary aims, therefore, are to assist in the enhancement of the quality of life for these people by means of liaison and effective communication with all concerned.

Why day care?

For most patients and their families, the diagnosis and treatment of malignant disease is a major intrusion into their lives. Many malignant diseases are chronic, and although the patients are better informed, and support is available to discuss and explain the aims of treatments, and treatment options, the future remains uncertain for many people.

Some of these uncertainties may be addressed by Macmillan/hospice home care nurses, or other professionals, thus enabling patients and their families to make realistic short and longer term plans. It is for those patients who are not actively dying but those ability to fulfil their usual roles is compromised, both within their families and society, that referral to day care is indicated.

Referral to day care

Referrals to day care are, inevitably, influenced by the locality and the existing services available, plus the needs and expectations of patients and families. By virtue of the wide diversity of needs of this group of people, a comprehensive range of services must be provided.

For many patients, referral is made to day care to provide peer group support, and mutual respite for patients and carers. Patients often feel isolated within their disease, with feelings of sadness and inability to cope due to lack of confidence. Many feel burdened by the responsibility of illness, and the impact that it has on their families. They describe themselves as being 'in limbo', as not being well enough, or confident enough to continue life as before. They are fearful and unsure of the future for themselves and their families. Support from a peer group may promote confidence and reassurance, and practical tips from other patients may be more welcome than advice from a professional carer.

Increasingly, patients are being referred for clinical surveillance of disease progression and symptom control, especially where there is a medical practitioner in palliative care on site or accessible. While the clinical responsibility for the patient's care remains with the community professional carers, specialist advice can be offered from day care.

Some patients may be referred to day care following discharge from in-patient units, and, in addition to the benefit derived from day care activities, the need to attend busy out-patient departments will be obviated.

From referral to acceptance

Day centres, generally, will meet the needs of the communities which they serve, and the criteria for acceptance of a newly referred patient being dependent on local policy. Where the demand for day care provision is high, the decision to accept a referral will be more discerning, with clear aims and objectives stated and understood by all concerned. Not all patients with malignant diseases need or want day care. Many people, particularly those who have multiple chronic medical conditions, and an incidental malignancy, may not meet some day centres' criteria for acceptance.

Most day centres require some kind of written referral which includes:

- the patient's name, address and telephone number,
- the patient's date of birth, and religion or belief,
- the name, address, and telephone number of the main carer, or next of kin,
- the name, address and telephone number of their GP,
- the name of their hospital consultant(s),
- brief details of diagnosis, treatments, current medication, prognosis,
- brief statement of the reason for referral, including the patient's knowledge or otherwise of the referral,
- statement of whether the GP is aware of referral (if the referral is not made by GP),
- any other relevant comment.

Assessment

An assessment of need for patients and families is usually necessary prior to the patient being accepted for day care. The assessment, again, will be determined by local policy and may be conducted in the patient's home or at the day centre. The professional making the assessment could be a member of the day centre staff or one of the extended team, e.g. a Macmillan nurse, but it is vitally important that the assessment is realistic and compatible with the services available. (For example, it would be pointless to set goals for physical rehabilitation where no physiotherapy is available.) However, once a patient has been accepted for day care, the importance of a visit to the day centre, prior to commencement of regular attendance, cannot be overestimated. This enables the patient and the carer to meet the team and other patients, and to allay any anxieties associated with the new and unknown.

It has been said that good hospice care is dependent on:

1. The creation of a caring environment.
2. The provision of time to talk.
3. Good symptom control.

Time set aside for assessment has shown to be worthwhile, as it allows the patient and family carer(s) the opportunity to reflect on their feelings, and voice their anxieties. It also provides an opportunity for the assessor to clarify facts, address fears and anxieties, and enable the patient and family to be better informed about the present status, if appropriate.

The interviewer needs to assess the physical condition of the patient, including the effectiveness of the current medication for symptom control, and establish whether he or she is well enough for day care. The patient should be able to travel comfortably, and be able to tolerate being away from home for up to 6 hours.

The interviewer may negotiate with the patient how day care can help with practical needs, especially those needs which are difficult to meet in the patient's home. Assessment will probably include seeking information regarding the amount and type of care and support that is being provided at home, and if the patient and family feel that it is adequate.

To complete the assessment, the interviewer will discuss the aims and objectives of attendance at day care with the patient, and identify expected outcomes. In cases where objectives are specific and short-term, and where the likelihood of achievement of those is high, the possibility of discharge from day care must be anticipated. 'Discharge planning should start on or before admission' (NHS Executive SSI, April, 1994).

Having met the criteria for acceptance for day care, attendance is dependent on the patient's willingness to do so. Some patients initially show reluctance, which may be a measure of their lack of confidence. Some people are naturally reticent and dislike being in company, therefore day care may not appeal to them. The patient makes the choice.

The interview is completed with the practicalities of attendance to day care being organised. A written report is usually made and notification of the assessment and its outcome sent to the referrer and other relevant personnel.

Day care centres

Day care in the British Isles is provided in a variety of settings. Some day centres are purpose-built, while others are converted, specially adapted houses. The majority of day centres are linked to hospice services or specialist teams. Some are funded and managed by the National Health Service, while others are independently managed by a board of trustees or council of management, and funded from charitable sources.

Day care operates on weekdays, accommodating between eight and 25 patients per day. Most patients attend on one or two days per week. Day centres vary in size, and in the number of rooms available. Most have a sitting area, space for creative activities, kitchen and dining areas, a bath or shower room, and toilet facilities. Some have a therapy room, hair and beauty salon, a medical consulting room and clinical areas, administrative office and access to secretarial services are desirable, but care must be taken not to allow clinical services and administration to dominate over the other facilities.

The art of day care

The strength and quality of day care is dependent on the personal and professional resources of the team members working together to create a relaxed and informal atmosphere. The day care leader has the responsibility for maintaining the ambience in the day centre, and facilitating the role of each team member. Each member's role will dove-tail with the other, and in some circumstances work in tandem with another team member. The roles are interdependent; therefore, no one should monopolise the situation, unless it is in their professional remit.

Programmes of activities and events are features of many day centres, but the level of activity or otherwise should be determined by the group of patients who are attending on the day. The art of day care is in the ability of the team being able to discern what is acceptable and achievable at the time. The objectives for each patient will be defined, and the expected outcome stated, so that each team member will be aware of the common goal. But if the physical, psychological or emotional state of the patient is unpredictable, the programme of activities that is planned for the day must be flexible enough to accommodate any needs of the patient.

Much has been taught and learnt about attitudes in the field of cancer care. According to Gagne (1985), 'an attitude is an internal state that influences the choices of personal action made by the individual'. Attitudes are commonly described as having three components:

(a)   a cognitive component or belief
(b)   an effective component or feeling
(c)   a motor component, or tendency to action.

Attitudes predispose an individual to act in a certain way towards stimuli, and are thus powerful influences. Many people have acquired a set of beliefs regarding cancer, plus a set of related feelings, e.g. shock, abhorrence or disgust. The action component may cause the person to withdraw or be avoided by others.

Thus, the day centre team must be able to create the kind of atmosphere that accepts the patient as he or she is, and by their attitude, influence the patient and his or her family towards accepting the situation.

It has been observed that patients learn from each other, and the day centre team as facilitators, should allow this to happen. Bandura (1977) who wrote about social learning theory said 'social learning or observational learning, occurs when an individual learns something by observing another person doing it' – in other words, it is learning by modelling according to social learning theory, behaviour is seen as a two-way interaction between an individual and his environment, that is 'both people and their environments are reciprocal determinants of each other'. Bandura identifies four processes involved in the observational learning situation, the fourth being motivational processes. He states 'modelled stimuli are more likely to be learned if the observer sees some value in them.' However, individuals who are lacking in self-esteem and confidence, and those who are dependent, tend to be more easily influenced by the behaviours of others who are obviously successful. Thus social dialogue may have a hidden agenda!

Humanistic theorists share a common view that involves the study of man as a human being, with his thoughts, feelings and experiences, including attitudes and values. Maslow (1954) was a major exponent of the humanistic approach to psychology, and has also made a significant contribution with his theory of a hierarchy of needs (Fig. 10.1). For the humanist, the goal is to assist the individual to achieve self-actualisation. Maslow describes this as 'helping the person to become the best that he is able to become'. When an individual is facing his or her own mortality for the first time, he or she may also be seeking and discovering his or her own identity.

Hospice philosophy recognises the physical, emotional, psychosocial and intellectual needs of the patient, and attempts to meet them in order that the life that remains is meaningful and of value. The prerequisite for meeting these needs is the provision of time, in a caring environment.

Day care personnel and services

Staffing requirements vary widely between day centres, but most of them are led by a qualified nurse who is responsible for co-ordinating and managing the service. In some instances, this person provides the clinical nurse specialist input, and is responsible for assessing, planning, implementing and evaluating the programmes of care for the patients in the day centre.

Although some day centres are managed and led by members of other disciplines, it is generally acknowledged that staff are required in the day centre to provide nursing care, and the skill mix varies according to local policy. In some organisation, the patients' nursing needs are met by an accessible nurse from in-

MASLOW'S HIERARCHY OF NEEDS

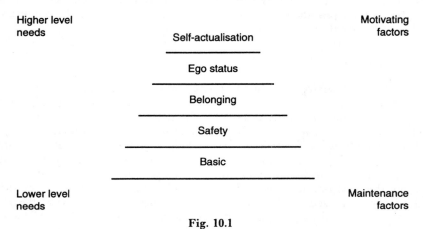

Fig. 10.1

patient facilities, but most day centres employ at least one nurse to assist with the care and comfort of the patients throughout the day.

Nursing care which has been prescribed by the community staff, can be continued when the patient attends the day centre, e.g. reloading syringe drivers, daily dressings to wounds or lesions, assistance with bathing, etc.

Creative, diversional and occupational therapies feature widely in day care, and many centres utilise paid and volunteer personnel to provide a whole range of remedial activities. The therapist will be skilled in initiating active and passive diversions with individuals or groups. Activities range from participating in art and craft work, gardening, baking, quizzes, outings to places of mutual interest, to reminiscence, socialising, debate and discussion. Many patients enjoy learning and developing latent skills, some will become involved in recreational activities such as board or card games, while others learn to relax. Day care should allow for passive involvement, especially for those patients who lack confidence, or, because of their illnesses, have a limited concentration or energy span. Their participation may be in appreciating the activities of other patients, including tasting the bakers' efforts!

Physiotherapy is recognised as an integral service within hospice and palliative care services in providing assessment and treatment for individuals and groups of patients. Patients who are recovering from spinal cord compression, can continue their programme of rehabilitation in the day centre, following discharge from in-patient services. Many patients with mobility difficulties, can be taught to move safely and confidently within the limitations of their diseases, thus enabling them to maintain their independence at home. The physiotherapist can also assist patients to overcome and manage acute attacks of breathlessness, by teaching them relaxation techniques, which obviate the need to call the emergency services. Gentle group exercise classes provide an enjoyable diversion as well as being therapeutic.

The relevance and importance of touch have been well recognised for many years, and complementary therapies have become valued in many aspects of health care. The provision of aromatherapy, reflexology, relaxation, yoga and visualisation, by qualified practitioners has a place in day care, to enhance the comfort and quality of life for those attending.

Volunteers

The skills and services of volunteers have always been utilised in day care, and without them, most day centres would not function. Many day centres employ a volunteer co-ordinator who is responsible for the recruitment and training, and support of volunteers, and who liaises closely with the day care leader.

Many volunteers are fundraisers, and provide a vital link with the community and other groups and organisations. Their roles in the day centre are varied, ranging from helping to transport patients between the day centre and home, assisting the therapists and staff with the patient's care and activities, to preparing and serving meals and drinks. They support the needs of the service, the staff, and the patients and their families, and are valued and loyal members of the day centre team.

Many day centres provide continuing support for bereaved families of patients who have attended day care, especially where there is no formal hospice bereavement service. It is not unusual for family members of a deceased patient to return to the day centre to thank the staff, and sometimes other patients, for the care and companionship afforded to the patient and themselves. Bereavement counselling requires the skills of qualified and experienced counsellors, within a framework of support and supervision, but the day centre may provide a venue for bereaved people to meet as a mutually supportive group, as well as offering a more formal bereavement service.

Many hospice and palliative care services, including day care have extended their remit to include the care of patients with other life-threatening diseases. Patients suffering from motor neurone disease, or acquired immune deficiency syndrome may derive much benefit, especially during a crisis, from day care facilities.

Conclusion

It is acknowledged that day care is a fast developing service. In the interests of the future of day care services, day care leaders and their teams need to be addressing audit measures, research initiatives, quality assurance and standard setting.

For may years, hospices and day centres have been teaching the science and art of specialised care to students from all health-care disciplines. There is a growing interest in learning about day care, and exploring its future potential as a major provider of palliative care.

The implications of the 1993 Community Care Act, will thrust day care services, together with nursing services to the forefront in the provision of hospice/palliative care for patients who choose to be cared for at home.

Finally, a quote from a patient who had been a girl-guide leader, when asked by her daughter what she did on her first day at the day centre replied, 'I cannot remember anything that I *did* – all I know is that my ribs ache from laughing!'

Acknowledgement

I am indebted to Mrs Beryl Howard, MBE, manager of Department of Palliative Medicine, Michael Sorbell House, Mount Vernon Hospital, for her invaluable help and support in compiling this chapter.

References

BANDURA, A. (1977). *Social Learning Theory*. Prentice-Hall, Englewood Cliffs, NJ.

GAGNE, R. (1985). *The Conditions of Learning and Theory of Instruction*, 4th edn. Holt, Reinhart & Winston, New York.

MASLOW, A. (1954). *Motivation and Personality*, Harper & Row. Also, see Table 1.

MASLOW, A. (1971). *The Farther Reaches of Human Nature*. Penguin, Harmondsworth.

ROGERS, C. (1951). *Client Centred Therapy*. Houghton & Mifflin, Boston; *Freedom to Learn for the 80s*. Merrill, Ohio (1983).

Further reading

FISHER, R. and McDAID, P. (1995). *Palliative Day Care*. Edward Arnold, London.

11

Spiritual care

The Reverend David Stoter

'For everything there is a season, and a time for every matter under heaven –
– a time to be born and a time to die,
– a time to weep and a time to laugh,
– a time to mourn and a time to dance,
– a time to keep and a time to lose,
– a time to love and a time to hate,
– a time to keep silence and a time to speak.'

Ecclesiastes: Chap 3. v. 1–7

The nature of spiritual care

Spiritual care is one of the most overlooked aspects of palliative care, probably because it is so often ill-defined and misunderstood, and for many of us fraught with unanswered questions and difficulties. Because of the many surrounding misconceptions some professionals tend to 'back off' and 'leave it to the clergy'. Nurses may ignore it apart from recording the patient's stated religion as part of the nursing process record (Faulkener, 1985). So often spiritual care is seen as religious care for the few who request it and therefore becomes dismissed as a footnote, just for the report. While it is important to recognise and meet the needs of those from all cultures and creeds, to see spiritual care only as religious care trivialises and diminishes its true nature. This perception may lead to paying lip service to meeting spiritual needs, but in reality giving it a low priority.

It is not only those of us who are involved in the day-to-day aspects of practical care who find this a difficult subject. Surprisingly, in research studies considering the care of the dying person there are very few references clarifying the nature of spiritual care, although our own hospice movement has its roots in Christian foundations (Owen *et al.*, 1989). This omission has been recognised during an international conference of experts at Yale University, when they faced difficulties in searching for a definition on the nature of spiritual care.

What is spiritual care?

The uncertainties mentioned above make it important to clarify the positive aspects of spiritual care from the beginning of our explorations. Spiritual care involves valuing individuals for themselves, each person having his or her own values and beliefs with the absolute right to be an individual needing affirmation of the person they are, and acceptance of their personal views and attitudes to life. Every person is a spiritual being having a spiritual dimension, only a few however have a specific religious dimension.

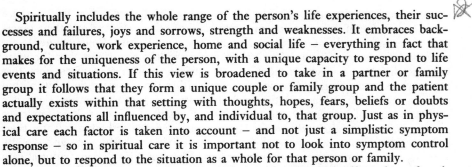

Spiritually includes the whole range of the person's life experiences, their successes and failures, joys and sorrows, strength and weaknesses. It embraces background, culture, work experience, home and social life – everything in fact that makes for the uniqueness of the person, with a unique capacity to respond to life events and situations. If this view is broadened to take in a partner or family group it follows that they form a unique couple or family group and the patient actually exists within that setting with thoughts, hopes, fears, beliefs or doubts and expectations all influenced by, and individual to, that group. Just as in physical care each factor is taken into account – and not just a simplistic symptom response – so in spiritual care it is important not to look into symptom control alone, but to respond to the situation as a whole for that person or family.

This means acceptance of that individual in totally, and affirmation of each person just as they are wherever we find them. It means accepting their range of beliefs, doubts, fears and anxieties as valid expressions of where they are, and affirming them with no preconditions of our own. This is a sound starting point from which to approach spiritual care, which is a gift of love with no preconditions, reflecting as it does the highest forms of human love, and for some a belief in God's love and acceptance of each of us as we are.

This then is our positive approach and starting point – that everyone has a spiritual dimension, and we need to differentiate between this and a religious dimension; that each individual is unique with personal values and needs, and each responds to a situation and to care in an individual way. This was summed up in a nicely defined statement at the above mentioned conference at Yale – 'it is the patient who defines the territory (for spiritual care) not the caregiver' (Fiefel, 1986). What is important is to recognise the potential of the spiritual dimension as a healing force for the whole person, body, mind and spirit.

The spiritual needs of the individual

Before looking at ways of offering spiritual care appropriate to each individual it helps to identify what the specific needs are, rather than embarking on a programme from our own perspective. The starting premise that each individual has a spiritual dimension, with certain values and beliefs that are unique, indicates that it is difficult to give an easy overall definition of spiritual need. However, we can say that it will vary between individuals, and that needs manifest themselves in several ways. Sometimes they are openly expressed, at others felt and not expressed. They are also relative to other conditions and, as such, may change at different times (Bradshaw, 1972).

It is, therefore, important to avoid sweeping value judgements and making assumptions about what people 'need' and thinking that there are set answers to questions asked. The discussion on spiritual care highlights the general factors which can help in meeting needs, such as recognising that there is a universal need for affirmation and unconditional acceptance, and a need for an opportunity to discover the way forward in a safe and caring environment, acknowledging that everyone is at a different stage on a personal spiritual or life journey.

The religious aspects of spiritual care

An important component of spiritual care is religious care, which needs to be related specifically to the individual's preferences and needs. For this purpose some knowledge of different denominations and of other religions and their practices is necessary to bring understanding of their complexities. Religious needs are discussed further in Chapter 00. Although it is widely recognised that there are obvious differences when considering other faiths, it is important to note that there are denominational differences not only within the Christian faith but within all religions. Even within a particular denomination, Christian or other, there is a wide spectrum of beliefs and attitudes with a diversity of practices. It is important to recognise that although some 'immigrants' remain orthodox within their culture/faith origins, others absorb from western living and education and thereby express more complicated transcultural needs. Therefore, if religious/cultural care is to be approached with sensitivity, it is important to understand these perspectives and find out what is acceptable and comfortable for the individual patient or family.

In the multiracial and multicultural society of today the range of religious beliefs may present a confusing variety of different approaches and practices, and it is helpful to have some information available on the wards or units for reference. For example, a list of denominations and other faiths outlining attitudes, practices or specific needs would be useful, together with local contacts who can be approached for information if required. Frequently in large hospitals the chaplain's department will act as a resource base for reference purposes. A practical example may illustrate the reason for the need to understand these differences. Nursing staff in a special care baby unit were concerned when they found a small dagger under the sheet of a baby in an incubator. They were considering calling in the social worker to follow up a perceived threat of non-accidental injury until they were reassured by the information that a dagger is one of the five religious symbols with significant meaning for Sikhs, and as such was placed close to the child's body.

There are several reference books available giving clear descriptive accounts of specific beliefs and practices, which will give the carer valuable insights into religious and cultural preferences relating to food, privacy, worship, and especially to death. An understanding of any of these can make an important contribution to the patient's general well being and quality of life (McGilloway and Myco, 1985; Neuberger, 1987).

Who gives spiritual care?

The comment has already been made that some professionals see spiritual care as the responsibility of the clergy or religious people alone, but when viewed in its true dimension it becomes clear that it involves the whole team and not any one person. However, sometimes one particular person may emerge or be selected by the patient or family as the key person to facilitate their own support, and with whom they feel comfortable. The contribution of the family should also be recognised, together with the need for the back up support of the rest of the team and any necessary specialist input.

The implications for the care giver will be considered more fully later, but at this point it should be noted that often the nurse, because of the nature of the work involved and time spent with the patient, is responsible for the majority of spiritual care. The nurse has a very special relationship with the patient and family making possible an input of spiritual care of the highest quality, especially if there is a willingness to remain open in the relationship and not try to give predetermined answers. Although the observations made in this chapter are addressed primarily to nurses, the principles considered are applicable to any professional involved with palliative care.

Some approaches to spiritual care

Spiritual care poses many questions where few answers are on offer, which may make it seem a threatening aspect of care. It deals with the kind of questions often appearing with the onset of serious illness – questions which need to be explored for each individual in a safe environment starting from where the person is in their own belief and experience, and allowing the discovery of answers when the time is right. Questions are raised like 'Why? 'Why me?' 'What have I done?' 'What has he or she done to deserve this?' 'What is happening to me?' 'Is there life after death – if so what is it like?' 'Is there a God – if so what is He like?'

Other expressions often heard are 'I've done nothing worthwhile with my life', 'Who will remember me when I'm gone?' or 'Why should anyone care about me?' To these questions or statements there are no direct answers or responses which can be handed out in the way pills or medicine are given for specific ailments. An even more complex situation may appear when the patient has a different religious origin from the professional carer, or more difficult still has no faith at all, or views death as oblivion, or has a particular faith when the carer has none or considerable doubts. A useful starting point is to begin by listening and receiving the questions and doubts as they are presented, and allowing the person to *be* who they are, as they are. This is the baseline from which to move forward – just to be alongside, in a non-threatening, non-authoritarian relationship which is not demanding or invasive of the patient's personal world of belief. This may present difficulties for some nurses as it is a relationship which requires some departure from the more traditional nursing role of 'delivering care'. It is important to be sensitive however, to the fact that the patient may not wish to enter into any relationship other than the professional one.

The 'history taking' approach using a question and answer method can have a depersonalising effect, giving a preconceived stereotyped photo-fit picture leading to false assumptions about the kind of care to offer. Such direct questions may be intrusive and a more 'oblique approach' is often more rewarding. For example, instead of using a question like 'Have you any children?', a more suitable approach could be to make a comment like 'That's a lovely picture of your family', an approach which may open up a relaxed conversation giving a sense of warmth and trust.

It is natural and desirable to talk about family life and this may well lead on to the patient sharing details about themselves, their families, fears, preferences and beliefs. The essential ingredient is for the patient to become aware that someone is willing to share their humanity. This should not be used, however, as an opportunity for the professional to work out personal problems in this relationship, or project personal needs onto the patient.

The patient may need to 'test out' the nurse to see if he or she has been really 'heard'. For many, once they are assured of being heard the opportunity comes for release of fears and doubts and the 'felt' anxieties and needs are openly 'expressed' as the patient takes the nurse into the darker areas of experience. Some may need to focus on impending death, and its nature, and projection into what it is like to be dead. These are powerful areas of pain and distress which are related to the unknown. Other frequent fears relate to burial, cremation, or being in a coffin; fears are often associated with dying alone, losing control of oneself or suffering pain, or anxieties about the family. Another common fear is associated with forms of loss, in terms of dignity or personal identity, loss of role, or loss of control over personal destiny. All of these are powerful fears especially for the younger patient, where loss of body image may be particularly important. Some of these fears may well find an echo in the carer.

The professional carer in the team

Personal skills needed

It is very clear that the nurse or any professional carer does need to have good listening skills to enable the patient to share these painful areas fully. Such a relationship can create a very exposed situation for the nurse, particularly when there is an expression of despair, as the patient enters into and shares the darkness. The situation may well be so threatening that the temptation is to stop the process to avoid becoming completely lost and deal with one or more aspects through a problem solving model. This feels safer but is less helpful to the patient, who is looking for someone to be with them on the journey as far as they feel able to go – to stay close without judgement or ready answers that could trivialise the situation and need. The professional carer may experience a strong temptation to reinforce their own security by comforting the patient through trite sayings such as 'Don't be frightened' or 'Don't worry, we will look after you'.

This may be a particular area of difficulty for those trying to express comfort in religious terms. It is easier to do something positive to fulfil the nursing role by attempting to bring hope or relief of pain and distress, at a time when the patient is aware of the situation which has to be faced but wants to express it to someone who can hear and accept the rawness and weakness of pain and darkness. It is helpful to know that others do not have the answers to death and dying and that professionals have their own fears and uncertainties about these issues.

The response of the carer then is not in words, but to stay and listen, to hear, and to be eyes and ears to the person expressing the pain as they enter the darkness. With this accompanying hand and presence in the shared experience they may be enabled to express the depth of their distress. Having been heard and accepted in the deepest place of darkness or despair they may find their hopelessness begins to lift as they discover that they feel heard in that most threatening place of all, and now know that in future it is safe to share at depth with that person. This may be followed by a change in perspective as a glimmer of hope comes. An example of a similar kind of experience familiar to most of us is when travelling through a long tunnel where the darkness deepens and becomes more oppressive as we approach the centre. After that point the darkness is always behind and whenever we look ahead we are looking towards the light which, even if it is only a glimmer at first, is getting brighter all the time. The carer needs to accept that this glimmer may be very faint and may remain so.

Part of the process which brings relief to the patient is being given permission to express these feelings without being told they are silly or there is an easy way out. It is not the professional's role to give hope but to enable the patient to discover a meaningful hope for themselves. This may well be the point at which the patient knows the despair is understood and accepted but this insight is something which cannot easily be put into words. It is tempting for the carer to respond by saying 'I understand how you feel' which is never helpful or true – it is the receiving of the shared experience which brings reassurance where words may trivialise the moment. When the patient feels understood they may quietly say 'I'm glad you understand'. Perhaps this listening process is best summarised in the words of Dr Cicely Saunders – for her the phrase 'watch with me' epitomised her approach to spiritual care in hospice work, and she wrote, 'Watch with me, means above all, just "Be there" (Saunders, 1965).

Skills of co-operation in the team

The whole process and relationship for the nurse in this experience is rather like being strapped into a roller coaster at a funfair. The harness needs to be fixed at the beginning of the ride and the passenger must stay harnessed until the end of the journey and not try to get out. Trying to side step or solve the problem is like an attempt to remove the harness, and to fail to reach the end of the journey. The professional needs to 'fix the harness' and stay in until the end. This may present practical difficulties in terms of continuity of care and is a problem that needs acknowledgement, and hence the importance of teamwork and support. It is important for most people to have one key worker whom they can trust – very few can reveal themselves at this depth with more than one or two people. It is not always advisable or necessary for more than one person to hear the whole life story, and this means there is a need to develop trust between members of the team, and more senior staff may need the humility to value the contribution of less experienced members of the team. No one person can be effective for everyone at all times.

A difficult issue may arise for the team where confidentiality is concerned. By definition the sharing of deep feelings should be recognised as confidential as it is threatening for the patient to feel that his or her personal revelations are common knowledge. There is a fine line to be negotiated between sharing confidences within the team or holding them absolute. Some kind of contract or agreement may be necessary with the patient and the family where information needs to be shared for very good reasons. This is a very important area for the professional who needs to be aware of personal limitations and when to call in the specialist or a more experienced person, and at the same time to show a sense of discrimination about what can be shared.

There may well be a need for the professional to seek back-up and support in coping with personal insecurities and moving forward in a difficult relationship. It is important for a nurse not to pull out but to know where such support can be found and to have ready access to it, also that help is available to identify the problem areas and enable a return to the situation with renewed insight and confidence to see it through, while exploring new territories. It is preferable for a person with specialist skills or more experience to work with the carer, supporting and helping them to carry on rather than taking over the key role, which might have the effect of 'de-skilling' that member of staff in future helping relationships. It is sometimes necessary for a chaplain or other professional to come in for some aspects of the work which may remain confidential to them. Even in these cases it is important that the nurse retains a continuing responsibility for spiritual care.

The whole area of adequate preparation and available support for staff working in these areas of palliative care is one of utmost importance as it will ultimately affect the quality of care given. These issues will be discussed more fully later in the chapter. Professionals in this field need to be aware of their personal limitations and of the importance of receiving help in resolving these areas of difficulty and sharing their own pain, anger, doubt and helplessness.

The caring team

The patient in the family

In considering the provision of spiritual care it is central to the observations made thus far that the patient is not just the recipient of care offered, but rather a full member of the caring team (Owen *et al.*, 1989). The traditional terminology of talking about the delivery of care mitigates against the approach which involves the patient fully in all discussions about progress, nursing, medical and spiritual care. A more usual approach acceptable today sees the individual person within the setting of the family and environment, and as a partner or fully involved member of the decision making team. Thus it is an integral part of spiritual care to help the whole family to feel involved and accepted and to enable them also to question and express fears both with the professional and/or with the patient, which will facilitate open communications within the family.

Unresolved anxieties can create barriers and lead to negative communication – it is important that the legacy left for the family is a good one and not destroyed by premature disengagement or inappropriately expressed anger. Anger expressed at the appropriate time is unlikely to be remembered with bitterness after the death is over. Feelings openly expressed within the family maybe painful at the time, but if accepted in love and openness are likely to be resolved. On the other hand, where the patient feels alone and separated and unable to express feelings openly with the family or with a sympathetic professional, feelings of isolation may follow which may well be expressed in anger and bitterness.

The professional's role

The professional's role is therefore one of enabling and not of taking over. The patient and family need to remain in control of the relationship with one or two provisos. Firstly, it is unwise to enter a conspiracy to deceive which may often be set up in the early stages of illness when the family is shocked and vulnerable – such a conspiracy may well close the ability to relate openly, and disable family communication from the time of diagnosis or prognosis. Secondly, the patient needs to relate to the nurse in two different ways, both feeling confident there is a professional clinical control present for patient safety, and recognising that, in the spiritual dimension, the patient has the control.

Also the patient and family have the right to establish the parameters of what they are willing to receive and in whatever style and cultural form they desire. They have a right to have their own religious faith or no faith at all, to be individual or unorthodox in approach.

It is important to remember that no one has the right to set out to impose upon another their own way of thinking in this situation. It is one thing to attempt to share our faith with others by knocking on people's doors or preaching from a pulpit, but in these situations we cannot compel people to open their doors or listen to us, so we have no right to expect them to listen just because they are captive in bed and reliant on us for care. If we establish good caring relationships it is highly probable that the patient will ask for our opinions and will then be open to listen – we can then share, because, and as long as, we are invited to do so. We also have the responsibility to provide care for patients of every race, culture and creed – these principles are an integral part of the international code of nursing ethics.

One area in which the nurse may be helpful and have an educative role is in enabling the family to understand what the patient needs, helping them to see how inappropriate it is to deceive, and how this deception closes communication possibilities. It may help if they understand that many patients do know there is a strong possibility that death may not be far off and may not find it easy to express this knowledge in words. (See Chapter 16 on communication and Chapter 18 on counselling for further discussion.)

Some important issues for the professional

One issue which may present difficulty is accepting that some patients remain angry and never appear to come through to acceptance of their situation even with constant encouragement and support. This may be more apparent in the hospice approach to care where patients sometimes find the intensely caring atmosphere inhibits their need to express anger forcefully. Nurses need to beware of the danger of matriarchialism in palliative care – of overprotecting the individual from his or her stronger feelings by a 'cosseting' approach. While acknowledging the enormous contribution of the hospice movement (both past and present), for some people the gentle accepting aspect of their philosophy may present difficulties, when the patient feels unable to express the intensity of emotions and personal experience in an uninhibited way. Professional carers need to be aware of and sensitive to the sharp face of spiritual response, and the whole area of pain and harsh reality of loneliness in suffering as exemplified in the experience of Jesus in Gethsemane before his crucifixion (Luke, Ch. 22, v. 39–46).

Kindness and gentleness have a very positive input for some patients, and for most patients for some of the time. But many need harsh reality to be met with naked realism. It is most unsatisfying to thump a soft pillow when angry or thrown anger at a 'pillow-like' person. Professional carers need to accept the patient's right to die angry, or to die not accepting their illness or death – they have a right to continue to fight or to give up. The carer has no right to dictate how or when they shall die, but simply to affirm their right to be themselves.

Guilt for the professional

There is often much guilt created for professionals in palliative care, generated by the fact that they cannot give clear answers. This is especially so where it has not been possible to relieve pain or distress, or where there is not a demonstrable acceptance of the situation. Because of how we are it takes a great deal of maturity to realise that the expression of uncontrolled tears, anger or naked fear is an affirmation of our skills in providing spiritual care and not the reverse which is a negative and more traditional interpretation. These emotions need to be translated into a model which is acceptable to the patient. In the acceptance of the naked emotions, frequently healing and a sense of peace may well follow. There are some for whom these emotions will remain fraught up to the time of death and that is not to be seen as failure on the part of the professional.

Another difficult area arises for some concerning the individual's right to receive the kind of religious or cultural faith care in whatever manner, and from whom they wish to receive it, irrespective of how that may appear to the carer. This means that, at times, the nurse may need to bring in someone to give a form of care which is felt to be 'wrong'. This may mean calling in a priest or representative of another faith or religion. (One obvious exception to this is if someone is asking for some action which is against the law of the land.) There is a need for true humility in all carers, to acknowledge that while they know what they think truth is, others may well see things differently and have a right to do so.

Sometimes misunderstandings arise where lay and professional people use the same words to express different meanings, resulting in confusion. It is important to avoid the use of jargon which is not really applicable in the field of spiritual care. Another helpful area of preparation is for the professional carer to be assisted to identify and clarify his or her personal beliefs. This will encourage a sensitivity to the patient's uncertainties and explorations and also increase awareness of any possible prejudices arising from a particular personal perspective or belief.

Support in the professional role

There are many ways of offering support through existing networks within a particular organisation. These may include group settings or one to one relationships, in which the feelings of helplessness and questions arising in the palliative care situation may be explored in a non-threatening and non-authoritarian environment. Here the individual is in turn acknowledged, accepted and given care in his or her own personal pain or doubt. In some places programmes of self awareness and self development are available through educational channels and these are enhanced if they can be accompanied by adequate 'on the spot' back up and debriefing in the work place where real life experiences occur. Such programmes are valuable in helping individuals to be aware of their own personal humanity and therefore better able to accept the frailties of others and to become less afraid of failure.

While there may appear to be constant factors within the body of truth, if people look carefully back through their lives, truth is not a static commodity, but it develops and evolves, and most people have a broader and different perception of life and faith from that which they held ten years ago. While the core of a person's understanding of truth may remain essentially unchanged, their perception of truth develops when they make new discoveries on the journey through life. If it does not change they are not engaging with life in the world around them or growing within their own knowledge/faith/belief.

Preparation for the professional role

In looking at these aspects of spiritual care it is apparent that it requires a certain level of maturity and experience in situations which, at times, may feel threatening to the carer. This calls for a degree of adequate preparation and support provision that presents a major area for consideration, which cannot be fully explored here. However, it is worth indicating some ways in which carers can be prepared or equip themselves for this kind of work. It is helpful to build up as wide a personal knowledge as possible about various different religions, cultural and denominational groups, and to understand the thinking of agnostics, atheists and humanists (McGilloway and Myco, 1985). (See also Chapter 12.) This will help in meeting with the patient on a basis of mutual understanding. A knowledge of local resources and culture is also important so that one can learn to communicate effectively with the patient and family.

The team is an important source of support, where it engenders an atmosphere of trust and openness which acknowledges the threatening nature of the work and values each member's contribution. It should be remembered too that increasingly chaplains are involved in providing care right across the whole spectrum of care and many make a specific contribution to staff support as well as to patient and family care.

Summary

Good spiritual care then is never heavy or intrusive, but natural, human and warm. Above all else it is acceptance by a very human being of another very human being within a safe, affirming and loving environment. Although there are common responses and ingredients within the process of dying and bereavement (Kubler-Ross, 1969; Carr, 1982), and models of care are excellent for understanding the process of dying and grieving, they can be dangerous if used in a prescriptive manner to push or steer people along their journey. Each pathway to death and each personal grief is essentially individual and a unique experience for that person and therefore cannot be standardised in any way (Clench and Neville, 1982). The recognisable stages may not all be present or they may appear all at the same time or in different sequence. Therefore these models, while a useful aid to acknowledging the process, cannot be seen as a definitive statement (Sims, 1988). Good spiritual care demands a close empathy – a closeness and ability to touch and hold appropriately and one of the greatest skills is to use and value silence.

> 'Never speak unless you think you can improve upon the silence' (Archbishop Michael Ramsey).

References

BRADSHAW, W. J. (1972). The concept of need. *New Society* 30, 640–3.
BURNARD, P. (1990). Learning to care for the spirit. *Nursing Standard* 4, 38.
CARR, A. T. (1982). Dying and bereavement. In HALL, J. (ed.), *Psychology for Nurses*. British Psychological Society and Macmillan Press.
CLENCH, P. and NEVILLE, M. (1982). *Introducing Nursing*, Series 1 34, 1475.

FAULKENER, A. (1985). *Nursing. A Creative Approach*. Baillière-Tindall, Eastbourne.

FIEFEL, H. (1986). Foreword. In *In Quest of the Spiritual Component of Care for the Terminally Ill*. Proceedings of a Colloquium, Yale.

KUBLER-ROSS, E. (1969). *On Death and Dying*. Macmillan, New York.

McGILLOWAY, O. and MYCO, F. (1985). *Nursing and Spiritual Care*. Lippincott Nursing Series. Harper & Row, London.

MORRISON, R. (1989). Spiritual health care and the nurse. *Nursing Standard* **4**, 28.

NEUBERGER, J. (1987). *Caring for Dying People of Different Faiths*. Lisa Sainsbury Foundation Series, Austin Cornish.

OWEN, G. M. *et al.* (1989). The dying person. In: *A Study of the Marie Curie Nursing Service*, pp. 14–16. Marie Curie Memorial Foundation, London.

SAUNDERS, C. (1965). Watch with me. *Nursing Times* **61**, 48.

SIMS, S. (1988). Cancer and ageing. *Nursing Times* **84**, 26–8.

Further reading

STOTER, D. J. (1995). *Spiritual Aspects of Health*. Mosbys.

12

Religious needs of the dying patient

Bill Kenny

'The Great Learning is rooted . . . in being still, in coming to rest in a perfect equilibrium.'

Confucius

All religious faiths have one common dimension; they always deal with the major events of the life–cycle such as marriage, the birth of children and death. While religious faiths have many different forms and also vary enormously in the extent to which they impinge on everyday life, they all contain special rites or rituals dealing with these events.

Some simple knowledge of different religious traditions can be especially helpful when caring for people who are dying. When equipped with such knowledge health-care professionals are better prepared to help people face the task of dying with the greatest degree of acceptance or equanimity possible. Our own understanding of our patients' religious feeling may often add something very important to its significance: when we offer someone our understanding of their religious faith, we may actually increase the degree of comfort that the faith can give them.

This chapter deals with some relevant features of the major religions that nurses and other health professionals may expect to meet in an increasingly multi-racial society: its content is best understood by additional reference to Chapter 11 on Spiritual care.

Religious needs and the nursing task

To introduce this subject it might be useful to notice some very important aspects of any declared religious belief. Firstly, people following religious faiths vary a good deal in their *attachment* to their declared religions: some are *deeply committed* while others are very *casual* (or even nominal) adherents. Nurses can never be sure that a person who declares him or herself as 'Church of England' on the hospital admission form has actually been to church since the day he or she was baptised as an infant. The same may be true of other kinds of declaration, since many people feel obliged to say something about 'their' religion on admission to hospital, rather than claim to have none. For this reason alone, the health professional should always be wary of making easy assumptions about the *personal meaning* of religious faith; we should remember that faith is always personal, that any faith is always worth of respect (even when we may disagree with its teachings), and that all *appearances* of faith (or its absence) can be deceptive.

Since most people are judged by their behaviours, unless great care is taken a person's feelings about religion may easily be wrongly assessed. When religious faith seems deeply held and obvious, for instance, health professionals may feel that they can help provide facilities for its observance fairly easily. This may be a false assumption however. One significant aspect of many religious traditions is that they help people feel a separate and perhaps special kind of *identity* that distinguishes them from others. This can manifest itself in a variety of behaviours (by patients and relatives) that cannot be otherwise easily understood. Since by far the commonest difficulty that health professionals face is to deal with patients whose declared religion is one of which they have no personal knowledge at all, some recognition of the idea of special identity defined by religious observances can be an extremely telling factor in a patient's judgements about the standard of care he or she receives.

Good nursing will try to attend to the needs of people whose faiths pervade all aspects of living: certain religious practices can determine the types of food, clothing, work, arrangements for hygiene and leisure activities that people keeping the faith can accept. In such cases there is no essential difference between sacred and secular activities. Then, virtually all daily activities have some religious significance. A patient with this kind of religious background will make judgements about good nursing care that are influenced by the extent to which he or she feels the religious aspects of his or her lifestyle are understood.

Alternatively, sometimes people can be deeply (and seriously) religious in some traditions, without any obvious demonstrations of their faith. Some religions do make very clear divisions between secular life and sacred practice. The correct religious observances for them may be confined to set times in the day, week or year carried out in complete privacy, and there may be few other behavioural clues to suggest how deeply held religious faith may be. To offer good care here, the carer may have to be exceptionally alert to a person's behaviour, constantly looking for clues as to whether or not this kind of person's basic needs for privacy and quiet are being met adequately.

Lastly, in thinking about people who seem to have little interest in religious expression, we should remember that many people facing death find that half-forgotten religious questions suddenly become significant again. These questions may sometimes have *frightening* as well as *comforting* aspects. Since most religious ideas are acquired in childhood, and because they may not have been developed or considered since that time, there may be a real need for some people to re-evaluate or to reaffirm something of their declared faith despite having ignored it for a lifetime. Nursing that recognises this kind of problem is clearly very sensitive and thoughtful, and may have considerable significance to a patient and his or her relatives.

Nurses, because of their constant contact with patients and their families, may be key figures in ensuring that their patients receive religious support that is really appropriate for them. Nurses' relationships with patients are such that the sparse information contained in admission forms can be expanded into insightful assessments of patients needs for religious care. To be able to do this well nurses may need to acquire a little specialised knowledge and some particular sensitivities. A good deal can be achieved, however, by remembering that it is always *difficult* for patients to practice their religions in hospitals.

Religious observances always need some form of privacy, some dedicated time in terms of opportunities for them, and may also need some special facilities. Good nursing care can usually provide the first two of these and may often be able to arrange for the provision of the third, by making some fairly simple arrangements.

Maintaining contact with hospital chaplains, and collection of literature on the requirements of major religions which is easily accessible to all staff who might need it, are two very practical things that nurses can do to meet the needs of patients. Above all else, however, it is nurses' traditional abilities for open-mindedness and their observational skills that create the greatest possibilities for ensuring that religious needs of patients are met. This is why nursing can make such a singular contribution to a neglected aspect of care for the dying patient.

Varieties of religious practice

In the same way that different levels of commitment are hidden within the simple statements in records, it is also clear that two people whose recorded religion is the same may practice different versions of the religion. All major religions have different branches whose practices may differ markedly from one another. In the short accounts of major religions that follow, only the themes common to all branches are mentioned. To learn more it will be necessary for readers to seek out and consult an appropriate leader from the religious tradition about which information is required.

Buddhism

Buddhist teaching is a prescription for ethical behaviour and spiritual well-being that informs all aspects of everyday living. Buddhists are not theistic; they do not believe in a personalised God but revere the Buddha as an example of right living. Buddha nature is said to exist in every person and is released by prayer, purification, meditation and virtuous conduct.

Buddhists respect all forms of life and follow a pathway of compassion for every living creature, of service to others and of generosity. All Buddhists believe in reincarnation and choose to live in a way which they believe affects the subsequent lives that may follow this one. Aspects of right living in the Buddhist tradition include practising selflessness, not killing, fasting at appointed times and developing unfailing compassion.

Buddhists are opposed to abortion, euthanasia and contraception that acts after conception. They do not usually object to transplants or transfusions. Diets vary according to climate, but many Buddhists are vegetarian. Fasting days occur on New Moon and Full Moon days. Festival days take place on Buddha's birthday and death day, his enlightenment, his first sermon and others. On such days Buddhists eat at the regular times, which means before 12 noon and not afterwards. A quiet place for meditation and prayer is a helpful facility for Buddhist patients: they will advise on the times when such a place is most helpful to them.

A Buddhist priest should be informed as soon as a Buddhist dies. The priest will say prayers over the body and will conduct a burial service, advising on its appropriate timing after the death. Since there are several schools of Buddhism, most Buddhist patients and their families will be happy to advise on a priest who should be contacted when they are admitted to hospital.

Major Asian religions: Hinduism and Sikhism

Hygiene is exceptionally important in Asian religions. All Asians will need water for washing in the same room as the WC itself. They will require a container of water if a bedpan has to be used and Hindus prefer free flowing water for washing (for example, a shower), rather than sitting in baths.

Asian women are very modest. They will prefer a female doctor and female nurses, will be uncomfortable in mixed wards and will need great care with hospital clothing, for example gowns, because of over-exposure of the body. Some men may prefer male doctors and male nurses.

Hindus

Hindu men have three names, a personal name first, a complimentary name second and a family name third. The family name equates to the surname, the personal name to the 'Christian' or 'given' name. Hindu women have a personal name and a family name.

Hinduism is an old religion with thousands of gods and goddesses who are thought by some to be different manifestations of one God. Hindu deities are hierarchic with three supreme gods – Brahma the creator, Shiva the destroyer and Vishnu the preserver. Hinduism is divided into many sects and according to Neuberger (1987) the majority of Hindus in Britain are Vishnavites, worshipping Vishnu principally and his incarnations as Rama and Krishna. Hindu religious literature includes the Vedas, the Upanishads and the Bhagavad Gita. Hinduism was responsible for the caste system which, although now illegal in India, may have some remnants in relationships among older Hindus. Brahmins (the priestly castle) were the highest order and Haridjans (untouchables) the lowest. Menstruating women and mourners are temporarily untouchable during the purifications required of them at these times.

There is no standard form of Hindu worship. Attendance at the temple ranging in frequency from twice daily to once weekly may be required however, dependent on sect. Worship may consist of meditation, prayer and yoga exercise. Central to all Hinduism is the belief in progressive spiritual development as life itself progresses so that early attachment to worldly necessities gradually gives way to loosening of physical and emotional ties to worldly things. Ultimately Hindus wait for death as freedom from the world and unification of the spirit with God. The idea of Karma is also central to Hindu thought: Karma indicates the extent of spiritual progression and return to earth in various life forms may be necessary (in higher or lower forms) for further spiritual development, dependent on conduct in the present life. In hospital patients will usually require privacy for meditation and prayer: this should allow them to be completely alone if they require it. They will also need space to keep small idols or pictures of gods, charms and flowers related to their worship.

Hinduism has its own science of life and medicine, ayurveda, which recommends practices for sleep, diet, defaecation, exercise, sexual activity and personal hygiene. Illness is believed to be a function of the life led and final illness may cause a Hindu patient to be concerned that his life was faulty and somehow causal of the illness. Death, however, may hold little fear because Hindus believe that death leads to oneness with God.

Hindu thought and ayurvedic medicine require that patients will need special facilities for washing and for their diets. Washing the body requires running water, and is part of purification rituals, but additionally washing the hands and rinsing the mouth are needed before and after eating. Diet is often vegetarian, has a total ban on beef which includes any suspected contamination of other foods by beef in any way at all. Many patients will prefer their food to be brought from home rather than risk breaking food taboos in a hospital setting. Fasting is common, especially among women and great care is necessary to overcome the religious need for fasting in circumstances where it might be dangerous to health.

Last offices for Hindus must be performed by Hindu priests, Brahmins. They will assist dying patients with acts of worship and will reinforce Hindu ideas about the meaning of death. Cremation is always required after death: Ganges water will be needed for the ceremony but priests will provide this. There are no taboos about handling bodies by non-Hindus following death.

Sikhs

Unlike Hinduism, the Sikh religion is monotheistic. It has no priesthood and is essentially organised by and identified with a Sikh community. The centre of religious activity is the temple or gurdwara. Sikhism has a strong tradition of hospitality (towards other Sikhs and non-Sikhs alike) and has no caste system. Sikhs follow the teachings of the 16th century spiritual leader, Guru Nanakh: these emphasise the importance of a virtuous life, and individual relationships with God. Sikhism stresses virtuous involvement with the world, stresses family, friends, community and service, instead of the ascetic practices and unworldliness of Hinduism. Both religions share beliefs in reincarnation, and cycles of birth and rebirth through which each soul must progress before perfection is achieved and unification with God is attained. Karma is also a feature of Sikhism, leading to belief in living a good life and so affecting the progression of the soul.

Sikhs have visible symbols of their faith which are extremely important to them. These are uncut hair (in both men and women) which men cover in a turban, a comb which must be retained at all times even when not worn in the hair, a steel bangle worn on the right wrist (except for left-handed Sikhs who wear it on the left), a symbolic dagger which is worn at all times and special shorts which are nowadays a symbol of modesty and sexual morality. Great care must be taken by nurses in dealing with any of these symbols: it may be exceptionally difficult to remove any of them from a patient for any reason.

Some food restriction are observed by Sikhs. Meat must be killed in the halal way (see p. 174) approved by Moslems, and some Sikhs will eat neither beef (following the Hindu tradition) or pork (following Islam). Many Sikhs are vegetarian and some will not eat eggs. Alcohol is forbidden and tobacco is found distasteful.

The Sikh holy book is the Guru Granth Sahib, written in Punjabi but in a special alphabet. Sikhs who are dying are likely to feel extremely cut off from their temple because it is the focus for all Sikh life. The local temple will usually send people round to a hospital to sit with a dying person if here is no family. Sikhs also have a tradition of private prayer which involves rising early to shower and to pray for one or two hours before breakfast. Privacy is greatly appreciated and assistance with washing before prayer, when the patient needs this help, will be welcomed. A dying Sikh's family will prefer to remain with him or her and the family may wish to be responsible for last offices. After death, nurses should not attend to the body other than by closing the eyes and wrapping the body in a plain sheet without religious emblems of any sort. The family will prepare the body for cremation by washing and dressing it. Cremation should take place as soon as possible after death.

There is an important point to note about Sikh names. All Sikh men have the middle name or title Singh, and all women the middle name or title Kaur. The order of names is as in Hinduism: personal name, Singh or Kaur (both of which are honorific titles) and then the family name. Sikhs prefer to be known by their personal name and the honorific name, which is why all Sikh men seem to be called 'Mr Singh'. Their wives are not 'Mrs Singh' but 'Mrs Kaur'. The correct name for identification purposes in official records is, however, the last or family name.

Islam

The religion based on the teachings of the prophet Mohammed is called Islam. Its followers are called *Moslems* or *Muslims*: they may come from all over the world but the majority come from Arab countries, from Bangladesh, Pakistan and North Africa. As Islam is so widespread, Moslems may speak a variety of languages including Arabic, Urdu, Punjabi and Gujerati. Moslems believe that Mohammed was the last in a long line of prophets which included Moses, David, John the Baptist and Jesus.

According to Islam, Mohammed completed the work of his predecessors. Islam teaches that Mohammed was a mortal man, not a mediator between men and God but was a special teacher of the message that everyone is called to the service of the One God, Allah and should try to live perfectly according to God's Holy Book the Koran (Quran). There are five religious duties imposed on Muslims, the five pillars of Islam. These are having faith in God, daily prayer, fasting during Ramadan (see below), giving alms to the poor and making a pilgrimage (hajj) to Mecca.

All Moslems say prayers five times each day. The times for prayer are, after dawn, noon, mid-afternoon, just after sunset and at night. The observance of these prayer times is affected by variations in daylight hours in Britain: so that the prayer day is extended in summer and compressed in winter. Moslems must wash before prayer, and prayers must be said on clean ground (or on a mat) while facing Mecca. Shoes are removed and the head covered before prayer begins. Friday is the holy day for Moslems: all males over 12 will go to the mosque. Women will either be provided with a private room in the mosque, or will stay at home for their prayers.

Washing the body is of great importance in devotions. Facilities to wash in running water are imperative and may create some difficulty for a bed-ridden patient, even though seriously ill people are technically exempt from these obligations. Moslems must also wash after urination or defaecation and cannot pray unless they do so. A Moslem patient may wish to be given a jug from which water can be poured in order to wash after using a bed-pan.

Modesty is exceptionally important to Moslems. Women's clothes traditionally conceal the shape of the body and Moslem women will expect to remain fully clothed even at night. Moslem men are also very modest: they are always clothed from waist to knee even in the presence of other men. Older Moslems, including men, may insist on keeping their heads covered at all times. Moslems will expect to be cared for by nurses and doctors of the same sex as themselves.

Moslems eat Halal food, meat from animals killed by a Moslem over which prayers are said. Pork meat and blood are forbidden and all types of alcohol are prohibited. This may include alcohol in drug preparations. Fasting occurs during the month of Ramadan (which occurs at different times each year, because the Islamic calendar is lunar) and may have special significance for a person who is dying because the observance of Ramadan will be an opportunity for personal reconciliation with God. During Ramadan food may be taken only before dawn and after sunset. Neuberger (1987) notes that even very ill people may insist on fasting and that the fast requires nothing to be taken into the body during fasting hours. This may include drugs and may therefore cause problems with pain control regimes.

Moslems believe in life after death, so that death may be accepted by relatives as only a temporary separation. The family will offer prayers for a dying patient and the dying person should be placed with his or her face turned towards Mecca. The local mosque will provide someone to pray over a dying person if there is no family. After death, the body should be buried as quickly as possible, and the body should not be touched by hospital staff. If touching by a non-Moslem is essential, disposable gloves should be worn to avoid actual contact. A family member (or perhaps someone from the local mosque) will attend to the body. Post-mortem examination should be avoided if legally possible: organs should be buried inside the body.

Judaism

Judaism considers that there is one universal God with whom Jews have a particular and personal relationship. Jewish religion and culture are closely mixed together. After centuries of dispersal from their land of origin, Israel, Jews have spread throughout the world and may be indistinguishable in appearance, dress and behaviour from any other member of their present home country. Nonetheless, many Jews feel that they have a separate cultural tradition which unites them with all Jews in other countries and transcends national boundaries. Religious practice is one important aspect of this tradition. Judaism is based on the Torah or Pentateuch (the five books of Moses) of the Old Testament. Orthodox Jews believe that God literally handed the Torah to Moses on Mount Sinai and dictated the Ten Commandments to him. Progressive (reform or liberal Jews) believe that the Torah is divinely inspired and was written down by different people at different times. The principal religious precepts of Judaism are to worship one God, to carry out the ten commandments and to practise charity and tolerance towards other human beings.

All Jews derive comfort from keeping the sabbath (from nightfall on Friday when candles are lit, to the sighting of three stars on a Saturday night) and observing the Passover. Orthodox Jews regard the sabbath as a day of rest: they will not write, travel (except to the synagogue), work, cook or switch on electrical appliances during the sabbath. The Passover, a celebration of Jewish freedom from Egyptian slavery, requires special food, unleavened bread, bitter herbs, cinnamon, apples and wine.

The centre of worship is the synagogue where services take place on Friday evenings and Saturday mornings. Orthodox congregations may hold discussion groups on the holy books, led by Rabbis, on Saturday afternoons. Other important Jewish religious festivals are Yom-Kippur, the day of atonement, usually falling in late September or October, when 24 hour fasting is required, and the Jewish New Year. Yom-Kippur is regarded by many Jews as the holiest day of the year and, if health permits, most would prefer to keep the day quietly in prayer and a mood of penitence, to set the path for the year to follow.

Jews are subject to many dietary restrictions. All meat must be kosher (fit) from animals killed in a humane way (with as much blood as possible drained from the animal) and prepared by soaking and salting by specially trained personnel. Pork is absolutely forbidden, as are shellfish, and most Jews will have considerable qualms about mixing milk and meat at the same meal. The ban on this mixing includes a requirement to keep utensils for milk and meat completely separate.

There are no last rites in Judaism. Orthodox Jews claim to believe in an after-life and the physical resurrection of the dead, but there are wide variations in actual belief. A dying person may, however, ask to see a Rabbi who may offer prayers including the Shema Yisrael, the first line of which the patient may be encouraged to speak – 'Hear O Israel, the Lord is our God, the Lord is one'. Judaism expressly forbids any form of euthanasia but allows the withdrawal of treatment when death is near, and so also obviously allows the control of pain and severe discomfort.

After death, the body is traditionally left for eight minutes or so with a feather over the mouth and nostrils to ensure that breathing has ceased. The body is prepared by washing and dressed in a shroud before being placed in a coffin. Mutilation of the body is not permitted except when post-mortem examination is necessary. The funeral usually takes place within 24 hours; cremation is forbidden. Family mourning of 7 days is required in Judaism, during which time prayers are said and mourners visit the household.

Christianity

Christians of all denominations believe that Jesus was the human embodiment of a loving, just and personal God. As the son of God in human form, Jesus has set all Christians an example of God's mercy in action and has provided a remedy for human sin through the personal sacrifice of the Crucifixion. The triumph of Jesus over death, through his resurrection from the grave, and ascension to heaven to be with God is the symbol of all Christian hope.

Virtually all Christians believe in an after-life, although their visions of this may vary considerably. Christians of a fundamentalist persuasion believe both in Heaven, a place of perfect existence in which God is revealed clearly, and also in Hell, a place of darkness and torment in which the souls of unredeemed sinners are cut off from God eternally. More 'liberal' but committed Christians may have different and less polarised views of the after-life. All Christian theologies, however, teach that a new spiritual birth comes about by accepting Jesus into one's life, as Saviour and example. All Christian denominations celebrate the festivals of Christmas, the birth of Jesus, and Easter, the death and resurrection of Jesus, although some traditions celebrate the festivals on slightly different dates from others.

There are some important differences in required last offices and burial rites between different Christian denominations. Roman Catholic Christians who are dying will wish to make confession (if they are able) and to have a priest administer 'the sacrament of the sick', sometimes known as 'last rites'. The priest annoints the patient with oil, prays to God to ease suffering, and administers absolution – a statement of God's forgiveness for past sins. After death Roman Catholic families may prefer that the deceased person's hands are placed in an attitude of prayer holding a crucifix or a rosary.

There is no universal equivalent to 'last rites' in the Protestant Christian tradi-tion; chaplains may pray with the dying patient or may administer communion if the patient is able to receive this. Some Anglican patients may however wish receive the 'sacrament of the sick' since certain branches of the Anglican chur are quite close in belief and practice to the Roman Catholic tradition.

Christians of the Orthodox tradition (Greek or Russian) may be comforted by having a small icon near them, in addition to the more usual prayer book, Bible and crucifix of other branches of Christianity. An Orthodox priest will be welcome to the dying person and may hear a last confession, anoint the patient with oil and given communion. There are no special difficulties about handling the body after death. Orthodox Christians are usually buried rather than cremated and there may be a formal lying-in-state in their church so that family and friends may pay their last respects.

The nurse's own religious views

Like anyone else, nurses and other health care professionals may hold religious views themselves or may have none. In one sense the meeting of patients' religious needs asks the greatest degree of professionalism possible from nurses, because it may be necessary for them to set aside their own religious views in favour of those of their patients.

Where nurses' own views are deeply meaningful and important to them, they may be tempted (reasonably enough) to offer them as a source of comfort to people in distress. Perhaps this should be guarded against. The argument throughout this chapter has been that, in offering care to dying people, the patient's own religious views are what matter most, simply because it is always difficult for a person from one religious tradition to understand the personal meaning of a different tradition. To this idea might be added, the thought that death is in some sense a summation of life: if religious belief has been any part of that life then the opportunity to deal with unresolved questions about belief is extremely important. By doing this well, a dying patient may find that the whole of his or her life suddenly makes perfect sense.

Robert Pirsig in his book *Zen and the Art of Motor Cycle Maintenance* expresses this thought clearly when he says, 'Sometimes when you look at where you're at and look back at where you've come from, a kind of pattern seems to emerge. Sometimes you can use the pattern of the past to see more clearly where you're going to next'. Good nursing that attends to the religious needs of patients can certainly help this kind of process along. To do this well is surely to see holistic nursing in action.

Reference

NEUBERGER, J. (1987). *Caring for Dying People of Different Faiths*. Lisa Sainsbury Foundation Series, Austin Cornish, London.

Further reading

Our Ministry and Other Faiths: a Booklet for Hospital Chaplains (1983). CIO Publishing, London.

13

The care of the patient near the end of life

Ann Newbury

'I shall live a year, barely longer. During that year let as much as possible be done.'

Joan of Arc

There are many people with a progressive malignant illness who have a year or much less to live. During this period realistic advice, attention and support can make a vast difference to their remaining life. Today there is increasing professional and personal interest in palliative care. On discovering that a disease is progressive and curative procedures are no longer appropriate, patients and their families may feel rejected, confused, frightened and lonely. Facing death is probably the most profound experience any one of us will ever have to cope with and, Hinton says that the emotions aroused by it are legion, the commonest one being fear (Hinton, 1991).

When considering the holistic care of the patient with a limited life-span, he or she must be viewed as a member of a wider circle of family and friends within the cultural and environmental setting. Therefore when planning and delivering care the needs of the whole family must be considered (see Fig. 13.1).

All patients with cancer have the right to appropriate care by experienced nurses wherever they are cared for.

Higginson observes that just as a person chooses to live in their own way so they will choose to deal with ill-health and die in their own way, and that services must be flexible enough to allow this (Higginson, 1993).

When a disease no longer responds to active treatment, It is important that the emphasis of care is placed on palliation, in order to improve the quality of the person's life. This includes monitoring and controlling symptoms, advising and offering support to both the patient and their family. Every nurse has a responsibility in respect to providing for or facilitating the general well-being of the patient, by the provision of effective palliative care, whether the duration of the illness is days, weeks, or months.

Ultimately the patient must be able to experience a dignified, peaceful death which is free from distressing symptoms, and hopefully in the company of those he or she chooses and not in imposed isolation.

Wherever these patients are cared for they will have similar needs throughout the illness, and if nurses are to be efficient in their caring role there must be a full understanding of these needs. Not only should the nurse understand the total care required and the needs of the patient, but also the role of relatives and friends

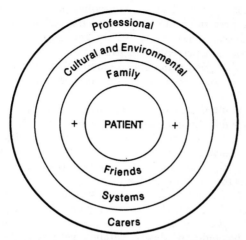

Fig. 13.1 Total care of the patient which includes care of the family and friends within their own cultural and environmental circle.

and the care which they may require, and the role of the nurse and the nurse's needs.

The total care and needs of the patient

Many patients receiving palliative care for cancer are not confined to bed until the final stages of the illness and, then, more in-depth nursing care may be required. Initially they may be comparatively well and able to enjoy a fairly normal life. The aim of care must always be to provide for the patient's total needs (see Fig. 13.2).

Physical care and needs of the patient

Relief of pain

Fordham and Drum (1994) claim that pain is an experience of the whole individual, and that chronic pain isolates by capturing concentration, making constant demands for attention and energy. They also describe it as an interior landscape or a separate world not populated by others, although the external world is

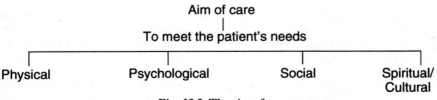

Fig. 13.2 The aim of care.

shared. O'Brien observes that Twycross describes pain as being a 'dual phenomenon' involving the perception of stimulus and the patient's emotional reaction to it (Saunders and Sykes, 1993). Fear, anxiety and unrelieved physical symptoms may intensify the patient's perception of pain.

Raiman observes that good pain control requires both sensitivity to the patient's needs on every level and the competence to meet them (Wilson-Barnett and Raiman, 1988).

Poor pain relief is often caused by inadequate or irregular medication. Administration of analgesia for chronic pain must be regular and the doctor will adjust the dose according to the patient's level of pain, increasing slowly until the patient is pain-free. The principle being to give the next dose of analgesia before the previous one wears off. More than one analgesic drug may be required. Those used will depend on the cause of the pain.

O'Brien observes that addiction, or psychological dependence does not appear to occur in patients taking opioids for cancer pain, although physical dependence can (Saunders and Sykes, 1993). If pain is able to be controlled in other ways then opiates can be reduced slowly without withdrawal symptoms. Fear of dependency is more of a concern to the professional carer than the patient. All too often opiates are seen only to be given at the very end of life and even today the full potential of their use is not realised.

Alderman (1988) suggests that the aim of pain control 'is to relieve the pain without compromising the consciousness'. Controlled pain will usually eliminate the fear of pain.

Twycross advises that attention should be paid to factors that modulate pain threshold (Twycross and Lack, 1990).

Raising the pain threshold

The professional carer can assist in raising the pain threshold to improve relief by ensuring the following.

- Medication regime is understood and followed.
- Other symptoms are controlled.
- Good night's sleep and adequate rest.
- Understanding to relieve fear and anxiety.
- Prevention of isolation and loneliness.
- That opportunity is given for expression using listening and counselling skills
- Relief of boredom.
- Comfort by the use of special equipment or treatment as required.

Other common symptoms

The symptoms mentioned are some of the more common ones which may be experienced by patients with a progressive malignant illness. Many other symptoms are discussed in detail in other chapters and works such as Twycross and Lack (1990).

Nausea and vomiting. These symptoms are under the control of the vomiting centre in the medulla and may be stimulated in several ways. Medical treatment will depend on the cause. Predisposing factors should be eliminated in addition to the use of antiemetic drug therapy.

The nurse's role should be to administer prescribed therapy, control nauseous odours, prevent unpleasant sights, eliminate constipation, ensure pain control and to see that an appropriate diet is provided. If diet is not tolerated soda water or cool fizzy drinks are often helpful.

Reassurance will be required as gastric symptoms are very distressing and exhausting to a person, especially to those who are already weak and anxious.

Constipation. This may cause other problems such as nausea, anorexia and abdominal discomfort if not adequately controlled. As the patient's condition deteriorates and he or she becomes weaker and less mobile, the risk of constipation can increase. It is aggravated by poor dietary and fluid intake which frequently occurs with the progression of the illness. Increased analgesic therapy may slow down the motility of the gut, but Thomas emphasises that this is one area where anticipatory care can alleviate much distress (Wilson-Barnett and Raiman, 1988). The nurse's role is to ensure the appropriate use of aperients, provide a suitable diet and to encourage an increased fluid intake if the patient can tolerate it.

If simple measures to control constipation are not effective the administration of suppositories or enemas may be necessary. In this case it is essential to minimise exhaustion and discomfort to the already weakened patient and care must be taken to preserve the patient's dignity.

Anorexia. This frequent symptom may cause fear. As the patient's disease progresses the inability to eat may be seen as a threat to life. Antiemetic therapy should be given as prescribed. This is very significant when the fear of vomiting still lingers, having been the original cause of anorexia. Fear may precipitate vomiting. Carers should do all in their power to encourage the maximum enjoyment of food, but as the person becomes more ill food often becomes less important to them. This is natural.

Meals should be served attractively. Small frequent meals or snacks will be appreciated, especially if the patient experiences gastric fullness.

Pain and nausea must be controlled. Unpleasant odours should be eliminated and it is helpful if offensive wounds are attended to at least half an hour before meals. This allows time for the patient to settle down and promotes comfort. It also prevents embarrassment. The use of charcoal-type dressings can help.

An alcoholic aperitif may stimulate the appetite. In the earlier stages of the illness the doctor may prescribe a trial of appetite stimulant, but as the person becomes more ill this is less appropriate.

Taste changes are fairly common and will affect the appetite and the desire to eat. Mouth infections and ulcers making it painful to eat, should be treated appropriately.

If the patient's desire for food lessens it may be beneficial to substitute one or more meals with a high-calorie drink. Reasonable fluid intake will prevent the distress of dehydration, and even when very ill, frequent sips of fluid will prevent thirst. The nurse has to be vigilant as the patient may be too ill to help him or herself.

Shaw observes that the loss of appetite is a source of conflict within the family as it is often their barometer as to the overall condition of the patient (Shaw,

1993). Thomas emphasises that the family may need to be 'relieved of their guilt' if they feel they are failing (Wilson-Barnett and Raiman, 1988). They may need help to understand and accept the patient not eating. Sometimes relatives feel that a person should be fed at all costs – 'the eat to survive syndrome'. They may even inappropriately request intravenous feeding.

Insomnia. Sedation is not necessarily the answer. Pain, nausea and other physical symptoms need to be controlled or else wakeful, restless periods will occur. When the person is near to the end of life they may be afraid to go to sleep in case they do not waken up, they may also become anxious and fearful during the night. The greatest need then is probably for a cup of tea and the opportunity to voice his or her fears to an understanding listener who will not brush aside the anxieties making light of the process of dying and just offer more sedation.

Sleep disturbances may also indicate depression but this must be recognised from the normal understandable sadness of the dying person.

Mouth problems. Patients suffering a debilitating illness are prone to develop sore or infected mouths. Regular oral toilet must be routine. Condition of the teeth may have deteriorated or dentures become ill fitting so a visit to, or from, the dentist may be beneficial and improve the quality of life. Infections must be treated. Medication in orobase, soothing gels or medicated pellets can give relief if ulcers are present.

Dry mouths can also be troublesome and may aggravate anorexia. Dryness can be indicative of dehydration, infection, mouth breathing, or may be related to medication or the person's deteriorating condition. Frequent mouthwashes, mouth care and attention to diet will help to minimise problems. Sucking boiled sweets, citrus fruit slices or pineapple chunks can be refreshing. Artificial saliva, special lozenges, frequent drinks, crushed ice or frozen tonic water cubes to suck may help. Medication should be reviewed with the doctor as this may be a contributory factor.

Pressure area care. Near to the end of life the patient may become debilitated and their skin may be friable from steroid therapy. There may be marked loss of weight, cachexia, and immobility. It is crucial the skin is kept clean and dry. Patients often appreciate a bath or shower even when they are very frail. Gentle massage may be comforting and aid circulation. The use of pressure relieving equipment plays a part in protecting pressure areas and should be used as a preventative measure for 'at risk' patients. Patients should be encouraged to change their position at regular intervals. As they become more immobile and perhaps confined to bed, it is the nurse's responsibility to provide adequate pressure area care.

Weakness. With the progress of the illness this may become one of the most frustrating symptoms. The mind is often willing and active but the body is too exhausted to respond to the demands made upon it. Uncontrolled symptoms will slowly weaken and distress the person, so effective symptom control is of paramount importance. According to Hoy at least 80 per cent of patients complain of weakness during their illness (Saunders and Sykes, 1993).

The realistic, caring physiotherapist may be able to assist in making the person feel stronger, become more mobile, and teach ways of doing things to preserve energy. O'Gorman emphasises the need to maximise each person's potential (Saunders and Sykes, 1993). Even in the last weeks of life a person may benefit from hydrotherapy because water gives buoyancy, is relaxing and enables easier movement. Rehabilitation is on-going and involves the person understanding their disability, regaining confidence, and incentive to do what they are able for as long as they can. They are encouraged not to be left out or forgotten. The person needs to be taught to reserve energy for the things they wish to do, and not to waste it on unimportant things. Alternating periods of rest with activity helps the person to live within their limitations. As they become more weak and ill the periods of rest usually need to lengthen and activity lessens.

When uncontrolled symptoms are severe the patient may wish to die but as they become controlled, even though the patient may be very ill, the desire to go on living is often revived. It is important to control physical symptoms so that the patient can invest the energy they may have in living until they die.

Psychological care and needs

Caring for people who are near to the end of life extends beyond physical care to supporting them emotionally as they adjust to an increasing physical weakness, and cope with grief.

Cancer is an emotive word and can conjure up many fears and anxieties especially when the patient becomes aware that curative procedures are exhausted. Having perhaps completed surgery, radiotherapy or chemotherapy, they may well feel that 'no more can be done', which may of course be applied to 'cure' but never to 'care'. This can leave the patient feeling anxious, frightened and disillusioned convinced they will suffer pain or die in the imminent future. Realistic hope must be restored and although cure is no longer an option, the patient must be assured that help is available and every effort will be made to control the situation, making the remainder of life worthwhile and meaningful. they need to understand and be reassured that all forms of palliative care will be employed where appropriate, such as radiotherapy for bone pain.

It may be at this point that the person considers complementary therapies (Chapter 15). Dobbs (1985) considers that alternative methods of treatment may enrich interventions and bring comfort and better health to patients with cancer.

A kaleidoscope of negative and potentially destructive emotions might be experienced (Fig 13.3).

Patients may well need to express any of the feelings indicated in Fig. 13.3 should they experience them, and should be given the opportunity to work through them. It is important to take the cue from the patient as to when, and how much they wish to discuss at a time. Twycross and Lack (1990) observe that there is no one right way of adjusting to a poor prognosis. Some people ask, want to know and be totally involved in all decision making, whereas others know but are not prepared to discuss the matter further and may not even be willing to make decisions. Some people live in a make-belief world where all is well, never acknowledging to themselves, let alone others, that they may be very ill. Morrison says that a person has a right to his or her defences by practising techniques such as denial. He also emphasises that this should be respected and that the person should be helped to share feelings at an individual pace. He also warns that there

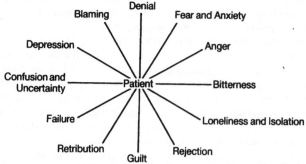

Fig. 13.3 Explosion of emotions which may occur in the cancer patient with a limited life-span.

may be a discharge of painful emotion when the time is right (Morrison, 1992). Denial may be a defence mechanism and the patient's way of coping until other positive coping strategies can be mustered. The decision must be the patients as to when he or she is ready to abandon denial. There are gentle ways of imparting the truth – it is not necessary to be blunt. Frequently given the opportunity the patient will answer his or her own questions.

Unexpressed fears may create anxiety and depression. There may be fear of pain and loneliness. Uncertainty, inability to cope with the process of the illness, and fear of lack of help from medical and nursing staff may all give rise to added anxiety. Patients need to be able to voice their fears, and work through their emotions with an understanding, empathetic person who is able to answer their questions, hopefully giving support, reassurance and encouragement. Summers and Young observe that everyone needs to be able to give and receive love.

Each person needs to be able to 'live' until they die, and wherever they are cared for this should be the nurse's prime consideration. The person must be helped to accept the things they cannot do and learn to set realistic goals for themselves, so there may be a sense of achievement. Encouragement to do the normal things of life, even dressing in day clothes when most of the day is spent resting, will improve the morale.

> Gill was a young woman who struggled valiantly to make up her face each day for her husband and children. When she was becoming too weak to manage this she taught her husband what to do. He continued to do this for her until she died so retaining normality, and for Gill, dignity.

> Ben was an independent, middle-aged man, who for a long time declined to attend the day centre. Eventually he came and began to develop latent talents. He continued to attend even after admission to the unit. He became very weak and ill but, late the afternoon before he died, he busily beavered away at making a plate for his wife. He worked into the early evening and saw it put into the kiln saying 'please give this to my wife'. He died that night but left his 'love gift' for his partner which she cherishes. It can be said of Ben 'he lived until he died' and was in control of the situation throughout, even though it took great courage.

In providing psychological care nurses' aims should be to use their listening, communication and counselling skills to support, encourage and give incentive to the patient hopefully helping them to feel fulfilled. Communication and counselling skills are discussed in other chapters.

Social care and needs

Social needs must be met so that the patient can remain as independent as possible, for as long as possible, preferably within their normal social setting. Fulfilment of social needs enhances safety and security and is an intrinsic part of total care.

Occupation within the patient's capability, even when frail or in hospital, helps to prevent boredom and withdrawal. It minimises feelings of uselessness and helplessness.

Each person needs to feel socially acceptable, of use to others, and that opinions and company are important. Life style and identity need to be maintained, and recognition of social status within the home and every other area of life, such as being a father, mother, chairman, business woman, sportsman, seamstress. Independence should be encouraged for as long as possible. Praising anything the person attempts or achieves will make them feel good and boost self-esteem. Investing in a new wardrobe of clothes when they have lost weight markedly, will improve body image and self-worth.

The ill person may experience financial embarrassment if they can no longer be the breadwinner, or perhaps it is the working wife whose financial contribution to the home has been essential. The nurse can direct them to the appropriate department for advice and assistance in making applications for allowances and grants such as attendance allowance or disability living benefit. The waiting time rule has changed fairly recently and immediate application can be made if the prognosis is thought to be up to approximately 6 months.

Smith suggests that the nurse perceives and responds to the human being who has become a patient, and that 'patient' is actually a label which may denote a stereotype if applied indiscriminately (Smith, 1981). Role stripping can be prevented by the patient always being acknowledged as a person with their own identity and specific place in society. Wherever they are cared for the title to be used by staff should be agreed. Not all patients are comfortable being called by their first name, equally so, it could be alien to some to be addressed more formally. The patient should decide. There must be recognition of the individual, respect of views, likes and dislikes, and they should be allowed to use their own clothing and be up and dressed if they are able. Clothes are a symbol of personal identity. People are quickly dehumanised by diagnostic labelling, such as the person in 'bed 2' with carcinoma of the pancreas instead of 'Andrew Green' who is still a person. It is important that each patient maintains their unique personality.

Social interaction is enhanced by early introduction to other patients, staff and volunteers, allowing freedom of choice as to whom the patient wishes to communicate. If a person is admitted for inpatient care they should be encouraged to make their own space personal, perhaps by displaying a photograph or cards which have a meaning for them as an individual. Maintenance of social role can be aided by the nurse showing a genuine interest in family, friends, job and hobbies, so keeping the patient in touch with the outside world.

Smith observes that there is something inherent in the make-up of the role of the nurse which fosters a dependency syndrome (Smith, 1981). This may be imposed unintentionally by the carer out of genuine fear for the patient's safety, or the need to feel needed. Every effort should be made to allow as much independence as is safe, reasonable and desirable to the patient. Views need to be recognised, acknowledged and permission asked of the person rather than 'taking over' by the carer imposing his or her own will. This is very important as the patient becomes weaker. When the person is admitted to any form of residential care it involves the transfer of the patient's 'home' for that period of time and the staff become an extended family.

Day centres

Day centres can complement the work of palliative care teams. Gibson suggests that because there is the support of a caring professional team, the patient has greater autonomy in making choices regarding remaining at home or being admitted (Saunders and Sykes, 1993).

Some day centres are essentially social, whilst others offer a full range of services. This was emphasised in the 1993 Qualitative Study on Day Centres (Help the Hospices, 1993). They can be a place for 'time out' from home or ward where people can be themselves, gain relief from boredom, loneliness, pursue hobbies and boost self-esteem. It may give the patient the opportunity to talk away from family and home, about the things that really concern them. They may not talk at home for fear of upsetting those whom they love. Attendance can be a means of developing latent talents, encouraging self expression, promoting social acceptance and interaction. Meal-times can be regarded as eating out. Socialisation can be enhanced by provision of pre-lunch drinks as an appetiser, and then meals being eaten round a dining room table. Outings are a great asset as they help to ensure that, patients remain a part of a wider society. Much satisfaction is derived from being able to help one another.

Many day centres now provide complementary therapies such as relaxation, aromatherapy and visualisation. Crowther (1991) suggests that patients with cancer have come to expect more than orthodox treatment can offer. Burke and Sikora (1992) suggest that if complementary therapies and orthodox cancer care are provided together then the consequent benefits could possibly be greater than the sum of the two.

Some day centres have developed lymphoedema clinics to give advice on skin care and specific treatments such as massage and compression techniques, also emotional support and counselling.

Day centres have an important role in providing care for patients with cancer whose illness is progressive, and respite care for relatives, but it must be remembered they may not be beneficial for everyone.

Spiritual/cultural care and needs

Spiritual care is that which is of the innermost being. It is not tangible or material. Every person has a need to feel fulfilled and an opportunity to work out their own beliefs, and confirm them for themselves. It may be a time when the person's thoughts on life and death are reviewed, re-evaluated and the things that matter often become more valued.

In multi-racial countries there are many religions and philosophies present. When caring for the patient with a short while to live it is important to be aware and acknowledge the needs of people of other cultures and customs, and to provide opportunity for them to fulfil these needs.

Hope is a part of spiritual care being revealed as a feeling that one's existence is in some way worthwhile and desirable which spurs on the will to live. Peberdy suggests that there is a failure to allow hopes to be articulated, such as a hope for a certain type of death. Or indeed they may be shared but heard as an expression of despair, whilst carers insist on an unrealistic hope for recovery (Dickenson and Johnson, 1993).

Spiritual care involves the nurse in helping the patient to cope with disappointment, losses, uncertainty and allowing them to talk of the meaning of life after death, if they, so wish. Some people experience a sense of meaningless-ness and this may be mistaken for depression.

For some people spirituality can be of great support particularly if they have a deep meaningful faith, but even people with an apparently unshakeable faith may question. Faith is not a guarantee against all the ills of life but hopefully will give support and meaning to the situation. Those with little or no faith may seek something deeper. Spiritual care and well-being is an important part of total care.

Throughout the illness the patient needs to feel that they are coping and in full control of the situation, with symptoms controlled and needs met. It is important that they participate in decision making. Within the community a variety of agencies provide services and support to enable people to enjoy a high quality of life, as independently as possible in their own homes. This has been greatly enhanced by the passing of the Community Care Act 1993 (Primary Health Care, 1993). This is particularly relevant as Neale observes that on average patients spend 90 per cent of their final year being cared for at home (Clark, 1993). It is important that the patient is encouraged to live life fully and not to be just waiting for death. Each day is a bonus to be enjoyed. Equipment needs must be met urgently as the patient's requirement is now, not next week or next year. That may be too late to bring the extra comfort and opportunity to maintain as normal a life as possible.

Sometimes during the course of their illness the person may need to be admitted for a period of assessment and stabilisation of symptoms, respite care, rehabilitation or more permanently for general care but at all times appropriate treatments should be employed. Sims observes the growing interest in comple-mentary therapies and emphasises the excellent position nurses are in to evaluate such non-invasive therapies when incorporated into patient care (Wilson-Barnett and Raiman, 1988).

It is desirable and advantageous that every patient has an individualised care plan which identifies needs, problems, action taken and outcomes. Recording goals and achievements are also important. This plan should be regularly evaluated and updated.

Where should the patient be cared for in the last days of life

The patient may have been deteriorating almost imperceptibly over weeks or months and then a change occurs and the process of dying is recognised. Hopefully discussions will have taken place between the patient, family and caring professional team, and desires for future care will have been expressed and wishes be known. It may be that admission to a palliative care unit or hospital is requested, or alternatively, the patient and carers may wish to continue at home.

Sometimes the patient who is actually in hospital may request to go home to die. It is all too easy to tell the patient that he, or she is too ill, and yet with the co-ordination of all the services available, and laying on of adequate caring facilities at home, it may be possible to grant that last wish.

Caring at home

Approximately 25 per cent of patients die at home but according to Hinton (1991) most people express a desire to die at home. Certainly admission is not necessarily best unless physical and emotional needs cannot be met at home. Where possible it should be the patient's choice. Field and James suggest that many people deem an ideal way to die as being comfortably in one's own bed in familiar surroundings with family and friends present (Clark, 1993). Home may be a more peaceful, relaxed informal atmosphere in which to die with those the patient cares about around him or her, and it encourages family participation.

Patients being cared for at home require adequate provision of the following.

- *Time.* Patients and families need to be given time to express their anxieties and fears. Nurses with good listening and communication skills are a valuable asset.
- *Personnel.* Community nursing staff are of prime importance in offering time, professional skills and support. In many areas the community nurses may be supported in their role by a specialist nurse who is experienced in symptom control, and the support of patients at home who have cancer. It is essential that all members of the caring team liaise closely with the patient's general practitioner. Night nursing services and Marie Curie Foundation services have an important contribution to make where they are available. Relief at night eases the pressure on relatives and ensures continuity of care.
- *Equipment.* Availability of loans are essential to aid the provision of quality care. The patient may require material items such as mattress covers, commodes, wheelchairs. urinals, bedcraddles, antipressure devices, and feeding cups.
- *Comfort.* Temperature must be maintained so extra heating may be required. Grants may be available to help finance this need. Sometimes the provision of extra bedding will be necessary and some areas have a laundry service.
- *Resources.* Caring for patients at home can make greater demands on available resources as more frequent visits may be required to ensure effective symptom control and care. Four hourly injections may be necessary, however, today in many areas the need for regular injection therapy has been almost eliminated with the advent of the 24–h syringe driver (see Chapter 3 for further information on syringe drivers).

Within the home it is especially important to ensure that drug therapy is readily available, with clear instructions and controlled drug records. As the patient's condition deteriorates and he or she is unable to take oral medication, a supply of intramuscular or subcutaneous analgesic drugs, such as diamorphine should be available in the home. It is also helpful to have a supply of

antiemetics, and some form of sedation for use as necessary in suppository or injection form. Hyoscine may be useful to minimise the 'death rattle'.
- *Professional carers.* The basis of good care at home is reliant on having an efficient, knowledgeable, empathetic team, who are communicating well and able to anticipate and so prevent problems. They must be able to work with and support the family.

Apart from specific needs associated with home, the care of the person at home, in a palliative care unit, or ward is very similar. Hinton observes that people dying at home are better able to maintain themselves as individuals and are still part of the family (Hinton, 1991).

Remaining at home may not be practical or possible for some people. Neale and Clarke (1992) observe that social rather than medical considerations have been identified as factors in the patients admission to hospital and consequent breakdown of informal care-giving.

Admission to palliative care unit or hospital

Reasons for admission include the following.

- Lack of provision of appropriate care and support.
- Inability of carer to cope physically
- Inability of carer to cope emotionally.
- Fear of the unknown.
- Patients request not to die at home.
- Difficulty in controlling symptoms.
- The need for 24-h nursing or medical care.

Timing for admission if carefully planned will allow the person an adequate period to settle in and become familiar with surroundings and staff. Leaving it too late may cause confusion and restlessness.

The move must be seen as both acceptable and desirable to the patient and the family, so as to minimise feelings of failure and guilt. This may prove a difficult time to the patient who has inevitably had to face many losses associated with the illness.

A rising proportion of people now die in some type of residential care and consequently have had to face the loss of their home, and now the prospect of losing life itself.

Admission – ward versus a single room

Patients nursed in single rooms may have increased psychological and physical needs especially if they are afraid of being alone. Equally it may be a comfort and less distressing if relatives are able to remain with them. Isolation can be a very frightening lonely experience. It may be desirable to move a patient to a single room for medical reasons, or if the situation is particularly distressing. The patients or relatives sometimes request it for privacy. Moves should only be made after careful consideration of the reason and implications. It is not necessarily in the best interests of the patient or those around them to remove them from familiar surroundings and companionship. For other patients it may conjure up an air of unease, suspicion and mystery if the person is suddenly removed, without explanation never to be heard of again. Most nurses have observed the fear of the person moved to a corner bed in a general ward, near the door or to a cubicle. The patient may recognise this as a final move and feel as though he or she is being shown the door before they are ready to leave. Sensitive explanation will avoid this and care must be taken to keep ward morale up, as other patients may fear this move for themselves. Fears of a distressing death may be eliminated by the observation of a quiet, peaceful death of the patient well supported by caring staff. It has been known for a patient to say 'if that is what death is like I am no longer afraid', and so a service to other patients may be done. However the repeated deaths of those with whom meaningful relationships have been established may be demoralising and depressing, so a willingness on behalf of the nurse to spend time with the remaining patients, encouraging them to express their feelings and fears In a positive way is appreciated.

It may be possible to provide a quieter, more peaceful atmosphere at home or in a palliative care unit rather than in a busy general ward.

The dying patient's needs

Dying can be a lonely experience and that loneliness can be increased if people avoid the patient because they don't know what to say or how to say things. Most people need some companionship. Loneliness can be worse in a busy ward where the patient is surrounded by hustle and bustle, and they see others getting well but their own life is slipping away.

Dying patients often become resigned to the approach of death but may need help to express themselves. The sensitive nurse can encourage them to talk and questions will often be of the type needing reassurance such as when and how they will die. Every nurse has a responsibility to face up to questions with quiet honest reassurance. Denying death will only bring more distress (see Chapter 2). Most experienced nurses can recognise when the patient is entering the final stage of the illness and is likely to die in the near future. Maintaining the comfort of the patient remains very important throughout.

Position. When patients becomes weaker and unable to move easily, frequent gentle massage and assistance to change position will relieve stiffness and discomfort and may well ease restlessness. Many patients prefer to be propped up a little with the head well supported and dislike the supine position intensely.

Skin. Some people perspire profusely and feel cold to the touch as peripheral circulation fails. The skin often becomes discoloured and mottled. Gentle sponging is helpful, also regular care to pressure areas. The use of appropriate pressure relieving equipment will aid care.

Thirst. This may be a last craving and can be eased with frequent small sips of water or by allowing the patient to suck fluid from a sponge. Keeping the lips moist is essential and protection with lip salve or a little Vaseline helps.

Mouths. Mouth care is essential to the end. They should be kept moist, dry mouths soon become dirty mouths, and unless attended to, dirty mouths will become sore and infected. Dry mouths can often be eased by giving drinks which increase the flow of saliva, such as citrus fruits, or sucking pieces of ice or frozen tonic water. Glycerine and lemon mouth swabs are comforting.

Treatment to the mouth should be carried out as often as required. Dirty mouths can be cleaned with a solution of sodium bicarbonate or hydrogen peroxide. Teeth should be kept clean, whether false or not. Infections should be treated and at this stage Nystatin suspension is often the easiest to administer.

Restlessness. There may be many causes of restlessness in the dying patient and before resorting to sedation the eliminatory care of the patient should be checked. Most patients hate being imprisoned by the bedclothes being tucked in too tightly and they may become restless in order to rid themselves of their burden. A change of position may help. A full bladder will aggravate restlessness. Pain must be controlled. Patients are more restful if they have put their house in order and it may be that, even at this late stage, if they are capable, they need to make a will, or repair a broken relationship.

Eyes. Frequent bathing with normal saline will help, especially when a patient is sleeping deeply or is unconscious with eyes part opened. If the eyes become sore installation of 'artificial tears' may help.

Spiritual. The chaplain or clergyman's visit may be appreciated and bring comfort to both patients and their families. The nurses' respect for the person does not permit them to impose their own faith or views upon the patient, but they may be able to bring comfort verbally or by unspoken presence and reassurance so helping the person to find peace of mind.

Support. When the patient deteriorates and becomes more ill, it may be that less time gets spent with him or her. On a busy general ward with other needs pressing, the entourage of doctors may pass by leaving the patient disillusioned. The visits of the doctor, however short, can be a great comfort to the person, as they realise they are still important and not forgotten.

At the end of life the dying person may appreciate a family member or friend sitting with them. If this is not possible a nurse or perhaps, volunteer should fill this role to ensure the patient does not die alone.

Medication. As the patient draws near to the end of life most medications can be discontinued with the exception of analgesia, antiemetics and some drugs made available for specific individual problems. The latter are usually given on an as required basis.

Analgesia should never be abruptly discontinued, even when the patient appears deeply unconscious. Restlessness and marked distress can occur if pain is allowed to break through. At this stage the patient may not be able to communicate, so unknown suffering can be caused if analgesia is thoughtlessly withheld. It must be remembered that the patient may have been taking opiates for pain relief for many months.

During the last period of life it may be useful to use a 24-h syringe driver (see Chapter 3) to administer regular medications, so abolishing the need for 4-hourly injections to a person who is probably very thin and frail. Diamorphine hydrochloride is often used for injections as 'its high water solubility allows small volume injection' (Regnard *et al.*, 1983) which is an advantage. The use of the syringe driver entails multiplying the single injection dose by the number of times it would be given in 24 h and administering that dose by the syringe driver over a 24-h period.

Death rattle. This is when secretions collect in the throat and oscillate with respiration. The patient no longer has the strength to expectorate and so a bubbling sound occurs. A change of position may alleviate this, or hyoscine given by injection at the earliest detection may prevent this situation from developing. Hyoscine may need to be repeated at regular intervals, but if the 'death rattle' is marked it is unlikely to be effective, because its action is to prevent secretions from forming, not to dry them up. The patient generally appears oblivious of the situation but it is the relative who becomes distressed and needs explanation and reassurance.

'Cheyne Stoke' breathing may occur and again may be worrying to the family so should be explained.

Senses. It is a well-known phenomenon to put curtains around a bed and nurse the patient in a semi-darkened room. However most patients, when they are dying, have a fear of the dark and desire gentle light and fresh air. They have a need to experience quiet feelings of life around them. Throughout the final period of life there is a need for contact. Sims comments that touch is one of the first senses to develop and is a basic way of communicating (Wilson-Barnett and Raiman, 1988). If the patient lingers he or she may be aware who is with them although unable to communicate. Care must be taken in regard to what is said in the presence of the apparently unconscious person as hearing is one of the last senses to be lost.

At the point of death most people are unconscious and have been for some time. There are a small number who drift in and out of consciousness and, although weary, are usually peaceful, relaxed and seem accepting of the situation. Most people wish to die in their sleep. Sedation may be necessary for the restless person when other causes have been excluded.

When death has occurred the relatives may appreciate a few quiet moments alone with the patient to pay their last respects. Simple prayers, said at the bedside after death, with the family if they so wish, may bring great comfort.

The role and care of relatives and friends

Relatives and friends are not patients or clients of the patients' professional carer in their own right. Therefore their needs are not always met.

Twycross and Lack (1990) suggest that the care of the family is an integral part of the care of the dying.

Many events cause stress in a family, because every member interacts with each other, so any problems will affect them all. Equally the patient's response will be affected by the carer's reaction to the illness. Clark (1993) considers that no two carers' needs and activities are the same, and that the closer the relationship, the greater the emotional strain is likely to be.

The average person encounters and copes with many stresses in a 'normal' life and it is worth remembering that most people do cope. A very stressful time for the family is being told of an unfavourable diagnosis or prognosis. This may be done at visiting time when they must remain composed to visit the patient. This may further inhibit questions, which in turn may lead to confusion over already revealed facts. An area of discord is where the patient is given information optimistically, and they pessimistically. Twycross and Lack (1990) consider there is much to be said for joint interviews where the patient and carer are seen by the doctor in the presence of a nurse, who will then be available to clarify the doctor's statements and deal with the on-going situation.

Faulkner (1993) suggests that one of the major hurdles for the family is when treatment regimes are seen not to work. Until this point, and actually being told, the carer can hope the patient will get well. Now they have to reconsider their goals.

It can be a particularly distressing time emotionally for the family as they travel along the road with the ill person unable to alter the direction. This may increase any feelings of helplessness and vulnerability. Throughout the illness the fears of the patient, family and friends are intertwined. They may experience the same emotions but frequently not at the same time, so are out of step with each other. Anger, anxiety and depression may all be a part of the process of adjustment, although it seems that patients appear to experience anger less often than their carers. Clark (1993) observes that researchers have rated anxiety as the greatest problem faced by a carer. There may also be feelings of guilt, which is understandable as no relationship is perfect and people can always find something to feel guilty about. Social isolation of the carer caused by restriction on their life, due to their caring role, may lead to resentment and later guilt. Some people try to justify their existence, whereas, for others there may be secret relief at the expected demise of the person. They will naturally feel guilty about that and may even feel responsible if at some time they wished the person dead.

Faulkner (1993) observes that even when the whole family is involved, difficulties in adapting to the fact that the person may die still arises. There may be conflict over whether a person should or should not be told. The reason for the carers resistance may initially be their own disbelief, or anxiety over their own ability to cope. Talking of death is still avoided by many people.

Families may need to be helped to see that if the patient is asking and genuinely wants to know, then it is important not to lie, but in telling hope must not be destroyed.

A woman who was told her husband's diagnosis, was also told she should not tell him. She kept this secret for 2 years even though he asked, but eventually when he became more ill it was impossible to keep up the pretence and he was told. This man was not angry or bitter, only hurt. Hurt that his wife had kept this secret from him all that time, when their marriage had previously been loving, open and shared. For the last 7 months of his life they were able to share again, both the good and the bad spells. His wife was a very capable lady who set goals with her husband and together they achieved many things. However, the experience of hurt has never left this woman.

All carers have needs and throughout the person's illness it is important to try and meet these. There will be need for practical help and information on all aspects of care, including financial benefits that are available. It is important that they as well as the patient are supported emotionally throughout the duration of the illness. They may need relief in the form of respite care. This may entail a sitting service at home or admission to some sort of residential care for a period of time. Throughout the illness it is reassuring for the family to know that the professional is caring for the whole person in the fullest sense. The family need encouragement and recognition in their caring role.

As the patient's condition deteriorates withdrawal from the person by the relative may occur, which is understandable as they now lead different lives, and the relative has to think about a future that does not exist for the patient. Equally there may be withdrawal by the patient. Both the patient and the family need to be helped to accept that this is natural. Quiet support and just being together is important. However, one must remember that not all family relationships are close or loving. Some families find it hard to let go, they may not be ready to do so.

Families are not guests but an essential part of any caring team and as key members should be encouraged to take an active role in decision making and care. They need to feel useful and helpful.

It must be remembered how easy it is to unintentionally neglect some relatives if they are reluctant to bother apparently busy staff, but they need time and support as much as anyone. When talking to relatives silences must be tolerated as these give them opportunity to collect their thoughts, and think through what has been said. It is the nurse's role to help them to find their own meaning in the situation but not to impose their own views.

The relative may find it hard to cope with the illness, especially when the patient is acting out of character. Their own anxieties and fears may cause physical manifestations such as weight loss, sleep disturbances, anorexia and lack of concentration, being unable to settle to anything. They will need extra support through this difficult period.

The latter period of time leading up to the death may be particularly distressing to the family. It is frequently a time when they need added support and reassurance. Over the telephone a little personal information and reference to the patient by name can be comforting. This may be a time when they do not really appear to be comprehending what is happening. A friendly welcome makes the relative feel needed and wanted. They may need encouragement to show natural affection and maintain contact by touch. Even in the last stages of life they have an important role to play, a job to do, perhaps sitting holding a hand, moistening a mouth or helping with practical care.

They need to witness a peaceful death, and be reassured that they have done all they could if that is so.

If the relative wishes to stay the nurse should not misguidedly discourage them from this last caring act by urging them to go home and get a good night's rest. This may be the last opportunity to give of themselves to the patient. Where possible an overnight room should be provided.

If the relative was not present at the death it is often helpful to reassure them of the comfort and peacefulness of the patient. It may be helpful to remind them that they were there when the patient could enjoy their company.

After death a quiet chat over a cup of tea can be helpful. The grieving one should be allowed to cry even though it may be uncomfortable to observe. Time to listen to the relatives is essential. Time to share the grief, the memories, the good times and the bad. Even sharing in silence can bring comfort to the grieving one. All too often people feel they must talk and sometimes this can be inappropriate and cause more distress. Support is very important at this time and the need to be busy and leave the person can be hurtful. A caring person can give more help than is realised.

If the death is to occur at home the family should be warned what to expect in the time preceding death. They need to know to call the general practitioner as soon as possible after the person has died. The doctor will visit to confirm death, and may write the medical certificate of death at the house, but if not, the family may be asked to collect it from the surgery later.

If the person was in hospital the attending doctor will sign the medical certificate of death. It is important that the family or next of kin understands about the collection of the death certificate and personal belongings of the patient. It can be helpful if there are written instructions because people often forget when stressed.

Once the doctor has confirmed the death and issued the appropriate certificate, the death can be registered. This is usually done by a near relative, at the registrar's office of the district in which the patient actually died. After certification of death a funeral director can be contacted to make arrangements for the deceased to be removed to a chapel of rest, but until registration takes place he can proceed no further. Funeral directors act on behalf of the family, making all necessary arrangements and are usually very helpful and caring, paying attention to detail. The family can be sure they will guide them through this difficult period. See Chapter 17 on bereavement.

The role and care of the nurse

It is important to summarise the role of the nurse in caring for patients with a limited life span. The nurse's role is to assist the person to live life as fully as possible, within the limitations imposed by the illness, until they die, maintaining hope, achieving goals and coping with the everyday situation.

Nash discusses the need for the nurse to journey alongside the family in their struggle rather than allowing the protective urge to take over (Wilson–Barnett and Raiman, 1988).

The nurse should be a provider of quality care, using his or her knowledge, expertise and skills at the appropriate times throughout the person's life. Holistic care which entails fulfilment of physical, psychological, social and spiritual needs can be better understood if the nurse understands the hierarchy of needs (see Table 13.1) formulated by Maslow (Quinn, 1980).

The nurse's role involves being a care giver, advisor, facilitator, enabler and educator to both patients and their families, bearing in mind that they may come from different cultural backgrounds with their own traditions. The nurse must be able to co–ordinate services and communicate effectively with the patient, carers and the whole caring team.

The nurse has a responsibility to share his or her expertise with colleagues and others. Counselling and facilitating are important roles. The nurse needs to be a positive listener, giving the person encouragement to identify problems, and find their own acceptable solutions, by knowing available resources. Counselling also involves dealing with feelings and the nurse must control the natural response to console and calm, but rather encourage the person to express the feelings they have. Negative feelings may have to be dealt with. It is crucial that nurses do not take over and impose their own views.

Table 13.1 Hierarchy of needs (special emphasis on those with a limited life-span)

Physiological	basic survival and comfort needs
Safety and security	confidence in carers receiving explanations and information
Love and belonging	being understood and accepted for themselves as a unique human being. Feeling needed – family unity
Self-esteem	recognition of need for independence and dignity achievement of goals
Self-actualisation	finding a meaning in death and working towards acceptance and disengagement from environment

Relatives must be kept fully informed and the nurse must have the ability to involve them in care as appropriate. This will be much appreciated and may well help to minimise social loss and separation anxiety.

The support role involves many other roles and will bring much comfort. It is said that just being there, willing to listen, share and show concern is all that matters, but support must not be a prop, which when taken away, causes everything to collapse.

This is a time when the nurse is permitted to share a very personal part of that person's life, when barriers are stripped and the real person is apparent. This is a great privilege for any nurse but also a responsibility. The effect on a nurse when a patient dies can be one of grief as though a friend has been lost. Professional people are often expected to be detached and uninvolved (Summers), but nurses are ordinary caring people with feelings like everyone else. They too may feel helpless, upset, moved or even relieved when a person dies. They also need to express their feelings and find an outlet. Shame should never be felt at a damp eye. Caring for these patients is intensive personal rather than curative care (Summers and Young).

Nash warns of the danger of the nurse losing sight of the role due to over-work, over-commitment and over-involvement without sufficient support (Wilson-Barnett and Raiman, 1988). So it is important that the nurse looks at herself, her philosophy of life and death, her feelings, and how and why she reacts as she does. In so doing, she will hopefully understand those she cares for better, and be able to help them look at themselves and share with them. It is important that the nurse knows how, and from where to obtain her own support, that she develops her own coping mechanisms and has a balanced life outside caring for these people, in order to prevent stress and 'burnout'.

'Let as much as possible be done'. Caring for the patient near to the end of life is a great challenge, and, if nurses provide holistic care and support, the patient will achieve much in their limited life-span.

References

ALDERMAN, C. (1988) *Controlling Pain. Nursing Standard*, pp. 31–2. Scutari Press.
BURKE, C. and SIKORA, K. (1992). Cancer – the dual approach. *Nursing Times* 88, 62–6.

CLARK, D. (1993). *The Future for Palliative Care.* Open University Press.
CROWTHER, D. (1991). Complementary therapy in practice. *Nursing Standard* 5, 25–7.
DICKENSON, D. and JOHNSON, M. (1993). *Death, Dying and Bereavement.* Sage.
DOBBS, B. Z. (1985). Alternative health approaches. *Nursing Mirror* 160, 41–2.
FAULKNER, A. (1993). Helping relatives to cope with a diagnosis of cancer in a loved one. *Journal of Cancer Care* 2, 132–6.
FORDHAM, M. and DUNN, V. (1994). *Alongside the Person in Pain.* Baillière-Tindall.
HELP THE HOSPICES (1993). *Hospice Day Care – A Qualitative Study.* Trent Palliative Care Centre.
HIGGINSON, I. (1993). *Matching Services to Individual Needs.* National Council for Hospice and Specialist Palliative Care Services. Land & Unwin (Data Sciences) Ltd, Northampton.
HINTON, J. (1991). *Dying.* Penguin, Harmondsworth.
MORRISON, R. (1992). Diagnosing spiritual pain in patients. *Nursing Standard* 6, 36–8.
NEALE, B. and CLARK, D. (1992). Informal care of people with cancer: a review of research on needs and services. *Journal of Cancer Care* 1, 193–7.
PRIMARY HEALTH CARE (1993). Countdown to April. *Primary Health Care* 3, 9–11.
QUINN, F. N. (1980). *The Principles and Practice of Nurse Education.* Croom Helm.
REGNARD, C. F. B., DAVIES, A. and RANDALL, F. (1983). *A Guide to Symptom Relief in Advanced Cancer.* Drogher Press.
SAUNDERS, C. and SYKES, N. (1993). *The Management of Terminal Malignant Disease.* Hodder & Stoughton, Sevenoaks.
SHAW, C. (1993). Appetite and appetite stimulants. *European Journal of Cancer Care* 2, 121.
SMITH, J. P. (1981). *Sociology and Nursing.* Churchill Livingstone.
SUMMERS, D. H. *Staff Support.* St Christopher's Hospice Leaflet.
SUMMERS, D. H. and YOUNG, J. N. *To Comfort Always.* St Christopher's Hospice Booklet.
TWYCROSS, R. G. and LACK, S. A. (1990). *Therapeutics in Terminal Cancer.* Churchill Livingstone.
WILSON-BARNETT, J. and RAIMAN, J. (1988). *Nursing Issues and Research in Terminal Care.* John Wiley, Chichester.

Further reading

BUCKMAN, R. (1988). *I Don't Know What to Say.* Papermac.
CLARK, D. (1993). *The Future for Palliative Care.* Open University Press.
DICKENSON, D. and JOHNSON, M. (1993). *Death, Dying and Bereavement.* Sage.
FORDHAM, M. and DUNN, V. (1994). *Alongside the Person in Pain.* Baillière-Tindall.
HINTON, J. (1991). *Dying.* Penguin.
MACPAC (1992). *Helpful Essential Links To Palliative Care.* Centre for Medical Education, University of Dundee.
SAUNDERS, C. and SYKES, N. (1993). *The Management of Terminal Malignant Disease.* Hodder & Stoughton, Sevenoaks.
TWYCROSS, R. G. and LACK, S. A. (1990). *Therapeutics in Terminal Cancer.* Churchill Livingstone.
WILSON-BARNETT, J. and RAIMAN, J. (1988). *Nursing Issues and Research in Terminal Care.* John Wiley, Chichester.

14

The special needs of children and adolescents

Denise Hodson

'To cure sometimes, to relieve often, to comfort always'.
M. Strauss (Familiar Medical Quotations)

Background

The last 20 years have seen great advances in the diagnosis, treatment and survival of children with cancer. Each year, approximately 1200 children are diagnosed as having a malignant disease in the UK. Childhood malignancies differ from adult cancers. Childhood tumours are commonly sarcomas or blastomas, unlike those of adults which are principally carcinomas. The most commonly treated childhood cancer is lymphoblastic leukaemia. However, childhood cancer is rare. Only 1 child in 10,000 per year under 15 years of age develops a malignant disease. The rarity of these diseases led to the development in the UK of regionally based paediatric oncology units in the 1970s, to facilitate research, diagnosis, treatment and the evaluation necessary in order to provide the optimal chance of cure for this small group of children. Seventy-five per cent of children with malignant disease receive all or part of their therapy in these units. Over 60 per cent are now expected to survive. The reduction in mortality has seen cancer as a cause of death in childhood (OPCS, 1987) fall from second to third, after accidents and congenital abnormalities (Fig. 14.1).

The intensive treatment regimes necessitate repeated hospitalisation for many children, with their parents, sometimes for lengthy periods. For most children, frequent out-patient visits are necessary, travelling to the oncology unit which may be many miles away. Oncology units may 'share-care' with district general hospitals to alleviate some of the problems caused by distance, to promote communication and establish confidence in the care-givers in the patient's own community.

Paediatric oncology units employ a multidisciplinary team approach, involving health visitors/liaison nurses, social workers, psychologists, dieticians and others, in caring for the child and his or her family. Spinetta and Deasey-Spinetta (1981) have shown that the whole family is affected when a diagnosis of cancer is made in a child. The unit's aim is to help families in whatever way they feel appropriate, to be able to understand and cope with their child's illness, enabling them to continue their natural role as primary care-givers and support them through the treatment and the uncertainty of the eventual outcome (Koocher and O'Malley, 1981). It is

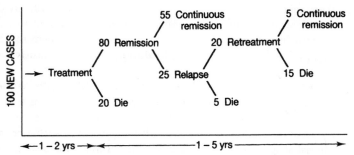

Fig. 14.1 One hundred typical paediatric oncology patients.

the aim of the units to adopt an honest and realistic approach from the time of diagnosis, an approach that facilitates discussion and understanding between parents, children and staff.

Although the outlook for most children is encouraging, there remains approximately one-third for whom a cure will not be achieved. A small number of these will die in the earlier stages of treatment from their disease, from infection or complications of the drug therapy, usually in hospital. For others, relapse or failure to achieve a remission may have meant further treatment programmes. Advancement of the disease necessitates a reassessment of aims and values and a change in expectations, that a cure will not be achieved and a period of palliative care is beginning.

Decision to end curative treatment

The decision to end attempts at curative therapy is not one made lightly. Where there is a progression of disease or the adverse effects of further treatment outweigh the benefits which can realistically be achieved, the need for on-going open communication between the parents, the child, if he or she is old enough, and the oncology unit is essential. It is important that all aspects of the treatment and the progression of disease are discussed so that the subsequent decision that active therapy has no further value is understood and made jointly with the professional carers. Open communication allows the older child or teenager to participate in these discussions, so that he or she too can be helped to decide if he or she wants to try new drug treatments or, if they wish, to set their own agenda in making new goals for their future. No family should be left to make the decision alone.

Children and parents develop close ties and relationships with carers in the oncology units over many months, often years. Once the decision to end therapy has been made, there is a real need for the assurance of continuing support and expression of the carers concern for the child's continuing quality of life. Fears of being 'abandoned' or no longer part of the unit's immediate priorities are real anxieties many parents experience, with fears of what the future will hold and worries about their abilities to cope. The goals set for future care will involve re-establishing and making new contacts at home, symptom control and to help the family resume a normality of family life. There is a need to help them make plans and to 'invest' in the time left and make this final time of caring a positive one for living.

Regional oncology units encompass many districts and health authorities. Families may live in densely populated industrial areas or in rural districts. It is the practise of oncology centres to establish communication with community carers at an early stage of treatment. Contact with the general practitioner is made at the time of initial diagnosis, by phone and letter. Links will also have been made by the unit's health visitor or liaison nurse to those already involved with the family at home – their health visitor or school nurse and the teachers. The first contact is important not only to establish a link, but to allow the exchange of relevant information. The rarity of childhood malignancies means that most general practitioners will only see one or two cases of cancer in a child throughout their career. Opportunities to meet and discuss cases are usually welcomed by both hospital and community staff.

It is at the time of relapse of the disease and the decision to end attempts at curative therapy that the framework of contact made at diagnosis establishes its importance. By building on the lines of communication, the feasibility of care that is needed can realistically be offered. Martinson *et al.* (1986) and Chambers *et al.* (1989) have demonstrated that by working together, the hospital and community carers can establish a plan of joint care to support the child and family in any way the family deems appropriate to enable them to care for their child.

The availability of carers and facilities differs widely from district to district. Health visitors, district nurses, paediatric community nurses, Macmillan or Marie Curie nurses are but a few of the appropriate professionals whose skills may be sought, but of course not all are available as a resource in any given area. The resources of oncology units also differs. Most can offer visits from liaison nurses/health visitors and social workers. Hospital doctors may also visit. For some units, distance may mean the majority of contact with families and home carers is made by phone. The most important factor is that appropriate care and support is given by those most acceptable to the family.

Establishing the pattern of care

Where the needs of the dying child and his or her family are best met has been the subject of much discussion and research (Wilson, 1985; Armstrong and Martinson, 1980). At the turn of the century home was the natural and obvious place to be born and to die, with family and friends around. Medical advances over the years changed expectations as treatments were developed for many previously life-threatening illnesses. The specialist care centres for children with cancer were presumed to be the most appropriate place for these children to be. Now, however, options other than the acute busy hospital setting are considered. Dying children especially want to be cared for at home (Armstrong and Martinson,

1980), care which can be given by parents in familiar surroundings, if they are helped by nursing and medical staff, even though they are living with the knowledge that their child will die soon (Martinson *et al.*, 1984).

Many factors can influence the decision: duration of terminal illness, distance from the hospital, availability of local support and the immediate medical/nursing needs of the child are but a few. There may be anxieties expressed by parents about their own ability to deliver adequate care, about the response of other children and fears of uncontrolled symptoms especially pain. They may be reticent to discuss these fears unless specifically given the opportunity to do so. Parents and children who choose to remain or return to hospital should not be left with feelings of failure – it may be right for them and it is important they feel they have done the best for their child.

Whatever the outcome, parents should know that no decision is irreversible and that an open-door policy is maintained, so that children can be cared for in the most appropriate way and place at any given time. For most families home is preferable, where family, friends and the familiar surroundings provide the comfort and support throughout this difficult time.

For some children hospice care may provide the alternative to home/hospital care. The concept of hospice care for adults is well established, with emphasis on the quality of life and symptom control to enable the person to live their life with dignity, control and fulfilment. There are few children's hospices in Britain. The first to be established to care for children who were dying was Helen House in Oxford. A retrospective study of 25 families who attended the hospice examined their perceptions of the care offered and of the impact of a life-threatening disease on the family (Stein *et al.*, 1989). Most families felt they were greatly helped by the individualised family-orientated care and atmosphere. However, the fact that the care was delivered in a setting solely for terminally ill children was considered a drawback. The home-from-home atmosphere where all the family could be together was deemed particularly appropriate for those whose child or children suffered a degenerative condition, and for whom periods of respite care could be offered. The impact experienced by families, caused by illness, was substantial and felt by all members. This included psychological difficulties, worries about symptom control, emotional and behavioural difficulties of siblings, financial and employment problems.

Figures show the largest group of children to benefit from the care of Helen House in its first year were those with central nervous disorders, followed by those with mucopolysaccharidosis (Burne *et al.*, 1984). Children with a malignant disease formed a much smaller group. Most children were admitted for respite care either as a planned admission or as a crisis-situation intervention.

The duration of terminal illness in children with malignant disease differs widely from those with degenerative disorders. For most, the time span can be measured in weeks to short months, establishing care at home as a feasible option. The role of the children's hospice should remain an option to be considered when care for a child is being planned.

Caring for a dying child is one of the most difficult and emotional times in which professional carers are all involved. For nurses and practitioners in the community their previous experience will probably be limited. Many have expressed their feelings of anxiety in caring for a child and in their ability to deliver appropriate care and symptom control. The initial reaction is often that children are 'different' and that they lack the necessary expertise. The actual principles of caring for the terminally ill are similar no matter what the age of the patient. The practises may differ when the patient is a child, but community carers have a wealth of experience and skills to offer.

Over long months or years the parents have become 'specialists' in their child's disease and treatment and have usually participated actively in general procedures, treatments and care. Their dependence on the oncology unit has already been described. Feelings of inadequacy experienced by some carers are understandable as families may bypass their general practitioner or nurse and contact the hospital unit directly. This can lead to feelings of 'exclusiveness' and make involvement seem difficult. If pathways of communication are kept open and contact is freely made by both hospital and home carers some of these difficulties can be minimised through active discussion and sharing of problems.

Principles of care

The principles of palliative care remain constant.

To continue meaningful communication with the child and family

Research (Norman and Bennet, 1986; Martinson, 1980) has shown that the majority of time spent in the child's home is spent listening to worries, fears and feelings expressed by families and in providing a 'listening' support. To be able to sit and listen is probably the most valuable contribution any carer can make. It asks carers to question their own attitudes to the process of dying and death, and to acknowledge the grief felt within this family.

Symptom control when necessary

As symptoms arise through the progression of disease it is important that they are not considered in isolation but that the physical and emotional needs of the child as a whole are considered. There may be more than one specific cause and younger children may have difficulties explaining how they feel. Various tools (Eland, 1985; Jerret and Evans, 1986) are available to assist us in assessing symptoms especially pain. Parents will describe changes in physical or emotional needs or abilities which often provide a valuable guide.

To respond appropriately to their on-going needs

The needs of the child and family can change quickly as palliative care evolves. The duration of care is variable and input in practical terms is dependent on the advancement of disease and the symptoms experienced. Subjects discussed may relate to other family members or friends or to practical issues such as finance, heating, bills or other needs. It may be appropriate to draw on the particular skills of other carers in the hospital or community to address specific problems.

Effective liaison and sharing of information between hospital and community carers

Throughout this time and after death the oncology unit will maintain contact by phone calls and visits to the child and family. Joint visits with community carers can reassure parents that everyone is working in close cooperation for their child's comfort and support. Maintaining contact between the hospital and community can lessen the feelings of isolation for staff and families alike.

Communicating with parents

The families of dying children are generally more extended than those of adults in similar circumstances, including grandparents, relatives, close friends and the child's peers in their family unit. Younger members may not have experienced death before and the experience is made more intensive and felt more strongly when the death is that of a child (Wilson, 1988). The needs of the family and their child have been identified as similar to, but not identical, to those of dying adults and their families (Wilson, 1985).

Parents may again feel all the emotions that surrounded the time of initial diagnosis; those of shock, anger and of disbelief, 'Perhaps the doctors have made a mistake, perhaps the scan is wrong, or not my child's'. For many these feelings are entwined in a deeper knowledge gained by living with his or her disease and its treatment over many months or years, and an acknowledgement that the grief began at diagnosis and has only been suppressed. A general observation is that mothers may be more pessimistic throughout treatment and fathers more optimistic. This may be a result of more mothers being resident with their child in hospital and forming close relationships with other parents. They seek information, not only about their child, and share good and bad times with other parents. Fathers may prefer to remain optimistic for their child's recovery, as they continue to work and organise normal activities at home for other children, and prefer to concentrate only on their child's progress.

Parents are individuals in their own right and their needs will differ throughout this time. They may find it difficult to relate to one another, as the impact of their differing emotions falls on the person they are closest to. They need to be given time to talk freely together, and individually, with carers. A common reaction is to blame either themselves for not preventing the disease or the impending death, or to blame others for not diagnosing the disease earlier.

Their hopes and expectations are forced to change direction, from the hopes of a cure to being able to give their child a peaceful, happy and painfree time to come. In a study to try to identify the needs of families with a terminally ill relative, O'Brian (1983) noted (i) their need for information and (ii) the need to be assured of their relatives comfort and that appropriate care was being given. The same opportunities to talk to medical and nursing staff should be open to the child's siblings and relatives, as they may have questions which they feel are inappropriate to be asked of the parents at this time.

In conversation with parents, some have said that their relatives make the situation more difficult to cope with. They seem entwined in their own grief and their need to 'put things right' and in expressing false hopes. Repeated explanations about changes in the child's condition and treatment become tiresome in the battle of maintaining a normality of family life. Parents express a need to talk to people who understand what is happening and for whom explanations are not necessary.

All parents will ask when their child will die, 'How long do we have with him?' A question that is impossible to answer in absolute terms. We can only answer in the very broadest sense in the light of our past experiences. No-one can answer in definitive terms of weeks or months, only maybe in the final hours.

Other questions will explore the way in which death will occur, 'Will it be sudden?' and, most importantly, 'Will he be in pain?' The professional carer is more able to discuss the answers to these questions at length, with knowledge about the most likely developments of their child's particular disease. It is difficult to describe these developments as options which may or may not happen to families, but parents feel better prepared to deal with symptoms or situations as they arise. They know that individual possibilities have been anticipated and that measures have been planned that will ensure their child's comfort.

Communicating with the patient

Childhood encompasses a wide age-range, from babies up to adolescence. The individual's age, development, both physically and psychologically, and experiences are all important factors to be considered. During illness and hospitalisation the child's need for his or her parents increases as he or she fears separation from the people and places they knows best. Children are happiest in their own home, with the normality of family life providing a secure environment (Armstrong and Martinson, 1980). Concepts of death are directly related to age and to personal experiences, and one needs to know about the child's understanding of death to be able to hold a meaningful discussion with them.

Children

In healthy children aged 0–3 years, the word 'death' has little meaning. The most frightening thought is that of separation from their parents and of being left alone. Between 3 and 5 years a curiosity about death and 'being dead' develops. Seeing birds or animals who have died promotes the idea of not moving, or eating, maybe sleeping? Whatever – it is not permanent. They feel invincible. Children will associate death with heaven. Heaven seems a real place where dead people go to be with others. The concept of not being able to visit, or of those who have died not returning at some time, seems strange.

From 6 years there is a gradual understanding that being dead is permanent, although for many, games played or television programmes watched reiterate the fact that their heroes recover to fight another battle next week or they can 'begin again' in a different game. Death can be thought of as a 'ghost' or associated with acts of violence or being 'bad'.

The development of children from 10 years upwards and the wider experiences they have gained leads them towards a more adult reasoning of dying and death and an awareness that one day they too will die and that it will be permanent.

The ages and above outline are very broad and generalised. Children will vary widely in their understanding of death, as in their physical development and their intellectual ability at any age. Children who are very ill and have experienced repeated hospitalisation, traumatic procedures and possibly the loss of a friend through death will experience a much greater awareness of the meaning, possibly at a younger age than most of their peers.

It was thought that ill young children had little or no concept of their own death, but research (Spinetta *et al.*, 1974) has shown much higher anxiety levels and feelings of isolation, possibly as parents seek to protect their child by avoiding addressing the issue or by changes in their normal attitude toward the child. Parents may have prepared themselves, however subconsciously, for the time when curative treatment ends. This preparation has been defined as anticipatory mourning, a set of processes that are directly related to the awareness of impending loss, to the emotional impact and to the adaptive mechanisms whereby emotional attachment to the child is relinquished over time (Futterman and Hoffman, 1973). The depth and degree of this mourning period will vary in intensity between families and between the individuals involved. Difficulties arise when a child dies suddenly in the early stages of his or her disease or during treatment, where parents have not had this time to prepare themselves and their families. Research has shown more long-term psychological, behavioural and physical problems are experienced by parents and siblings following the sudden death of their child. Children can also demonstrate this distancing from those around from a young age. They want to protect their parents from answers or situations they perceive will cause distress.

It is not unusual for a child to choose a person with whom they will discuss what is happening to them, their fears and thoughts, and then deny the reality with others by their silence. Not all children feel the need to have their impending death confirmed. What is important is that children are listened to, that statements they make may be questions to be answered and that they are answered as honestly, sensitively and openly as possible. A lie or concealment will prevent further open communication and increase feelings of loneliness and isolation.

Parents and carers express their anxieties about what to tell a child and when. They are understandably frightened about saying the wrong thing or not being able to answer because of their own emotions. Children did not commonly ask outright if they were going to die. This has changed over recent years, possibly as children have become more involved and more knowledgeable about their own illness and treatment. They may make a statement, draw pictures which can be discussed or ask a series of questions over a period of time which will provide a telling picture of their knowledge of their disease and of dying. When answering children one need only answer what is being asked. If one is unsure of the question then a simple return of the question to the child may clarify the thoughts behind it. It is better to say an honest 'I don't know' to a question than avoid the issue or make up what appears to be a suitable answer.

It should be remembered that children are most concerned with living. When they feel well, however weak, they want to resume their normal activities. For some this may mean a return to school for all or part of the week. They need to have their siblings and friends to play with or just to be with them. They also need the discipline that is the norm within their family unit. Where acceptable boundaries of behaviour are lifted the child becomes more uncertain of his role and limits within the family and feels insecure.

Adolescents

It is difficult to define an age-range which totally encompasses the adolescent years. For most, it includes the ages of 12–19 years. It is a time of great change in the physiological, psychological and social development of the individual. 'No two individuals are alike and at no age are these differences more apparent than during the adolescent years' (Crow and Crow, 1965). They are not yet adults but neither can they be treated as dependent children.

Life for a teenager becomes a challenge. It is a time of questioning the limits enforced by parents, schools and society in an effort to establish their place and identity. Their appearance assumes a great importance as they become heavily dependent on the approval and acceptance of their peer group, and as new personal relationships are formed. In the process of establishing their identity and independence, moods swing to extremes. They can be sad, uncertain, rebellious and argumentative (McCallum and Carr-Gregg, 1987).

Cancer and its treatment has a enormous impact on the teenager's self-image, identity and on their relationships within the family and with their peers. The necessity for repeated hospitalisation increases their dependence on parents when normally they would be moving away from it. Schooling is interrupted frequently, often when the most important study programmes for examinations are to be undertaken. Long or frequent spells in hospital result in a loss of one's place in the peer group. This is enhanced with changes in appearance: alopecia, weight gain or loss, all reinforce feelings of worthlessness.

Teenagers may regress emotionally and display more childish behaviour. Others may exhibit a maturity and more adult understanding. Many want to take on new experiences and opportunities 'to put themselves on an accelerated track for experiencing life. Denial can be part of this race with time' (Johansen, 1988).

Carers come face-to-face with their own attitudes towards death and dying especially when faced with a teenager who is dying. 'For health professionals to successfully work with dying adolescents they must first confront their own mortality' (Blum, 1984). Knowing that adolescent dreams and ambitions for the future will not be fulfilled, life seems unfair and unjust. Carers may be close to the patient in age or have teenage relatives, and the situation can become more personal.

> 'Dying adolescents grieve not only for the life they have lived but also for the life they have not lived. Grieving over their lack of future involves a process of discarding their unfulfilled dreams, expectations and goals' (Papadatou, 1989).

Questions such as 'Why me', 'What did I do', 'Why can't I be . . .' can be bitter and painful and have no answers. Anger and resentment for lost opportunities may follow. Very ill adolescents know they are dying but will fluctuate between acknowledging this, either to themselves or others, and denial. The knowledge doesn't mean that they accept it. However, by being able to express their worries to a chosen person, they may gain a freedom to live their lives and reassert their independence (Papadatou, 1989). Figure 14.2 demonstrates how two teenagers chose to describe their feelings in writing, in a letter and a poem. Adolescents especially need to be involved in open discussions about their disease, symptoms and care, to be given control and share in decision-making. Free communication between family members may be difficult to facilitate where parents try to protect their son or daughter (and themselves), and a conspiracy of silence and isolation can develop. Opportunities for communication that is honest and caring allows the adolescent to express his anxieties and concerns. Research shows much of their concerns are with the actuality of dying – 'Will I be in pain? How long?' and 'When will it be?'. These questions are most likely to be asked of medical or nursing carers, with their professional knowledge, than of their family. Again, these questions will only be asked where there is the trust and confidence that an honest answer will be given. Opportunities for the teenager to talk alone with medical staff should be made. This can sometimes be difficult to achieve as parental wishes must also be acknowledged, but sensitive exchanges can help them to understand their child's need for independent discussions. The individual may have certain tasks he or she wishes to complete: to say good-bye to friends, give presents, make a will or decisions about his funeral. Adolescents need reassurance that they will not be forgotten by their friends and that their life has made an impact on others.

Communicating with other family members

Siblings

Many parents describe real difficulties in approaching the subject of death with their child and his or her siblings. They may be anxious not to say too much too soon, or, of leaving explanations and the chance to talk too late. One can only offer the advice to answer questions honestly, as and when they arise. Teenage brothers and sisters will be more aware and involved than younger children, and need to talk about their feelings. Where siblings are encouraged to participate in their brother or sister's care, questions may arise more naturally over time.

'I am writing about this because I daren't talk about it. My tumour had gone – the Chemo had killed it off, but what if my new tumour doesn't respond to treatment and grows. I keep thinking about Tracy and then about this tumour. I might die as well. I know I shouldn't think about this but I just can't help it.'

Lynne

Reaching the limit

Got to go fast,
Head for the hill,
Don't seem to move,
Feeling ill.

Want to drop,
Feet do ache,

Have to stop,
Just can't wait.

Getting close,
Nearly there,
Reached the limit,
People stare.

John

Fig. 14.2 Letter and poem by two teenagers.

Questions may be asked more than once by siblings. This may relate directly to their age, understanding and concepts of death. There may also be changes in their emotional and behavioural responses, relating to the perceived anxieties of their parents. Where the sick child becomes the focus of the parent's attentions and where his or her needs and wishes seem paramount, siblings may feel left out, unimportant and isolated. Their behaviour may change to being clinging, attention-seeking or withdrawn. In promoting a more normal family life, one can encourage parents to include siblings in care-giving, in planning treats or visits for the whole family to participate in and enjoy.

Grandparents

The needs of grandparents should not be forgotten in caring for the family. Their grief encompasses many losses. They grieve for the impending loss of their grand-child's life, and for their own child's sadness. One does not expect one's child to die first, certainly not one's grandchild, who should have many years before him or her. There is a loss of hope and investment in their future.

Many will have played an active role during the hospitalisation and treatment of their grandchild, either in relieving parents by the bedside or in caring for other children at home. The relationship of grandparents and grandchildren can be a very special, close one.

It should not be assumed that returning home and re-establishing day-to-day living when a child is dying is always fraught with difficulties and communication problems. The belief that open communication about dying was an essential task for the family – held by health professionals – has been challenged (Northouse, 1984).

'Not all families need to communicate about death, especially those who have comfortable, agreed upon patterns of not discussing feelings within the family system' (Lewandowski and Jones, 1988).

The families who are identified as needing help are those who want to talk, but are uncertain of how to approach the subject, or those where the needs of one member are at variance with the rest of the family. This should not however provide an excuse for carers not to explore the need to talk as the palliative care stage progresses. Over time and as symptoms change, carers may become aware of changes in the needs of individuals in the family.

For many parents they now have the opportunity to give the ultimate care that any parent can give. The long periods in hospital or throughout treatment may have felt safe with support from other parents and professionals around, but when the therapy has ended, home with its comforts and familiar belongings can offer its own respite.

Symptom control

Pain: identification and assessment

In the past there have been many myths and misconceptions relating to a child's ability to feel pain. Many assumed it was not experienced with the same intensity as that perceived by adults. Subsequent research shows this assumption to be unfounded no evidence being available to substantiate it (Reape, 1990). The child's age, development, behaviour and ability to express his or her feelings are some of the factors which must be taken into consideration when assessing and managing pain control.

Various age-related tools are available to assist in this management. One of the most reliable is the Eland colour tool (Eland, 1985), where children use different coloured pens to draw on a body outline (Fig. 14.3). They choose their own colours to describe different intensities of pain felt in different parts of the body. Other scales used utilise colours, a range of 'smiling to sad' faces, numbers and visual linear analogues, where points are drawn on a straight line indicating 'least' pain at one end and 'worst' pain at the other. Results have shown varying degrees of reliability associated with the age and development of the child when using some of these methods (Eland, 1985).

The language which children employ to describe pain, varies considerably with age. The actual word 'pain' may not be understood by over half the children aged between 5 and 8 years (Eland, 1985). It is important that specific words used by the child and family are known in order to help communicate at the child's level of understanding. For example, some of the words more commonly used may include 'owie', 'sore', 'little hurts', and 'big hurts', also specific noises made by some children. Mothers naturally identify cries made by their babies or toddlers as being 'hungry', 'tired' or in 'pain'. Studies show us that children can and do express pain but in their own way (Jerret and Evans, 1986). They do not imagine or pretend to have pain but difficulties can sometimes arise in identifying its intensity.

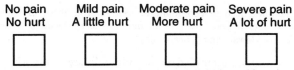

Pick the colours that mean *No hurt, A little hurt, More hurt*, and *A lot of hurt* to you and colour in the boxes. Now, using those colours, colour in the body to show how you feel. Where you have no hurt, use the *No hurt* colour to colour your body. If you have hurt or pain, use the colour that tells how much hurt you have.

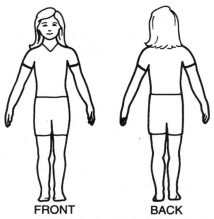

Fig. 14.3 Body outline – tool to describe pain intensity and sites for children.

The behavioural changes of young children, often described by parents, such as sleeplessness, irritability, anorexia and general unhappiness at being moved or touched may all indicate that the child is in pain. These symptoms of course may also be described in older children and teenagers. One must always listen carefully to what is being said by parents, the issues which cause them concern may be indicative of pain in their child. Professional carers should also be aware that older children and teenagers can be reluctant to say they are in pain, if they are anticipating a return to hospital or injections as a consequence. When the decision of where palliative care is to be given is being made, the major cause of anxiety for parents is the fear of uncontrollable symptoms, especially pain (Kohler and Radford, 1985). Children who are terminally ill do not all experience severe pain and do not require strong opiates. Personal experience has seen, for example, that many children who have brain tumours require little or no opiate treatment although other symptom control is often necessary. This contrasts sharply with some children who have bone or soft tissue tumours for whom opiate drugs are usually needed in large doses for long periods of time.

If the care of these children is to be effective in ensuring their comfort, the professional carer must learn to listen, recognise their symptoms then treat them appropriately and quickly.

The principles of assessing pain are well known. Pain may be related directly or indirectly to the disease or to previous anticancer therapy, and can be experienced in more than one site. The difference between these pains can be difficult to describe especially for a child.

It is possible to anticipate some of the types of pain which can be attributed directly to the nature and progression of disease (Miser and Miser, 1989). Severe headaches, with nausea and vomiting especially on rising, is most often seen in children with brain tumours and in leukaemia patients who have infiltration of the cerebral-spinal fluid by blasts cells, both giving rise to raised intracranial pressure.

Bone pains are commonly experienced by children with leukaemia or metastatic neuroblastoma. The pain results from invasion of bone and bone marrow and may be described as dull, aching and constant, progressively increasing in its severity. Invasion of bone and bone marrow also occur in Ewing's sarcoma and osteo-sarcoma. Occasionally this may lead to a pathological fracture. Very sharp severe pain may be indicative of rapidly growing tumour or of an intra-tumour bleed. The spread of tumour from soft tissue into adjacent nervous tissue results in a localised pain, described as sharp or burning, or in a more diffuse pain along the affected nerves pathway.

Pain: treatment

Each pain requires separate consideration and assessment of its history, severity and nature before a diagnosis can be made. Any treatment previously prescribed and its efficacy must also be noted. When treating the pain, it is vital that an adequate dose is prescribed for the individual child.

Most drugs for children are prescribed on a 'milligram per kilogram' basis, but it must be stressed that when opiates are prescribed, this guide only provides a baseline. Drugs may need to be increased quickly to maintain pain control. The dosage increase should also be appropriate, increases of 50 per cent or more may be necessary to regain control of symptoms.

Where pain is constant then analgesia must be prescribed regularly. There is no place for 'as required' doses for any patient in pain. Co-analgesics will often be necessary and will be described briefly later.

The most careful assessment, diagnosis and treatment is of little value if it is not monitored and reviewed often, with empathy and understanding. This may initially necessitate return visits to the home within short hours or of regular telephone calls to establish the effectiveness of the treatment. A contact, no matter how brief, is always reassuring and welcomed by the family. Where an immediate control of symptoms is necessary, contact that is once or twice weekly is insufficient and may result in panic calls or return visits to hospital which could be avoided. It can be a very demanding time for community nurses and practitioners. The decision of which analgesic agent is most appropriate should not be difficult if pain control is commenced early and in effective doses. There is a wide choice

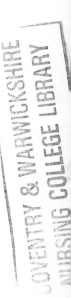

of drugs available but a useful recommendation is that one should restrict ones choice to a limited number, with which one becomes familiar (Oakhill, 1988).

The widely used 'analgesic staircase' provides a useful reminder that when one form of analgesia fails, when changing from one non-opiate drug to another will not regain pain control, and that to progress to a weak opiate is the next logical step.

The practise of our unit is to obtain pain control, initially, in younger children by prescribing paracetamol elixir, usually in one of the well-known proprietary forms such as 'Calpol' or 'Calpol 6 plus' (Wellcome Foundation Ltd). These are more acceptably flavoured and usually well known to the child. Where stronger analgesics are needed, progression is made to dihydrocodeine then to morphine elixir 4 hourly. Care should be taken when flavouring any medications that favourite acceptable foods or drinks are not used in an attempt to disguise the taste. This may only make the foods unpalatable with the result they are rejected totally.

Tablets should not be discounted by physicians because of the age of the child. Many children from a young age may prefer to take tablets, whole or crushed, and have become accustomed to doing so throughout their chemotherapy regimes.

The use of buprenorphine (Temgesic) as a moderate strength opiate tablet which is absorbed sublingually would appear to be suitable for some children. Pethidine is not appropriate for patients who have cancer as it is short-acting and therefore not suitable for chronic pain. In addition, patients may experience loss of control and hallucinations.

Many children aged 5 years and upwards when requiring strong opiate therapy have found MST Continus (controlled-release morphine) tablets more acceptable. Where this is prescribed, morphine elixir should also be available to control any breakthrough pain until the appropriate MST Continus dose is achieved, as there is a delay of up to 4 hours before peak plasma concentrations occur. It is our experience that MST Continus tablets need to be prescribed 8 hourly for children under 10 years of age and 12 hourly for older children and teenagers. The drug appears to be metabolised faster in the younger age group. For children on relatively long-term opioid therapy this can significantly simplify their drug taking and allows for longer periods of rest, especially through the night, for both child and parents between medication. MST granules are now available in a range of strengths, in sachets. These are mixed into a suspension in water and provide slow release pain control, without the need for tablets, and may prove useful for some children.

For the majority of children, utilising oral morphine preparations provides good pain control throughout their palliative care. However there are a small number of children for whom the oral route becomes inappropriate or insufficient. An alternative method may be necessary where the level of consciousness of the child deteriorates, where difficulty in swallowing for other reasons exists, for uncontrolled pain or where large repeated doses of oral drugs become difficult to tolerate. Failure to comply with any form of oral medication by the child is also a possibility!

Pain relief may be obtained by administering morphine as a suppository. With the exception of a few drugs such as anticonvulsants, the rectal route is not one commonly used in the UK. It is effective, but requires careful explanation to the child and parents for it to be accepted. Parents will often learn to administer the suppositories when shown by a nurse. Consideration of the child's diagnosis and condition must be taken into account where this method is to be used. Thrombocytopenia in a child with leukaemia, especially where episodes of bleeding have already occurred, may demand an alternative method of drug delivery. Morphine suppositories are available in 15 and 30 mg strengths, but pharmacies may be able to prepare other strengths should they be necessary.

In the past, lack of adequate pain control necessitated a return to hospital for intravenous analgesia for many children, with their families, usually hours or short days be fore the child's death. Anxiety at the child's condition, the urgency of the situation and failure to comply with the child and parents wishes to remain at home have all led to feelings of helplessness, lack of control, anger and extreme sadness by parents and carers at this already stressful time.

Over more recent years, parental administration of opiates at home by subcutaneous or venous routes have become more widely used. This method of drug delivery has been utilised for many years for adult patients and the principles for care remain the same for children. Some of the children for whom this method is appropriate will already have a venous access device *in situ*. Skin-tunnelled catheters, e.g. 'Hickman or Broviac lines', or implanted devices, e.g. 'Portacath' or 'Implant-a-port' are widely used in oncology centres for the administration of chemotherapy, blood products, parental feeding and for blood sampling so negating the need for repeated venepunctures and re-siting of infusions (Hollingsworth, 1987; Speechley, 1986).

A strictly aseptic procedure is essential when these devices are to be accessed. Parents are taught how to clean, dress and flush, with heparinised saline, the skin tunnelled catheter at home, in order to maintain its patency between use (Clarke and Cox, 1988). When chemotherapy is discontinued the lines are usually left *in situ* to provide immediate access should some supportive intravenous therapy be needed.

The administration of diamorphine utilising the central venous line and a battery-operated syringe driver is a very effective method of controlling pain. Despite the very slow delivery of the drug, it is rare for these lines to occlude. Should this occur, advice should be sought from the oncology unit.

When changing from oral morphine to intravenous diamorphine, the dosage should initially be titrated to one-third of the oral daily dose, although personal experience had noted that a subsequent increase in dosage has often been required quickly. It may be more appropriate to titrate opiates to at least half the oral daily dose, especially where there is increased pain.

When introducing new and more technical methods of drug administration the health professional must always be aware of the increased stresses experienced by families. In our experience, with the support of hospital and, most especially, community carers, parents increasingly take over much of the care associated with drug preparation and changing of syringes. It is of course essential that parents and community nurses have full knowledge and confidence in the equipment and techniques used. Sharing information and resources between oncology units and community carers can only increase this knowledge and so benefit the child.

Where a central venous line is not available, subcutaneous diamorphine by infusion is a viable alternative, using a fine-gauge 'butterfly' needle. To help allay anxieties relating to the use of needles in hospital are accustomed to (and demand) the application of a local anaesthetic cream (EMLA) (Maunuksela and Kolpela, 1986) under an occlusive dressing, applied an hour before the needle is inserted. This practise is recommended prior to needle insertion into subcutaneous sites. The sites most commonly used are abdominal or chest wall. A transparent dressing over the needle can then be applied to secure the needle and provide easy observation of the site. Sites should be changed immediately there is any sign of inflammation or if the child complains of any discomfort.

Most children and teenagers will tolerate the use of syringe drivers well, where the need for this method of administration has been fully explained. It is not unusual to see a child or teenager who has previously appeared withdrawn, un-comfortable or in obvious acute pain, become alert and interested in his or her surroundings. Syringe drivers which have a 'boost' control of a preset bolus dose allows the child or parent to administer an isolated increased dose should there be an acute episode of pain. For those less able to participate in family life, it is comforting for them and for their family, to be able to hold and cuddle them without causing signs of distress. There is no need or reason for repeated, painful intramuscular injections of opiates, when other methods of drug administration are available. Figures 14.4 and 14.5 are brief case histories of two children, describing their different needs and the ways in which pain control was achieved.

Pain control using opiate therapy is ineffective when symptoms are not recog-nised or there is a failure to prescribe adequate doses. The question of addiction to these drugs does not arise where pain exists. Children, like adults, will become tolerant of the drugs over a period of time and for this reason dosage must be increased to achieve the same level of good pain control as before. Reluctance to prescribe large doses may be expressed by some practitioners who are concerned about depression of the respiratory centre. This is not a problem as tolerance develops in the same way as the analgesic effect. Parents may also be concerned about increasing the treatment, sometimes by substantial amounts. Children can tolerate high doses of opiates and it is a difficult and very different concept for parents that there is no real upper-limit to the dose, only that which controls their child's pain (see Fig. 14.6).

Time should be spent by nurses and physicians to explain how the drug works and in what amounts it should be increased at the time. The social and media implications of opiate drug taking have great impact on the general public. Parents may have to be reassured that the drugs are most effective and appropriate for their child.

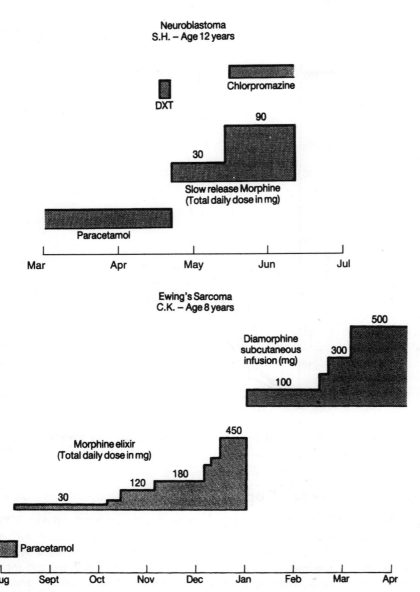

Figs 14.4 and 5 Case histories with diagrams of pain control for two children.

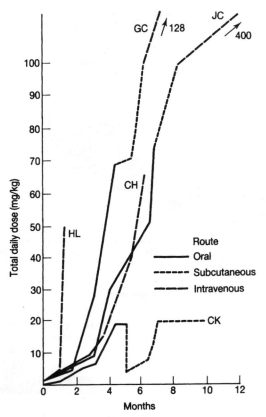

Fig. 14.6 Dosage and method of opiate administration for five children.

Adverse effects of opiate therapy

A side-effect of opiate therapy which is to be anticipated in all patients is that of constipation. Appropriate laxatives should be prescribed in conjunction with opiate drugs, for example, lactulose, Senokot or co-danthramer. Advice should be given to parents about active measures they can take with diet. Most children and teenagers will become drowsy when opiate drugs are begun. This is usually temporary, decreasing after a few days as they become more tolerant of the drug. It is essential that children who are old enough and parents are advised of this. It can be frightening for parents who are not informed, as death may seem to be more imminent when they are faced with a sleepy, less-responsive child. It can also be frightening for the child who may relate it to his or her own death or to previous experiences of chemotherapy, where antiemetics and sedatives give rise to the same feelings and memories of impending nausea. For both reasons they may be reluctant to start opiate treatment.

Nausea and vomiting caused by morphine preparations may be experienced by some children, where it is directly related to opiates, drugs such as metoclopramide or cyclizine can be effective in relieving symptoms.

A more common side-effect is that of pruritus. Children may complain of severe itching which can be very distressing. This again will last only a few days and the prescribing of an antihistamine will offer relief over these first days. Unfortunately, a side-effect of most antihistamines is drowsiness.

Adjuvant therapy

Analgesic agents form the basis of pain control but other drugs may also be used for specific symptom control.

Corticosteroids, e.g. dexamethasone, are frequently used to reduce cerebral oedema and thus relieve raised intracranial pressure caused by tumour. The reduction in pressure may relieve headaches, nausea and vomiting and may also cause a raising of the conscious level of the child. Corticosteroids are also effective where nerve pressure or soft tissue involvement gives rise to 'burning' symptoms. These drugs should be prescribed with care, as the features of Cushing's syndrome and overt weight gain are distressing, disfiguring and increase nursing problems. Dosage should be maintained at the lowest possible level at which the drug is effective for the child. Non-steroidal anti-inflammatory drugs (NSAIDs), e.g. naproxen and ibuprofen, may be indicated where bone pain or soft tissue infiltration exists.

Nerve pain may be experienced as burning and tingling or as sharp, shooting pains. The use of tricyclic antidepressants, e.g. amitriptyline, or anticonvulsants, e.g. carbamazepine, have proved effective in reducing these symptoms. The use of antidepressants for children or teenagers for psychological reasons may be questioned, but for an individual child they can be beneficial, in small doses. The need to look at reasons why the child remains depressed once his or her general condition is improved should not be forgotten, and time should be spent in helping the child communicate his or her anxieties. Chronic pain, tiredness and past experiences are some of the factors which may occupy much of the child's mind. Relieving painful symptoms and improving his or her quality of life will help the child to regain a feeling of well-being.

Sweating can be a major problem for some children which may or may not be associated with a raised temperature. It is more commonly seen where there is increased tumour load as the disease progresses and can be distressing. It may be helped by a low dose of corticosteroid (prednisolone or dexamethasone) or by naproxen.

Dyspnoea, which may be experienced by the child with lung metasteses, is probably one of the most distressing sights for parents and carers to witness. The use of opiate drugs is invaluable as the child, whilst conscious, is unaware of his or her struggle for breath. There is no obvious respiratory depression where dyspnoea exists and opiates are used. Persistent coughs are often relieved with the use of methadone. Antibiotics may be appropriate to treat chest infections where the child's general well-being will be improved. Where the child is unconscious this may be questionable. Oxygen therapy may be indicated to help distressed breathing and ensuring an adequate supply is essential. Helping the family cope with this situation asks for empathy and understanding.

It is possible to administer co-analgesic drugs in conjunction with opiates via a syringe driver. Figure 14.7 gives some examples of antiemetics, sedatives, bronchodilators and antispasmodics which can safely be mixed with diamorphine, so relieving the child of further oral or intramuscular medication.

Fits, caused by cerebral metasteses, are not uncommon and can be difficult to manage. They are distressing for families to see and naturally cause great anxiety. Occasionally these can easily be controlled at home, utilising oral anticonvulsants or rectal diazepam. They remain, however, one of the commonest reasons for a child returning to hospital for care or control of symptoms.

Radiotherapy and chemotherapy both have a place in palliative care. Bone pain caused by tumour infiltration and painful pressure symptoms caused by tumour bulk can be effectively treated by a single fraction or a short course of radiotherapy. Intrathecal drugs, e.g. methotrexate, hydrocortisone and cytosine are used where children who have raised intracranial pressure symptoms, caused by leukaemic cell infiltration, are experiencing severe headaches. Both forms of therapy necessitate a return to hospital for a brief period, which may be upsetting for the child – one must be sure the benefits outweigh the necessary procedures.

Where nerve pain is localised and unresponsive to drug therapy, nerve blocks using local or phenol anaesthetic agents or long-term epidural anaesthesia may all have a role. Experienced anaesthetists who have a special interest in pain control,

ANTIEMETICS
  Haloperidol (Haldol,
Serenace)
  Metoclopramide (Maxolon)
  Cyclizine (Valoid)

SEDATIVES
  Hyoscine (Scopolamine)
  Haloperidol

BRONCHODILATOR
  Salbutamol (Ventolin)

ANTISPASMODIC
  Hyoscine

EXCESSIVE NOISY
SECRETIONS
  Hyoscine

Fig. 14.7 Drugs currently used in syringe drivers compatible with diamorphine.

usually in symptom control clinics within hospitals, will advise and employ the most appropriate method of nerve block. Opiate drugs can often be reduced after this treatment and sometimes be stopped. The experience of using nerve blocks in children is very limited.

Transcutaneous electrical nerve stimulation (TENS) (Meyerson, 1983) is not widely used for palliation of nerve symptoms in children. It may be useful as a non-invasive procedure but, as it involves self-control by the patient and its effect on pain is often brief, it is probably more suitable for a teenager experiencing intermittent nerve pain, to whom its method and effect can more fully be explained.

The use of blood products may enhance quality of life and treat distressing symptoms in some children. Transfusions of packed cells may be given to a child who is generally well, but where anaemia is resulting in tiredness and weakness. Platelets should be infused where thrombocytopenia is resulting in distressing or persistent bleeds. To see overt bleeding is upsetting and causes great anxiety for parents and children, measures should be ensured that this is treated actively.

Nutritional needs

There is a natural need for parents to provide food, warmth and comfort for their children, and it can be difficult for them to accept their sick child's lack of interest or appetite for food. The progression of disease, sore mouth or gums and alteration of taste sensation caused by chemotherapy are some factors which will increase the child's reluctance to eat. Some children may 'pick' at small amounts of food then decide they have had sufficient, others will have 'fads' where one food is requested constantly. Feeling they are not providing sufficiently for the child can cause much anxiety for parents. Food may be an issue on which they can focus their attention when they feel they can do little else to help.

It takes time and gentle encouragement from carers to establish realistic expectations of their child's needs. The ambulant, active child may be encouraged with high-calorie drinks or ice pops, and a low dose of corticosteroids may stimulate his or her appetite. The child who is less mobile, or sleeping for lengthy periods, will have different intake needs. His or her condition will determine when fluids alone may be sufficient.

Children and teenagers themselves may express their own desire to eat, and worry about their lack of appetite. Their nutritional intake may have been a focus of attention throughout their treatment. Special attention to their needs and calorie supplements to food or drinks can alleviate some of their anxiety.

Oral care

The pain and discomfort which is experienced where the child has a dry or sore mouth, ulcers, gingivitis or candid will enhance his reluctance to eat. Particular attention to oral hygiene should be made and any ulcers or infections treated. Soft toothbrushes will help where gums have a tendency to bleed and measures such as tranexamic acid mouth washes may also be useful. Mouth washes containing a locally-acting analgesic, e.g. Difflam (Riker Laboratories) may help the child to eat when a 'numbing' effect has been achieved.

Oral care packs, or soaked gauze wrapped around fingers should be used to cleanse the mouth when the child is unable to do so.

When the child is drinking, fruit juices will encourage the mouth to feel fresh and will encourage salivation.

Skin care

As children become progressively weaker and less mobile, care of the skin is important. A small child is easily lifted and position changed, but this can be difficult for parents of older children and teenagers, or where the child is unconscious. Advice on techniques for lifting or rolling the child will be appreciated. They may also need help with bathing.

If the child is thin and wasted, the use of a Spenco or ripple mattress is indicated.

It is much less common to see fungating lesions in a child than in adults, but where this is the case, the appropriate cleansing agents and dressings should be used. Pressure sores may be a problem and specific care to these areas must be given.

Parents are usually very willing to participate in caring for their child's physical needs, and advice is often welcomed from nursing carers.

Responding to on-going needs

The therapeutic effect of maintaining as normal a family life-style as possible should not be underestimated. Children enjoy playing with other children, or having stories read to them in quieter moments. Their attention can be diverted as their symptoms become controlled. When they feel well, it may be appropriate that they return to school for all or part of a day. When this is not possible, friends and teachers should be encouraged to visit and to include them in their daily life.

As the child becomes weaker, their room may become a central place for family and friends. Where there is space, a downstairs room may be converted into the child's bedroom, so that he or she is not isolated from daily events. Being able to participate in games or conversation may help distract the child and re-establish a sense of well-being.

Equipment

Parents have identified a particular area where help in practical terms is welcomed when caring for their child at home (Kohler and Radford, 1985). The provision of home nursing equipment has occasionally proved difficult, but community nurses are expert in mobilising available resources. The most commonly required items include mattresses, sheepskins, bedpans and urinals, commodes, backrests and bedcradles, wheelchairs or buggies and syringe drivers. Most oncology units have a small supply of equipment which is available for home use. One item which we have found some parents have appreciated is a baby-listening device which can be moved from room to room. This allows the parents to leave the child knowing they will hear him or her, should they be needed.

Employment

Caring for a child who is dying is the most stressful time for any parent. It imposes enormous physical and psychological strains on the individual and is a time when most of those in employment feel the need to be at home, to participate in care and share the time left together as a family. Many employers are sympathetic, but there may be a need for a sick note to be obtained from an understanding general practitioner during this difficult time.

Finance

Caring for a sick child at home over what may be a prolonged period of time is expensive. Whilst this may seem of lesser importance, real financial hardship can be experienced where there are increased heating and phone bills and loss of earnings if parents are at home.

It may be possible to obtain an attendance allowance from the Department of Social Security, although application of the criteria may seem to be variable. Charitable organisations will often give direct financial assistance, the most well known are the Malcolm Sargent Cancer Fund for Children, the Joseph Rowntree Family Fund and the Leukaemia Care Society.

It is important that the family is aware of all allowances and grants available to them.

Contact, communication and liaison

Throughout this chapter the need for on-going contact and communication between carers has been stressed. Where disciplinary boundaries and roles are minimised and the channels of communication established early and then maintained, then optimal care for the child and family can be provided. The 'shared-care' management approach is most effective where there is continuing flexibility, good communication and close cooperation between oncology units and community teams (Fig. 14.8).

Death

Caring for a child who is dying is an emotionally and physically exhausting time. The 'anticipatory mourning' of parents from the time the child no longer receives active therapy encompasses knowledge of their impending loss with hope, that it

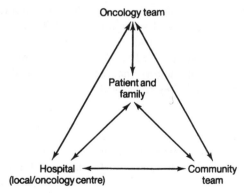

Fig. 14.8 Flexibility, co-operation and communication.

will not happen, and despair that it is inevitable (Futtermnan and Hoffman, 1973). Families grieve at what is inevitable, then may reconcile themselves with thoughts of what their child has meant, and given to others. The emotional detachment from the child as death becomes imminent is a recognition of the inevitability of death, that their child's life will end soon, with no hopes of a future. The final stage, described by Futterman and Hoffman, is of memorialisation where parents develop a mental picture of their dying child, which may be idealised and not actual, but a picture which will remain with them.

The duration of palliative care of children with cancer is variable, usually lasting weeks or short months. Where this time is prolonged, the time of waiting by parents may be fraught with other emotions. Parents have described how they mentally plan what will happen at the time of death, their plans for the funeral and what will happen afterwards. But when death does not happen immediately they may feel guilty for 'wishing it would end' and empty of sadness or 'lost'. The waiting may seem endless. Others may feel a comfort in knowing that it would all end, that they could prepare for life again, with a different normality (Kubler-Ross, 1969). The need for parents to know what will happen when their child dies has been well described (Martinson, 1980; Kohler and Radford, 1985). 'How will it happen', 'will I know when the time comes?' are common questions. They fear that it will be traumatic, a struggle or that it will be sudden with no time to prepare themselves and their family. The medical issues relating to the progression of disease and its effects should have already been addressed, but parents may want to know what happens when someone actually dies. It has been found helpful to have someone explain the physical changes, changes in skin colour and of breathing patterns (Martinson, 1980). These are the issues which many fear and for which most are unprepared. At the time of death, some parents may ask that a nurse or doctor is with them.

It may also be appropriate to describe the practical measures which need to be taken: the certification of death by a doctor, the registering (an event which may be traumatic) and the arrangements to be made with funeral directors for burial or cremation. Some units may have a prepared booklet or letter which describes the procedures to be undertaken.

The wishes and needs of parents, at the time of death, remain very individual and must be respected. Some will want the formal procedures to begin immediately. Others may want to keep their child at home, to wash and dress them, cuddle them or sleep, holding them. They should be encouraged to do whatever they feel is right for them, to say their own good-byes.

For siblings, to be able to be with their dead brother or sister and touch them or give them presents and to see that death is not frightening or a mystery may help to allay their fears or fantasies, and so not feel excluded from the adult's grief.

Bereavement

The death of one's child has been described as the 'ultimate loss' (Wilson, 1988). It is a loss of part of one's self, of an individual and of hopes and dreams for the future. No-one expects their child or grandchild to die before they do. Many emotions may be experienced during the months and years after the death by an individual, but it may be more helpful to describe the tasks of mourning which must be accomplished before any person can adjust to their personal bereavement.

To accept the reality of their loss

Families may initially experience feelings of relief, and release from the stresses of their child's illness. This is often followed by numbness and shock, as they begin the formalities of funeral arrangements and of informing relatives and friends. The practicalities serve to reinforce the issue of the child's death, and allows for a time of saying good-bye and shared emotions.

To experience the pain of grief

The aching and longing for their child will be intense. Many parents describe their need to hold, hug and cuddle their child, but there is an emptiness which can only partly be filled by holding their other children. No-one can replace their child who has died. The pain of grief can express itself in physical symptoms; anxiety and panic, breathlessness, lack of energy, insomnia and loss of appetite are just some of the symptoms described. Some will describe themselves as 'going mad'. They need the reassurance that their grief and feelings are being acknowledged and that these feelings are normal, that it will pass with time and to be encouraged to talk about themselves and their child.

To adjust to an environment in which their child is missing

This task is one that cannot be completed early or easily. The daily reminders of their loss are with families constantly: Favourite music or television programmes, the child's school friends growing up, an empty chair at a table, birthdays and anniversaries all enhance the grief which is never far away. One of the most difficult questions parents have to answer is 'How many children do you have?' Do they give a long explanation of why there are now two children, not three, or just say 'I have two children', and experience all the feelings of sadness and guilt at denying their dead child's existence. The process of adjusting to a new normality of family life may take years to accomplish.

To withdraw emotional energy and reinvest it in other relationships

The need to take up, and enjoy, life again may seem impossible. Parents may cling to the memory of their child, anguish when they feel unable to picture his or her face or to remember his or her voice, and to feel they can never truly enjoy life again. The differing needs of other family members can be difficult to cope with, when grief can be expressed in so many different ways. To smile or laugh may seem disloyal and parents feel guilty when they realise a period has passed when they have not thought about the child. Talking about the child, remembering happy times and being able to acknowledge and share emotions are part of the healing process. As time passes they are able to enjoy life again without displacing their memories.

It seems natural that one should try to protect children from the sadness around, but we must recognise that they too have lost a family member, and must also grieve. At a time when they need the closeness of their family most, it may be that other members are not able to fully respond, that their own grief is too intense. Research has shown that when a child has been cared for in his own home, families cope better as a unit because they have shared the experience (Lauer *et al.*, 1989). There is less guilt and they feel more able to share their sorrow with the rest of the family. This had led to a more positive and cohesive attitude for the future as a family.

Children will also express their sorrow in many ways. They too are individuals whose feelings must be acknowledged. They may be anxious or worried about being left alone, their security being threatened or about their own health – are they too going to die? Insomnia, fear of the dark or nightmares and sleepwalking are not uncommon, neither is a regression to more childish behaviour, tantrums and bedwetting. Parents have sometimes said that their other child may never talk about his or her sibling. 'It's as if he never existed, he only wants his toys to play with'. They may recognise the need to keep something of the child who has died, but not so easily recognise other behavioural problems as being related to the sibling's personal bereavement and grief.

Children must be encouraged to share their feelings, to know that it is alright to cry, to be angry or sad. When parents try to hide their own sadness, children feel they too must deny it. They may feel responsible, that death has happened because of something they said or did, or less important and unloved, as attention has surrounded their dying sibling for so long. They need the reassurance and closeness of their family to know that they are loved for themselves and that their feelings are important too (Fig. 14.9).

> *Still there, but gone*
>
> To see him there,
> When he's not,
> Although he's there in my Mind,
> I still Miss him alot.
>
> I can just imagine him there to say
> "Go away,
> leave me alone,
> I want to play"!
>
> When treatment time then came,
> You could always hear his name,
>
> It was Peter this,
> Peter that,
> Oh sigh!
>
> It was like the talk of the World,
> Envy and sometimes hate, you'ld
> think he had Enough on his plate,
> All the Attention.
>
> But he is my brother,
> And will be forever,
> And I'll love him like never before.
>
> *Michael*

Fig. 14.9 Poem by bereaved sibling.

School teachers and friends are a major part of a child's life. The death of a classmate affects them all. Some children may be reluctant to return to school after their sibling has died. On return they may be easily distracted, disruptive, withdrawn or display what seems to be inappropriate emotions, all of which may be signs of inner distress and grief. A sympathetic teacher and close peer group can give the child support and security to talk about his or her feelings, or just be there when the child feels alone.

Bereavement following the death of a child is longer than after the death of an adult. One study reported that more than 20 per cent of families were experiencing most intense grief at 2 years, after their child's death (Corr *et al.*, 1985). Another 25 per cent said their grief was most intense in the 1 year to 18 months period. In many cases, the grief of siblings was experienced for longer periods than that of their parents.

It can be difficult for carers to know how best they can support families through this time. It is the practise of most oncology units for someone who has been closely involved with the family to attend the funeral. Families do appreciate the presence of someone who has helped them care for their child and who is showing that the child also meant something to themselves.

Maintaining contact by telephone calls and visits is essential. Strong bonds develop between carers and the family as they share a unique experience. Families lose much of the regular contact and input from those around in the months after the death and need to share their feelings with those most closely involved. Where contact is not maintained, families experience a 'double loss', they need to feel that they and their child are still part of our thoughts and that we do care.

More obvious times when contact should be made are birthdays and anniversaries of the death. These are very personal dates which belong only to their dead child, and are usually seen as a great hurdle to be got over. Christmas is another difficult time where there are mixed emotions of the need to have a day which the other children will enjoy and yet be able to grieve for the child who is not there. Families will have many individual ways of spending these days, acknowledgement by carers that the anniversaries are important may help them feel less isolated.

Families are invited to come back to the oncology unit, usually a few weeks after the death, to talk to the physician who cared for their child. Most will welcome the opportunity to be able to talk about their child's illness, treatment and death. There may be many questions to be asked, some will come with lists prepared as they did whilst their child was receiving treatment. The impact of actually returning to the hospital should not be underestimated, it can be very traumatic to pass all the places they so often took their child. For some an alternative office may need to be found, to enable them to take the first steps of returning. They are encouraged to repeat the visit as often as they feel the need and have questions to be asked. Many will visit 'socially' for coffee and a chat, by which they are able to maintain their links.

Families will often focus their attention and energies into fund-raising for the parents groups and hospitals, finding a positivity in working for the benefit of other families. Some units may have groups for bereaved parents where they can meet others and share their experiences with people who can truly say 'I know how you feel'. Others may find locally run groups such as 'Compassionate Friends' helpful.

The reactions of other family members or friends can be difficult for parents to cope with. They may meet unhelpful comments, avoidance in the street, refusal to mention the child's name or meet people who are unaware of their loss. Parents reactions will differ to each situation, relating to how they are feeling at any one time.

It is helpful for those visiting to show that they care and to allow parents to talk about the child as freely as they want. Parents need the reassurance that they did everything they could for their child. Over time, visits and contact will naturally lessen, but even after many months, if carers should think about the family for any reason and wonder how they are, a phone call will always be welcomed.

Caring for ourselves

To have a child die in one's community is a rare occurrence, even more so when that child is dying from a malignant disease. The experience is a very personal one, where we may question our own feelings about death and its meaning. We may relate the child and parents to our own families and how we would cope with such a situation. In sharing some of their anxieties and fears we often feel inadequate and awkward. But it is in this sharing that carers have much to offer. It can be difficult when one feels one must be offering practical advice and performing tasks but the majority of help that we can give is by being with the family, establishing trust and being ready just to listen.

Resources are available from the oncology units to help manage specific problems which may be encountered and we must seek to strengthen these links. In working as a team, our own feelings of isolation lessen. During the palliative care and after the death of the child, it is important that we can also talk about our experience and our loss. It does help to share it with others both in our immediate unit and with others who have been involved in the care. Despite the sadness of the situation it can be a very positive and rewarding time.

Acknowledgements

The author is grateful to Dr C. C. Bailey, Dr J. Lewis and Mrs P. Fidler. And to the UKCCSG for permission to publish Fig. 14.1 – 100 typical paediatric oncology patients from the report on Cancer Services for Children, March 1987.

References

ARMSTRONG, G. and MARTINSON, I. (1980). Death, dying and terminal care: dying at home. In: KELLERMAN, J. (ed.), *Psychological Aspects of Childhood Cancer*, p. 306. Charles C. Thomas, Springfield, IL.

BLUM, R. W. (1984). The dying adolescent. In: BLUM, R. W. (ed.), *Chronic Illness and Disabilities in Childhood and Adolescence*. Grune & Stratton, New York.

BURNE, S. R., FRANCIS DOMENICA and BAUM, J. D. (1984). Helen House – a hospice for children: analysis of the first year. *British Medical Journal* 289, 1665–8.

CHAMBERS, E. J., OAKHILL, A., CORNISH, J. M. and CURNICK, S. (1989). Terminal care at home for children with cancer. *British Medical Journal* 298, 937–40.

CLARKE, J. and COX, E. (1988). Heparinsation of Hickman catheters. *Nursing Times and Nursing Mirror* 84, 51–3.

CORR, C. A., MARTINSON, I. M. and DYER, K. L. (1985). Parental bereavement. In: CORR, C. A. and CORR, D. M. (eds), *Hospice Approaches to Pediatric Care*. Springer, New York.

CROW, L. and CROW, A. (1965). *Adolescent Development and Adjustment*, 2nd edn. McGraw-Hill, New York.

ELAND, J. M. (1985). The role of the nurse in children's pain. In: COPP, L. A. (ed.), *Perspectives on Pain*. Churchill Livingstone: London.

FUTTERMAN, E. J. and HOFFMAN, I. (1973). Crisis and adaptation in families of fatally ill children. In: ANTHONY, E. J. and KOUPERNICK, C. (eds), *The Child in his Family: The Impact of Disease and Death*. John Wiley, New York.

HOLLINGSWORTH, S. (1987). Getting on line. *Nursing Times* 83, 61–2.

JERRET, M. and EVANS, K. (1986). Children's pain vocabulary. *Journal of Advanced Nursing* 11, 403–8.

JOHANSEN, B. B. (1988). Care of the dying adolescent and the bereaved family. *Loss, Grief, Care* 2, 59–67.

KOHLER, J. A. and RADFORD, M. (1985). Terminal care for children dying of cancer – quantity and quality of life. *British Medical Journal* 291, 115–16.

KOOCHER, G. P. and O'MALLEY, J. E. (1981). *The Damocles Syndrome*. McGraw-Hill, New York.

KUBLER-ROSS, E. (1969) Parent care. In: *Living with Death and Dying*, pp. 95–159. Souvenir Press.

LAUER, M. E., MULHERN, R. K., SCHELL, M. J. and CAMITTA, B. M. (1989). Long-term follow up of parental adjustment following a child's death at home or hospital. *Cancer* 1, 988–93.

LEWANDOWSKI, W. and JONES, S. L. (1988). The family with cancer – nursing interventions throughout the course of living with cancer. *Cancer Nursing* 11, 313–21.

MARTINSON, I. M. (1980) Dying children at home (occasional paper). *Nursing Times* 76, 129-32.

MARTINSON, I., NESBITT, M. and KERSEY, Y. (1984) Home care for the child with cancer. In: CHRIST, A. E. and FLOMENHAFT, K. (eds), *Childhood Cancer*. Plenum Press, New York.

MARTINSON I., MOLDOW D. G., ARMSTRONG, G. D., HENRY, W. F., NESBITT, B. E. and KERSEY, J. H. (1986). Home care for children dying of cancer. *Research in Nursing and Health* 9, 11–16.

MAUNUKSELA, G. L. and KOLPELA, R. (1986). Double-blind evaluation of a lignocaine–pilocaine cream (E.M.L.A.) in children – effect on pain associated with venous cannulation. *B.J.A.* 5, 1242–5.

McCALLUM, L. and CARR-GREGG, M. (1987). Adolescents with cancer. *Australian Nurses Journal* 16, 39–43.

MEYERSON, B. A. (1983). Electrostimulation procedures – effects, presumed rationale and possible mechanisms. *Advances in Pain Research* 5, 405–534.

MISER, A. W. and MISER, J. S. (1989). The treatment of cancer pain in children. *Paediatric Clinics of North America* 36, 979–8.

NORMAN, R. and BENNET, M. (1986). Care of the dying child at home, a unique co-operative relationship. *Australian Journal of Advanced Nursing* 3, 3–17.

NORTHOUSE, L. (1984). The impact of cancer on the family – an overview. *Int. J. Psychiatry Med.* 14, 215–43.

O'BRIAN, M. E. (1983). An identification of needs of family members of terminally ill patients in a hospital setting. *Military Medicine* 148, 712–16.

OAKHILL A. (1988). Terminal care. In: *The Supportive Care of the Child with Cancer*, pp. 238–57. Wright.

OPCS (1987). *OPCS Monthly Statistics – Cause*. HMSO, London.

PAPADATOU, D. (1989). Caring for dying adolescents. *Nursing Times* 85, 28–31.

REAPE, D. (1990). Children and pain (pain perceptions). *Nursing Standard* 4(16), 33–6.

SPEECHLEY, V. (1986) Intravenous therapy: peripheral/central lines nursing: add-on. *Journal of Clinical Nursing* 3, 95–100.

SPINETTA, J and DEASEY-SPINETTA, P. (1981). *Living with Childhood Cancer*. C. V. Mosby, St Louis, MO.

SPINETTA, J. J., RIGLER, D. and KARON, M. (1974). Personal space as a measure of a dying child's sense of isolation. *J. Consult Clin Psychol.* 42, 751–7.

STEIN, A., FORREST, G. C., WOOLLEY, H. and BAUM, J. D. (1989) Life threatening illness and hospice care. *Archives of Disease in Childhood* 64, 697–702.

WILSON, D. C. (1985). Developing a hospice program for children. In: CORR, C. A. and CORR, D. M. (eds), *Hospice Approaches to Paediatric Care*. Springer, New York.

WILSON, D. C. (1988). The ultimate loss: the dying child. *Loss, Grief, Care* 2, 125–30.

Further reading

DENT, A. *A Child is Dying – Care of the Family in Illness and Bereavements*. Professional Pack. Macmillan Education Centre.

HILL, L. (ed.) (1994). *Caring for Dying Children and their Families*. Chapman & Hall.

OAKHILL, A. (1988). *The Supportive Care of the Child with Cancer*. Wright.

Coping strategies

15
Complementary therapies

Jenny Penson

'There are more things in Heaven and Earth, Horatio, than are dreamt of in your philosophy.'

Shakespeare (Hamlet)

It appears that people who are facing the challenge of cancer are increasingly seeking ways of taking more control of their illness and its treatment. They are looking for more information, more choice and for different kinds of support. Among the options which are available to them is a bewildering range of potentially therapeutic approaches which a few may choose as alternatives to orthodox medicine and many may wish to try in addition to conventional health-care systems. (See Table 15.1 for a list of current complementary therapies.)

Therefore, this chapter will consider the use of therapies which are thought to be complementary to orthodox medicine. Its main focus will be on what Wells with Tschudin (1994) term 'supportive therapies', being approaches which may be incorporated into nursing care in order to enhance holistic nursing practice.

One of the problems is in defining what can appropriately be fitted under the 'complementary' umbrella. The boundaries between what may be considered to be orthodox, what may be truly alternative systems and what can be used to complement conventional care can be blurred. It is even more difficult to know how to group therapies together. One way is for complementary therapies to be categorised according to the potential change they achieve in the patient after their use. These changes can be:

1. Psychological: concerned with the mental state of the person.
2. Physiological: related to the structure and function of the body.
3. Psychophysiological: where change in the mental state may bring about physiological change which can then act as a feedback mechanism to the mental state (see Table 15.2).

Each category shown here contains examples which are usually acceptable to orthodox medicine and which are known to be of practical benefit to the patient. In the psychological category examples include counselling and psychotherapy while in the physiological domain osteopathy and acupuncture are becoming widely accepted. However, it is in the psychophysiological areas that complementary therapies have the greatest potential, for it is in these that the link between mind and body is strongest. It is accepted that thinking patterns can alter physiology and affect the health status of the individual or the progress of a disease. It is probably no accident that these are the therapies most widely used by nurses.

The common ground between, at least, the principal complementary therapies is that they all carry a belief that the body has the power to heal itself, although this

Table 15.1 Current complementary therapies: some possibilities

Acupressure/shiatsu	Drama	Osteopathy
Acupuncture	therapy/psychodrama	Pets as therapy
Alexander technique	Guided imagery	Psychotherapy
Allergy therapy	Herbal medicine	Radionics
Aromatherapy	Homoeopathy	Reflexology
Art therapy	Hypnotherapy	Reiki therapy
Biofeedback techniques	Iridology	Relaxation techniques
Chiropractice	Kinesiology	Rolfing
Colour therapy	Massage	Spiritual healing
Counselling	Meditation	T'ai-chi ch'uan
Crystal healing	Music therapy	Therapeutic touch
Dr Bach's flower	Nature cure	Visualisation
remedies	Nutritional medicine	Yoga

may be defined in different ways. They all recognise that the mind and the emotions play a part in the maintenance of health and the causation of disease. They all see health as being about wholeness and balance, the experience of being at peace with ones internal and external worlds. They are all considered to be safer and gentler than many orthodox treatments, particularly in cancer treatment. However, it must be remembered that regimes that include, for example, drastic alterations in eating habits or the regular use of enemas or washouts, or the use of Chinese herbal concoctions which are extremely unpleasant to take, or the pain that may accompany manipulation of joints, may not always appear gentle to the recipient.

There is much evidence that the use of complementary therapies is increasing and, when one considers some of the reasons for this, it is easy to see why patients with cancer are likely to seek out such approaches in order to receive treatment and for support. They, like others with life-threatening or chronic illness, may feel, rightly or wrongly, that conventional medicine reaches a point where it can do no more. Faced with this possibility or coping in a system which may appear to be dehumanising the person with cancer may well look for alternative or additional help. Although they appear to be looking fundamentally for increased quality of life, there is likely to be a hope, though often unexpressed, for extra quantity of life or even for a cure.

Table 15.2 A categorisation of some complementary therapies according to potential change in the patient

Psychological	Physiological	Psychophysiological
Hypnotherapy	Acupuncture	Relaxation
Counselling	Osteopathy	Meditation
Psychotherapy	Chiropractice	Massage
Dr Bach's flower remedies	Herbalism	Aromatherapy
Crystal healing	Homoeopathy	Therapeutic touch
Guided imagery	Nutritional medicine	Reflexology
Art, drama, music therapy		Touch (PAT Dogs)

Certainly patients today are better informed than ever before. There is increased awareness of the nature of cancer and of options for treatment. There is less reliance on institutionalised knowledge and less passive acceptance of one person's opinion, even if he or she is an authority figure such as an oncologist or surgeon.

This change of attitude may be, in part, due to the changing ideology of our times which stresses individual responsibility and consumer choice, but it may also stem from a certain wariness or mistrust of the health-care system which, fuelled by the media, grew out of the Thalidomide tragedies of the 1960s. The public's confidence was shaken by the fact that this drug had gone through all the safeguards and was prescribed freely to pregnant women. Since then much attention has been given to the dangers of other medications, from opren to valium, from the use of cortisone to the over-prescribing of antibiotics.

At the time of writing, confidence in orthodox medicine has been shaken still further by publicity concerning the high mortality rate of women with breast cancer in the UK compared with other European countries. It has also highlighted the very different experiences of these women whose chances of recovery may depend, at least to some extent, on the willingness of their general practitioners (GPs) to refer them quickly and on the very variable skills and expertise of their local hospital.

Indeed, the women's movement encouraged the use of complementary therapies, for it was they who began to voice their dissatisfaction with the health-care system in general and with the quality of their encounters with their doctors in particular. At a similar time, there was a nostalgic move towards what was perceived as being natural, whether in food, clothing or lifestyle. This, plus an increasing awareness of environmental issues, led some to reject the scientific approach and to mistrust technology.

It appears that people are far more likely to turn to approaches that complement orthodox medicine than to choose therapies as complete alternatives. However, it also seems that people tend not to tell the health-care professionals that they are receiving complementary treatment, usually for fear of being ridiculed or of having orthodox treatment withheld from them.

Most complementary care takes place outside the orthodox setting, be it hospital or health centre, although this situation looks as though it is changing. A notable example is provided by the Hammersmith–Bristol project which is a joint development between the Oncology Department of the Hammersmith Hospital and the Bristol Cancer Help Centre. This is an exciting attempt to merge what Burke and Sikora (1993) refer to as two cultures whose practitioners have different styles, patterns of behaviour and hierarchical models. The supportive care model which has been created can be seen to provide a range and choice of approaches performed by practitioners, including the doctors and nurses who also provide orthodox care. Thus, this project provides an example of truly complementary and holistic care.

McCaffery is one of the most notable advocates of combining orthodox and complementary approaches; her highly acclaimed work focuses on the problems of patients with chronic pain (due to any cause). With Beebe (McCaffery and Beebe, 1989) she describes the benefits of using relaxation techniques, guided imagery, distraction and what is aptly referred to as 'how to cope with boring or strange days'. Their work is centred on the contribution of nurses to the care of patients in pain, and contains helpful suggestions and scripts that are patient-centred.

Palliative care, with its emphasis on a holistic approach, giving people choices and individualising their care, has the expressed aim of enhancing quality of life. Therefore, it is not surprising that it is in the forefront of the use of complementary approaches to care. The Help the Hospices survey (Wilkes, 1992) sent out a questionnaire concerning what it referred to as 'less conventional therapies', and received 108 replies. The four that were most used were massage, aromatherapy, relaxation and reflexology. Nurses carried these out more often than any other members of the caring team and were categorised as having an enthusiastic attitude to their use in 62 hospices, with doctors being keen in 30 of them. The limitations of this survey is that the research is on a self-selected group and the majority of the questionnaires were filled in by nurses.

Many hospices and palliative care units are now creating facilities to provide complementary approaches. Some are building new facilities for the exclusive use of complementary approaches whilst many more are making use of day rooms (see Chapter 10), treatment rooms, physiotherapy rooms. Some are also providing certain therapies for their home care patients.

The advantages of complementary approaches for the person with cancer are numerous. Probably the most important is the time, attention and skilled listening that a complementary practitioner gives. It is not unusual for an assessment visit to take over an hour, and we can all relate to the therapeutic effects of that individual attention, of really being heard by someone. If we have reached a point where we feel, rightly or wrongly, that nothing more can be done it can be encouraging to find that there are other approaches which may be tried. The confidentiality of the encounter may be a further incentive for those who wish to exercise their options over whether to inform their orthodox practitioners or not.

As cancer is a disease that, by its very nature, can make the person feel helpless and as if they are being taken over physically and emotionally, the act of seeking out a complementary therapist can lead to greater feelings of control. Exercising the ability to choose fulfils a fundamental human need (see Chapter 7) and can be an uplifting experience.

Touch in some form is part of many such therapies and can be a very effective way of conveying acceptance to a person who may be feeling isolated because of their disease. These, combined with the possible therapeutic effects of the particular one used, are likely to help the person with cancer to feel better and, as has been discussed earlier, provide them with some hope, whether this be for enhanced quality or quantity of life. Complementary therapies are considered to be safer, gentler and more free of side-effects than many orthodox cancer treatments and these are sufficient reasons for some people to choose them as alternatives.

Probably the greatest disincentive to trying complementary therapies is their cost. Some practitioners have tried to address this by providing assessment visits which are free or at a reduced cost. Others may make some concessions for those with a low income. People who have taken out private health insurance schemes will find that certain therapies are covered, providing they are recommended by the patient's GP. Homoeopathy is provided under the National Health Service at four homoeopathic hospitals, most notably at the Royal London Homoeopathic Hospital which offers a very comprehensive package of cancer treatments, well described by Hodgkinson (1994). As it has already been pointed out, the palliative care movement provides a great many complementary therapies for its patients in hospices, units and, sometimes, in patients' own homes. These are without cost to the patient.

It has been suggested that the largest group of users are middle-aged, middle-class women. If this is so, then empowerment is a crucial issue, with all it has to say about financial status, knowledge, expectations and social skills. People with cancer may feel, as we have seen, disempowered and it may be too demanding to be faced with choices and responsibility when feeling ill and vulnerable. Because complementary therapies are holistic in their approach, many advocate changes in lifestyle, and may recommend regimes which require a high degree of compliance. This may make them too daunting for an ill person, particularly if they also feel unsupported by family or the orthodox health services, in their choice. Furthermore, failure to carry out the advice and treatment prescribed, can leave the individual to cope with guilt and a lowered sense of self-worth which can cause much distress.

Those who do wish to try one or more of these therapies may find several obstacles in their path. Although there are more complementary therapists than ever before, there may not be any, or at least not the exact one wanted, available in a particular locality.

The features of different therapies can be very diverse and the range of qualifications is wide even within practitioners of the same therapy. These are usually difficult to recognise, unlike those of orthodox practitioners. There is also the possibility (although this does not apply exclusively to therapies which are outside the conventional health-care system) of misleading claims being made for the efficacy of the therapy offered.

A controversial aspect of complementary therapies is how far, if at all, they are associated with certain belief systems, not least with what is referred to as the 'new age' movement. It is, perhaps, a surprising misnomer in this context, because these approaches are based on very ancient ideas and practises and are, therefore, in this sense not new at all. Gennis (1992) wrote a provocative article about this issue in which she puts forward the view that practising such therapies is tantamount to performing un-Christian acts which could put a nurse in breach of clause 6 of the code of conduct (UKCC, 1992). Clearly, this aspect will be of concern to some patients and, as with all areas of nursing care, individual's belief systems must always be respected.

It seems appropriate here to refer to spiritual healing which is sometimes considered to be an alternative or complementary therapy.

Healers believe that they can become channels through which the healing force can be transferred to the patient. This may be described perhaps as energy, power, heat or light. This can be done via the laying on of hands or by simply being with the person or even by attending to them from a distance. Healers believe that the source of the healing is outside themselves, but may describe this in different ways, some seeing it as coming from God, others from some other form of Universal Consciousness. Most healers do not make claims to cure people, but see their work as being about helping people towards equilibrium and wholeness. In this process healing of mind and spirit can take place and this may sometimes be accompanied by physical improvement. Healing can be very therapeutic for people even when they are dying.

It may not always be appreciated that most healers undergo training courses and register with a professional body such as the National Federation of Spiritual Healers, thus protecting the public. Their code of conduct was drawn up in consultation with the British Medical Association, General Medical Council and the Royal College of Nursing (RCN).

Indeed, complementary practitioners are very much aware of the need to safeguard the public and to become credible by setting agreed standards of practice, and educating their members via training courses which are validated by their professional bodies. Nevertheless, progress is still slow although a first has been scored by the osteopaths, whose Osteopath's Bill went through parliament on 1 July 1993. Chiropractors and acupuncturists have bills which are waiting to go through parliament.

The other issue which is, perhaps, of more concern to orthodox practitioners than to the general public, is the absence of a scientific approach. Measurement of the effectiveness of complementary approaches is lacking, and claims of success rest on evidence which is largely anecdotal.

An attempt to address this issue was made by the Bristol Cancer Help Centre which was founded in 1979 by Penny Brohn who had, herself, suffered from cancer. It is used by those who turn to unorthodox treatment as an alternative approach as well as those who want to use both. It is not one system, but a cocktail of therapies which are individualised for each person. For example, nutritional medicine, herbal treatments, relaxation techniques, creative visualisation, meditation, counselling art therapy and spiritual healing may be used in different combinations. The approach, therefore, is holistic and aims to encourage people to take responsibility for their own health and promotes the idea that a healthy body and mind can reject cancer.

It took the courageous step of submitting its methods to scientific research and the study (Bagenal *et al.*, 1990) caused a furore when their findings indicated that the group of patients with breast cancer who attended the Bristol Centre, did worse than the set of controls. However, there now seems to be general agreement that the design of the study was flawed and, therefore, its findings were inaccurate.

There is some agreement that the approaches used in complementary therapies do not lend themselves to the rigid criteria of scientific research. The Research Council for Complementary Medicine is a central body for registering research and can provide help, advice and a database of current and completed studies. There is much research being undertaken now, particularly by orthodox practitioners trying to incorporate such approaches into their practice. Much of this has been instigated and carried out by nurses.

A further spur to the process of legitimising complementary therapies is the existence of the Centre for Complementary Health Studies at the University of Exeter, which ran the first degree course in this country. In 1993 Edzart Ernst became the first professor in the UK to hold a Chair in Complementary Medicine.

Nurses who wish to practice complementary therapies as part of their professional role need to have done a recognised course or period of study for the practice of the therapy and then can be covered by the United Kingdom Central Council code of conduct, clause 4. This states that the trained nurse must 'acknowledge any limitations in her knowledge and competence and decline any duties or responsibilities unless able to perform them in a safe and skilled manner' (UKCC, 1992) The problem here, of course, is that there is no agreement – as yet – about what may be considered to be a 'recognised' course. I have found that the period of study that nurses have undergone in order to prepare them to practice aromatherapy, for example, was very diverse and varied between 5 and 500 hours! It is necessary for there to be a standardisation of the competencies required and validation of all training courses by one professional body.

The way forward is for nurses to work closely with complementary therapists to plan and deliver courses in complementary therapies in nursing. The English National Board (ENB) course A49 provides a holistic pathway as one route to obtaining the BSc Hons/ENB Higher Award, which has the added bonus of ending up as either a nurse aromatherapist or a nurse reflexologist (Manchester University and 'Tenda' – the European Nursing Development Agency, Tameside). The Didsbury Trust are currently seeking validation by the ENB to provide post-basic courses in the Krieger/Kunz Method of Therapeutic Touch (also in association with Manchester University).

The RCN has a complementary therapies in nursing forum which now has over 2000 members. Its insurance covers nurses who practice complementary therapies providing they can demonstrate that they have the knowledge and skills to do so safely. It has, amongst other projects, produced some helpful information on what to look for when choosing a course. It would seem good advice to look for a course that involves hands-on practice and that requires case study work as part of its assessment strategy.

The British Medical Association report on 'non-conventional therapies' (British Medical Association, 1993) also focuses on the importance of sound training and emphasises the need for therapies to evolve enforceable ethical codes of practice. It also recommends, as does the RCN, that the patients consent should be obtained before using any therapy. So that this procedure does not interfere at the time that the therapy is decided upon, it may be best to have a form signed routinely on assessment.

Many health-care trusts are now putting together policies on the use of complementary therapies in their areas and documenting the training courses their staff have undergone in order to practise. One of the first was formulated by Bath District Health Authority (Armstrong and Waldon, 1991). The drugs and therapeutics committees are often involved in setting these standards for practice. But whatever the procedures and policies laid down for use by any staff in any clinical area, the trained nurse is always accountable for his or her own practice.

I will know turn to a consideration of the therapies which may most readily be used by nurses in their practice.

Touch

Nurses are well aware that much can be communicated to patients whilst they are involved in nursing procedures of many kinds. Attempting to meet the needs of someone who is incapacitated by illness is a demanding task and one which requires a willingness to share, to some extent, in the patient's experience. It can only be when a patient feels secure enough in his or her relationship with the nurse that he or she is able to ask the difficult question or share his or her deepest doubts and fears. Campbell (1987) describes this kind of nurse/patient relationship as 'graceful care' which he sees as 'not being about anxious people trying to earn love, but about sensitive people who release us from bonds of our own making in spontaneous and often surprising ways'. The use of complementary approaches are one way of working towards this quality of nursing care.

Nurses know that touch is an effective way of communicating warmth and acceptance to patients who are faced with cancer. Morris (1983) goes so far as to say that all individuals require a regular quota of body contact, 'the body quotient' in order to stay healthy. Barnett (1972) puts forward the view that becoming a patient increases the need for touch and it is easy to see that the elderly, the chronically ill and those with an altered body image, may have an unmet need to be touched. It can be concluded, therefore, that becoming a patient with cancer may indicate a particular need for touch. However, culturally the British are non-touchers and receiving a hug or having one's hand held may be felt as an intrusion. Nurses have to be sensitive to the cues from the patient as to whether this is a welcome approach. Those with defences against the intimacy of touch may find it easier to accept in the form of a massage because its purpose is clear.

Massage

Systematic touch, in the form of massage, appears to have originated in China and French translations of their texts mean that much of the terminology used is in French. It provides physical contact in what, for many people, is a very acceptable way. Brewer, a patient with advanced cancer is quoted by Pembrey (1989) as describing its effects as 'you unwind with the gentleness of the human touch. It would be marvellous if nurses could do it in hospital . . . with massage, as soon as the hands go on, you know she's there, she's calm, she has time for you . . . it helps you to think positive.'

When massage techniques are used for patients with cancer, the nurse must be careful to use only gentle touch and to avoid any areas where cancer is known to be present. It has been suggested that massage may promote tumour extension and metastases (Knapp, 1971). The hands and feet provide places where massage is likely to be safe, and stroking of the forehead and face may be especially relaxing. To do this only a very little oil, cream or even powder (unless the skin is dry) needs to be used.

Aromatherapy

However, the complementary therapy which has grown in use most in recent years, and has been enthusiastically taken on by nurses, is massage using essential oils – aromatherapy.

The use of such oils goes back at least 200 years and it is frequently mentioned in the Bible both as a treatment for illness and for religious purposes. From the 13th century onwards it has been used in England and Culpeper's famous work of 1652 classifies the aromatic properties of a large number of plants. The oil extracted from plants are usually referred to as 'essential oils' and are pure concentrated essences of plants, flowers, trees, fruits and herbs. They are considered to act not only on the body, by stimulating physiological processes, but also by either calming the emotions or restoring the mind.

Although aromatherapy is usually applied through massaging the oils into the skin they can be used in the bath or water used for washing. They can be inhaled by being disseminated into the air via a fan or a diffuser or by being heated in a burner, usually by floating a few drops on water which is heated by a candle.

Knowledge and care are needed when using such oils, because it is often not realised that these substances can be potent. The safety of the nursing staff as well as the patient needs to be considered, a particular point being that several oils should not be used during pregnancy. If oils are disseminated into the air in a hospital ward or department, then thought needs to be given to the safety of everyone who may inhale them. Some attention also has to be given as to whether the smell is attractive to other people who may come into contact with it.

Patients with cancer may have their sense of smell altered by the disease or its treatment, such as chemotherapy. Therefore, they should always be asked to smell the oil to be used first to decide if the therapists choice is attractive to them or not.

Essential oils are always diluted by mixing in a carrier oil and they can be diluted further if the person is particularly sensitive to them (for example, two drops of essential oil in 10 ml of a carrier oil such as almond).

A well-known study by Passant (1990) demonstrated that the need for conventional sedatives for elderly people in hospital was reduced when patients received aromatherapy. She found that using oils in baths and putting a drop on the patient's pillow also often induced a peaceful night's sleep. This reminds us of Florence Nightingale who used lavender to anoint patients' foreheads. Many of us will remember the comfort of this from our childhood. Perhaps this goes some way to explaining why lavender oil seems to be the one most commonly used by nurses. A very important reason is that is it one of the safest oils to use.

A trained aromatherapist will use oils in combinations which she blends together for an individual client. When knowledge is limited it is safest to use only one at a time.

Reflexology

Reflexology, also known as reflex zone therapy, is a form of massage which concentrates on the feet. Each part, or zone, of a foot represents a part of the rest of the body. Therefore, when massaging the feet, differences in tone, colour, temperature or sensitivity to touch may be found which reflect imbalances in other parts of the body. This can be used to diagnose problems and to help to eliminate them. If it is not possible to treat the feet, then hands can be used instead as they too correspond to other part of the body.

Massage, aromatherapy and reflexology are all therapies which are being widely used to complement nursing care. They all help to induce relaxation, aid sleep, enhance feelings of well-being and convey warmth and caring. They can also be used to complement the observations made during nursing assessments.

Relaxation

We are all familiar with the concept of relaxation. The word is often used loosely, to suggest times when one is socialising, or not at work. However, true relaxation of the body and the mind is much more than this. Watching television or dozing in a chair is not sufficient to reduce tension which has accumulated and will continue unconsciously.

Techniques for relaxation can be quickly learnt via groups or classes or by listening to tapes or reading guides. It is suggested that just 30 minutes devoted to this per day is all that is required, yet most people will say that they are too busy to spare the time to relax! Perhaps this is an area where it is particularly important to practise what is being preached, and nurses can benefit from learning the skill of relaxation and how to incorporate this behaviour into their lifestyle.

There are different kinds of relaxation techniques. Some people may find that the progressive type with its focus on clenching and then letting of each muscle group and on control of the breath, suits them best. This is the one that many women are familiar with, because it is taught in antenatal classes.

Others may find guided imagery helps to relax them and, for some, this may lead to the use of meditation to help to achieve a balanced mind and body. Some people may like to try biofeedback techniques as an aid to relaxation and to control physiological processes.

Guided imagery

Guided imagery makes use of the imagination in order to focus the mind and induce relaxation through pleasant thoughts, a form of planned day-dreaming perhaps. Words create a picture for the mind of some pleasant scene and the person visualises themselves travelling to a place which is special to them and which they can revisit at any time in the future. All the senses are called on to make the mind-picture come alive, with descriptions of, perhaps, the feel of the sun on one's face, the sound of the breeze in the trees, the taste of the salt air in ones mouth. If a tape is used it may contain music or the sounds of, for instance, the sea or of birdsong.

Visualisation

Visualisation techniques applied to the fight against cancer, are associated with the work of Carl and Stephanie Simonton in the 1970s. The underlying hypothesis is that physical processes in the body are affected by what the imagination creates and that, with training, the individual can learn to develop their powers of imagination and use them to combat their cancer.

People with cancer who are interested in this approach are helped to visualise their cancer and their immune system as if in a battle, the actual images used should be chosen by them. Brohn (1987) makes the important point that the cancer must be represented by something which is weaker then the image chosen for the immune system. The main picture is to be that of a strong, powerful force which is battling against a weak and feeble opponent. An important end to the visualisation is one of seeing themselves healthy and active in the future. This may have to begin by remembering when they were well in their past. It is usually suggested that the image should be used for a short period once or twice a day, and is combined with relaxation techniques.

Visualisation can give back feelings of control to the person with cancer, they are a positive approach which can counteract the negativity which surrounds the disease itself. It seems feasible that nurses could learn to assist people who would like to try this approach, though they need to be aware that for some people the regular focusing of the mind on the fact that they have cancer, could be detrimental.

Meditation

Although meditation may be thought of as a form of religious exercise it can also be viewed as another form of relaxation or visualisation technique, depending on the beliefs of the individual using it. The aim is to quieten the mind and body. This can be achieved by learning to concentrate, perhaps upon an object such as a candle or on a word which is special to the individual, their own mantra. Thinking about their breathing may be another way into this peaceful state. Then the person learns to let go of the busyness of the day and the incessant chatter of the mind, letting thoughts come and go until they reach a state of inner quiet, a silent space. Like other skills, this takes time to learn. Books, tapes or classes are available to help and scripts to guide meditation can be found in the book by Bond (1986).

Biofeedback

Biofeedback is a technique for learning how to govern body states which are not normally under the control of the conscious mind. It does not require regular supervision of any kind and some people may be able to learn it at home without more than an initial training session. The individual learns this by watching some kind of visual display or by hearing noises either of which act as signals which feedback the alterations which the body has made in response to his or her thought processes. An example of this is a stress monitor which issues a high-pitched bleeping noise when the person is tense. The aim then is to learn how to alter this to a low-pitched hum. They achieve this my practising relaxation techniques, which may be accompanied by imagery as they wish. Interested people can purchase these kind of feedback machines fairly inexpensively (for example, one sells for about £15) and can use them regularly without outside help. Nurses may find this useful to suggest to the person who values independence and prefers to try techniques which do not require regular visits to therapists either orthodox or complementary.

Therapeutic touch

Therapeutic touch is a term that may be confused with massage techniques. Here it refers to a specific form of touch, first used by Krieger (1975). She is a professor of nursing in the United States who was much influenced by, among others, the work of Rogers (1980) whose model of nursing contains the concept of unitary man who she sees as being an open energy system, in continual interaction with the energy fields of others. In other words, we do not end at our skin but at the boundary of the energy field which surrounds us and which is constantly changing. We may imagine that when we feel good our energy field is expanded and we feel open to others whereas when we feel ill our energy field contracts and we feel closed in.

In the United States, thousands of nurses have been trained to tune into the energy fields of patients, both to help to assess problems and to smooth them and help the patient to feel relaxed and calm. In order to do this, the nurse places her hands a few centimetres away from the body and runs them over the patient so that she has felt all surfaces. With practice, she can learn to detect subtle differences in the sensations she receives and to interpret them. She can learn to

em out, thereby helping to balance the energy field and enhance feelings
ion. This exciting and innovative approach that it being developed by
emselves can be learnt in the UK though the Didsbury Trust, and there
ing body of knowledge of the uses and effectiveness of therapeutic touch,
research by Kreiger and others.

These are a few examples of complementary therapies which may be incorporated into nursing care. They all require knowledge and understanding on the part
of the nurse so that they are completely safe for the patient and others who may
be involved. Well-developed interpersonal skills are always needed when putting
them into practice. An environment that is as quiet, calm and private as possible
is essential to optimise their effects. Although time is also needed, some of the
therapies can, in fact, be used quite quickly, for example a foot massage may only
take a few minutes, therapeutic touch can be done in 2 min, a drop of lavender on
the pillow may take a few seconds.

However, as we have seen there are important issues which have to be
addressed. These include appropriate and validated training programmes, the setting of standards for safe practice and the need for research studies to gain cred-
ibility and provide a sound knowledge base for nursing practice.

From this it can be argued that orthodox medicine as practised by the doctor
and complementary therapies as used by nurses as an adjunct to care should be
the path that palliative care should continue to pursue. The combination of these
two closely related disciplines will provide a model of holistic care that is
reminiscent of the ancient philosophies but is one that has relevance to modern
thinking. This model is shown in Fig. 15.1.

Nurses have a professional responsibility to respond to the wishes of the patient
and act as his or her advocate. By supporting the use of complementary therapies
as part of conventional nursing care, people with cancer can be offered the best of
both worlds by receiving care which is truly holistic.

References

ARMSTRONG, F. and WALDRON, R. (1991). A complementary strategy. *Nursing
Times* 87, 34–5.
BAGENAL, F., EASTON, D. and HARRIS, E. (1990). Survival of patients with breast
cancer attending the Bristol Cancer Help Centre. *The Lancet* 336, 606–10.

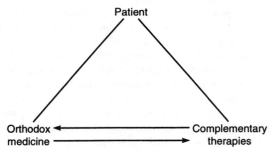

Fig. 15.1 A model of holistic care.

BARNETT, K. (1972). A survey of the current utilisation of touch by health team personnel with hospitalised patients. *International Journal of Nursing Studies* 3, 195–209.

BRITISH MEDICAL ASSOCIATION (1993). *Complementary Medicine: New Approaches to Good Practice.* Oxford University Press.

BOND, M. (1986), *Stress and Self Awareness: A Guide for Nurses.* Heinemann, London.

BROHN, P. (1987). *The Bristol Programme.* Century–Hutchinson, London

BURKE, C. and SIKORA, K. (1993). Complementary and conventional cancer care: the integration of two cultures. *Clinical Oncology* 5, 220–70.

CAMPBELL, A. (1987). *Moderated Love: A Theology of Professional Care.* SPCK.

GENNIS, F. (1992). Alternative roads to hell? *Nursing Standard* 6, 43–4.

HODGKINSON, L. (1994). Therapy with complements. *The Independent* 19 May.

KNAPP, M. (1971). In: KNUSEN, K. (ed.), *Handbook of Physical Medicine and Rehabilitation.* W. B. Saunders, London.

KRIEGER, D. (1986). *The Therepeutic Touch: How to Use Your Hands to Help or Heal.* Prentice-Hall, New York.

MCCAFFERY, M. and BEEBE, A. (1989). *Pain: A Manual for Nursing Practice.* C. V. Mosby Co., St Louis.

MORRIS, D. (1983). *Intimate Behaviour.* Bantam Books, London.

PASSANT, H. (1990). The holistic approach in the ward. *Nursing Times* 86, 24–6.

PEMBREY, S. (1989). The development of nursing practice: a new contribution. *Senior Nurse* 9, 8.

ROGERS, M. (1970). *An Introduction to the Theoretical Basis of Nursing.* F. A. Davies, Philadelphia.

UNITED KINGDOM CENTRAL COUNCIL (1992). Code of professional conduct.

WELLS, R. with TSCHUDIN, V. (eds) (1994). *Wells Supportive Therapies in Health Care.* Ballière-Tindall, London.

WILKES, E. (1992). *Complementary Therapy in Hospice and Palliative Care.* Help the Hospices Survey/Trent Palliative Care Centre.

Further reading

CHOPRA, D. (1989). *Quantum Healing.* Bantam Books, New York.

DAVIS, P. (1988). *Aromatherapy: An A–Z.* C. W. Daniel, Saffron Walden.

DAVIS, P. (1991). *Subtle Aromatherapy.* C. W. Daniel, Saffron Walden.

MACRAE, J. (1990). *Therapeutic Touch: A Practical Guide.* Penguin, Harmondsworth.

PEARCE, I. (1989). *The Holistic Approach to Cancer.* C. W. Daniel, Saffron Walden.

PIETRONI, P. (1993). Complementary medicine – its place in the care of dying people. In: DICKENSEN, D. and JOHNSON, M. (eds), *Death, Dying and Bereavement.* Open University.

RANKIN-BOX, D. F. (ed.) (1988). *Complementary Health Therapies: A Guide for Nurses.* Croom Helm, Beckenham.

The Reader's Digest Guide to Alternative Medicine (1991).

SIEGEL, B. (1989). *Love, Medicine and Miracles.* Harper & Row, New York.

SIMONTON, C., MATTHEWS-SIMONTON, S. and CREIGHTON, L. (1978). *Getting Well Again: a Step by Step Self-help Guide for Patients and their Families.* Bantam Books, London.

16

Communication

Sally Anstey

'Cancer patients who are well-informed seldom complain of being told too much.'

Hughes (1987)

Introduction

For the purpose of this chapter it is presumed that the reader will have a prior working knowledge of the basic skills of verbal and non-verbal communication. The aim of this contribution is to build on to these general communication abilities particular skills tailored to meet the needs of individuals and their families receiving active palliative care in a variety of clinical settings.

Research background

Why is a research background important? It is important to discuss past research for a variety of reasons. Nursing interventions and interactions should be made in a response to evidence from scientific research, rather than on the basis of the maxim 'We will do it like this because we have always done so'. Research also highlights the inadequacies of nurse training and, consequently, of the nurse's role in effective communication in the area of death and dying.

Communication needs of dying patients

Many studies highlight the difficulty professionals experience in communicating effectively with dying patients and their families and illustrate that poor quality communication adversely affects the psychological well-being of these patients. These studies broadly categorise the communication needs of dying patients as follows.

Social interaction

Brewin (1977) discusses the importance of humour and the small talk of normal social discourse as improving patients' morale and decreasing fear and isolation.

To discuss and work through feelings, fears and anxieties

Individuals with life-threatening disease, especially cancer, may experience a variety of feelings and emotions which are in need of expression (Vachon, 1988).

These people appear to expect us, as professionals, to show interest in; explain and provide non-judgemental information about any subject they are concerned with (Doyle, 1987). Interestingly, patients appear more satisfied when professionals are warm, concerned and empathetic, but not necessarily more practically skilled (Francis and Morris, 1969).

Family care

Treatment of the family unit has been identified as one of the most important elements of the psychosocial care of the terminally ill (Webster, 1986). However, in our society there are increasing numbers of homosexual and common-law relationships. Consequently, we should be aware that the term 'family' should refer not to the patient's relatives alone, but to encompass all others of significance to him/her (Henley, 1986).

Information, advice and explanation

Stedeford (1981), over a decade ago, identified considerable suffering directly resulting from poor communication, with patients generally wanting more information than they had been given.

It is this area of concern to patients upon which this chapter will seek to concentrate.

Communication and professionals

Over many years, a growing body of literature highlighting the difficulties faced by professionals in communicating with people who have life-threatening diseases, especially cancer, has been produced. It has been recognised that patients can evoke reactions in professionals that lead to various forms of direct or indirect avoidance, so that their communication and psychological needs are never appreciated or dealt with. The most intense avoidance responses are probably triggered by the circumstances of dying and death (Barton, 1972) and are, in part, influenced by individuals' own prior experiences of death which directly affect their attitudes and feelings.

A study by Maguire (1985) has suggested that many doctors and nurses consistently use distancing tactics with dying patients; this occurred when observations were made of their interactions in real, simulated or role play situations. The tactics were described as being used to protect the professional emotionally but, in practice, served to discourage patients from disclosing their psychological concerns, thus detracting from effective care in this area.

Studies concerning nurses specifically are rare, but Fielding and Llewellyn (1987) confirm that they also have difficulty in communicating with patients, especially those who are emotionally distressed or dying. These authors point to the importance of organisational issues, in that communicating with patients and relatives is often perceived to be of little value, and consequently left to the most junior member of staff. Such issues may, in part, explain the findings that nurses are more likely to respond to the expressions of physical rather than emotional distress, even when they perceive the latter. In an early study of communication between nurses and cancer patients by Bond in 1978, it was discovered that once a patient had been given a diagnosis of cancer, his or her care would deteriorate. Nurses were noted to become reticent in giving the patient information, and skilful at ignoring any signs of their distress.

Communication and nurse training

The teaching of professionals, particularly nurses, in communication skills specifically appropriate to the area of palliative care is now undertaken by many hospices or hospice-type organisations in the UK. Parkes and Parkes (1984) compared individuals who had died at St Christopher's Hospice with others who had died in general hospitals in the same part of London and found no difference in pain, symptoms and general distress between the two groups. This was in contrast to a similar study conducted 10 years earlier where hospice care was found to be universally superior. The change was attributed by the authors to the teaching work undertaken by the hospice to hospital personnel in the intervening years. Reisetter and Thomas (1986) in a Canadian study of hospital nurses, support the view that post-qualification education in the field of death and dying can improve the quality of palliative care provided.

However, few pre-registration nursing programmes adequately prepare students to care for the terminally ill. Webster (1981) identified as reasons for poor communication both a lack of skills and a practically useful knowledge base – the 'theory–practice gap'

Touch and other non-verbal skills are an important facet of communication but are sorely neglected in the training of nursing staff. Moy (1981) suggests that few nurses receive any formal instruction on the subject, but states that their ideas about touch in particular develop through gradual professional self-awareness. Most qualified nurses questioned said that the main intention of using touch was to convey caring; the most common response to it was that the patients or relatives further expressed feelings, or that there was an increase in verbal responses (Aguilera, 1967; Langland and Panniccucci, 1982).

Difficulties which affect effective communication

In the palliative care setting, the nurse, by the very nature of his or her role – be it in hospital or the community – has a direct, continuous and intimate relationship with the patients and their carers. Nurses' satisfaction with the quality of their care is related to the perceived openness or ease of communication with the patient and family (Wilkinson, 1988). However, most recognise that there are many barriers to good communication which should be explored, as they directly affect care/performance. The following is not intended as an exhaustive list and is not in order of importance:

- Difficulties imposed by *patient* and *family*.
- *External* difficulties, e.g. organisational issues.
- *Internal* difficulties, e.g. personal fears and anxieties.
- Difficulties imposed by the *ambiguities* in the nurse's role.
- Difficulties imposed by the *multidisciplinary team*.

Difficulties imposed by the patient and family

Wilkinson (1991) recognised that communication with the terminally ill will always be of a different nature to the usual interactive processes involved in the nurse–patient relationship. The physical, mental or spiritual condition of the dying patient may make communication more difficult.

Communication may often be poor, regardless of the nurse's attempts to improve it – this may be simply because the patient does not want to talk (Fielding and Llewellyn, 1987). Interaction may well be impeded by well-meaning family members who often withhold information from dying patients as a protective gesture (Maguire, 1985).

External difficulties

Time. There is a widely held myth that communication in whatever form is a process of considerable duration. Perhaps this is, in part, due to the fact that when communication does occur, it is in response to a crisis, when there is much about which the patient wants to talk. Nurses' time is seen as precious and there is a perception of constantly racing against the clock to provide patient care. In some instances, it is non-nursing duties, for example, in hospital, answering the telephone, ordering stock, accompanying *all* the doctors on *all* ward rounds, that takes their time; in the community it is paperwork, inadequately completed transfer documents, auditing of visits/journey times and the grey area of social versus clinical care.

Consequently, constraints of time often lead to the placement of more emphasis upon the completion of less time-consuming physical tasks, despite the perpetual need for the fulfilment of patients' psychological needs (Webster, 1981). Poor staff–patient relationships are wholly undesirable, yet recurrent consequences of the high patient turnover and task allocation on busy wards (Fielding and Llewellyn, 1987). The GRASP (Grace Reynolds' Application and Study of Peto) (Hiscocks, 1994) data on nursing workload in South Glamorgan Health Authority corroborates these findings.

Communication should be seen as an on-going process, and, as such, it may be regular short bursts of support or encouragement which meet some needs and ease distress. One gesture of physical touch – a cuddle or hand held, should not be underestimated as its therapeutic benefits are highly valued by patients. It is the 'quality' not the 'quantity' that counts.

Pressure from superiors and/or peers. The patient's physical needs, for example washing and the skilled tasks performed for patients, are perceived to be of paramount importance and are recognised by superiors as 'real work'.

Communicating with patients and relatives is seen as an easy option (which of course is not true); a sign of laziness and not part of the nurse's job. Such explicit disapproval and pressure from colleagues, peers and superiors influences practice, since it is important to be accepted as part of the team. Superiors influence professionally, complete appraisal forms and directly affect the nurse's career.

It is learning in the ward environment which has been suggested to be most influential, and junior nurses learning from role models in that environment are provided with a guide to determining future practice. However, in most instances practical tasks are shown and very rarely communication skills.

Nurse training. There is a wide disparity between the training school and the ward environment (see the earlier research section). In particular, training in the care of the dying patient is inadequate with regard to psychological and communication aspects. Talking to dying patients and their families is a frightening area of care upon which to embark, especially if it is untaught, viewed as unacceptable and unsupported. It may also be assumed that if something is a proper subject, then it will be taught as part of the curriculum; its exclusion implies that nurses do not need to venture into that area of practice.

The role of the nursing auxiliary is currently evolving to that of the more clinically involved health-care support worker. Although their work is increasingly involved with patients who are terminally ill, their preparation is far from ideal (and this puts understandable extra pressure on the trained staff). The National Vocational Training (City and Guilds, 1990) that the health-care support workers receive deals largely with physical care needs.

Organisation of ward work. The use of the nursing process, nursing models and theories and patient allocation has implications for nurses in that they are held individually responsible for the holistic aspects of patient care. Often the most junior members of staff are involved in the care of the dying, as it is regarded as 'basic nursing', whereas the more experienced staff are involved with those requiring potentially life-saving or technical skills. The stresses involved for junior staff who are unsupported, untrained and feeling vulnerable mitigate against them. Communicating ineffectively ultimately makes them less satisfied with their performance, but also renders them less likely to try to provide this facet of care.

Sanitisation of death (as first described by Buckman, 1988). We live in a society where dying is not seen as an acceptable part of living, it is not acknowledged or discussed in a natural way but seen as something alien or taboo. So, when a person is dying, the denial of death creates a barrier between them and the rest of society, isolating them when they most need support. The causes of this may include the following:

• The loss of the extended family, with more people dying in hospital. Fry (1983) presents national figures on the site of death, including sudden deaths:

    25 per cent occur at home
    64 per cent in hospital
    4 per cent in hospices
    7 per cent elsewhere.

When cancer deaths alone are considered, Fry estimates that seven out of 20 (35 per cent) occur at home – thus when death does occur, more often than not it is partially hidden in an institutional environment. This enables the nurse to avoid the prospect of death, viewing it as clinical and distant.
• Medicalisation: medicine is seen as being 'high tech.' with the emphasis on keeping alive and having power to stave off death, so the care of the dying may, in part, be seen as a failure of health-care.
• Society's acceptance of a materialistic way of life, placing more emphasis on possessions than the way life is lived, quantity not quality.
• Most people have never seen anyone dead or dying and so are afraid of the unknown, the horror of the unseen often being worse than the reality.

Internal difficulties

Internal difficulties are related to the health professionals' own personal fears and anxieties.

- Personal fears of illness and death are linked, in part, to the sanitisation of death discussed earlier, in that talking about death and dying is seen as a social taboo and beyond the realms of the carer's personal experience. In addition, psychologists suggest that some individuals become doctors or nurses to exorcise their own fears of death and dying by perceiving that they have a direct responsibility to 'keep individuals alive at all costs' – power over life and death. By avoidance of close contact with people who are dying, they do not have to confront the threat of their own mortality and consequently are not threatened.
- Fear of being seen as responsible for the patient's situation, or being blamed for the patient's impending death, the implication being that perhaps the doctor or nurse did not try hard enough, or possess appropriate skill or expertise to 'cure' him or her. This is linked to the general public's view of the omnipotence of the medical and nursing professions.
- Fear of the consequences of our interactions. Firstly, precipitating a reaction in the patient or relative, especially if it is emotional. What do we do if the patient breaks down and cries, or gets angry, abusive and shouts? This fear of an emotional reaction and being labelled as 'the nurse who upsets patients' may make people wary of embarking on some areas of communication.

Secondly, there is the fear of expressing their own emotions. Nurses are taught to behave in a professional manner, remaining detached and uninvolved, hiding behind their uniform but, in reality, becoming distressed when having to hide this. For patients, it is sometimes supportive and helpful if nurses show that they care about the patient's situation or distress, but not that they are accepting the blame for it.

- Anxiety about not knowing the answers: admitting that we do not know is seen very much as failure since medicine is expected to be an exact science. However, in palliative care 'don't know' is an honest response as the situation of death and dying is not clearly predictable. How long have I left to live? What will my dying be like? These are common questions for which inappropriate reassurance and an exact time limit are not helpful responses as they are not likely to be accurate. Often the questioner needs the nurse to listen to how they feel, what they think and what their problems are – rather than to provide them with the answers.
- Over-identification with the patients or their relatives by being reminded of a member of the nurse's own family or a past bereavement. It is important for nurses to accept limitations in the care which they provide, they cannot be 'all things to all men' and they need to remain effective, not overwhelmed by past and current emotions. There is no disgrace in admitting that a situation is causing anguish and asking to be relieved of caring for a particular individual: it takes courage but is important for the nurse's own welfare, and to ensure high-quality care that the nurse is unlikely to be able to give in such a situation.
- Relationship difficulties in nurses' professional lives are not unknown. In palliative care, there is the need to establish a relationship more quickly than normal

and, by necessity, it is more personal and less formal – if the relationship does not appear to be working on either side, there is no harm in withdrawing and handing over to a colleague. Ultimately, there is more harm to all parties in persevering and not establishing an effective quality caring relationship.

* For all nurses there are particular areas of care that they find rewarding and those they find either difficult or unsatisfying. It is important, therefore, to recognise that some nurses, for a variety of reasons, are not comfortable in caring for the dying and consequently should not be forced to become involved at a level they find difficult or distressing. This, however, is not a blanket absolution in allowing individuals to opt out of palliative care totally, as it unfortunately forms a very large body of nurses' work, but should encourage awareness of the problem by colleagues.

Ambiguities in the nurse's role

The changing role of the nurse. In the UK, the pressures internally and externally on nursing to redefine its roles and spheres of influence are increasing with the proposals of the English National Board (ENB) for Nursing, Midwifery and Health Visiting (1989) for Project 2000, relating to nurse training, those of the United Kingdom Central Council for Nursing, Midwifery and Health Visiting (1989, 1990) for post-registration education (the Post-registration Education and Practice Project, PREPP), and the shifting emphasis from the treatment of disease to the promotion of health.

Community. For community nurses, the implementation of general practitioners' contracts, the government's community care white paper, the suggestions of role re-alignment, numbers of practice nurses, nurse prescribing, and the extended role of the nurse with its ambiguities cause increased anxiety. On the positive side, the extended role of the community care assistant may release more time for the community nurse and his or her team to spend on skilled nursing care, including holistic palliative care. The evolution of the role of the Macmillan nurse from providing 'five star' clinical care to a small number of patients to the provision of education to enable primary carers to provide effective palliative care to the majority of patients dying from advanced cancer, has implications for the wider teaching of communication and other relevant skills.

Hospital. There have been vast changes in the role of the nurse within the hospital setting, the moves from task to patient allocation; the adoption of nursing models; the nursing process with individualised patient care; nursing development units; team and primary nursing; the change in roles for the enrolled nurse and auxiliary within the emerging multilevel health-care assistant. All these changes have implications for the evolution of the nurse's role. Individualised patient care has implications for improving communication skills at all levels – it is more difficult for a nurse to respond to the patient's questions by saying 'I will go and ask Sister', for each nurse has the individual responsibility to deal with the situation. This is particularly so in team and primary nursing, where the ward sister acts as teacher and facilitator rather than overall clinical manager and care provider.

Advocacy. The growing acknowledgement of advocacy as an integral part of the nurse's role is especially relevant for care of the dying patient and family. In this particular sense, advocacy implies respecting the human rights of patients, including the promotion and protection of their autonomy. The ultimate implication of this includes the patient's right to participate in decisions which affect them, either directly, or by using the nurse as a 'go-between' in their interactions with other members of the health-care team, or between their family and friends.

Active versus passive communication. Nurses have no obligation to involve themselves at every level of communication with their patients. In palliative care, communication needs can include the following:

• Normal communication on a wide variety of subjects, e.g. gossip/jokes.
• Relating to diagnosis and prognosis.
• Specific problem areas relating to the process of dying.

It is apparent that patients will select who they feel is appropriate to deal with a particular subject area. If chosen, nurses have to make the decision as to whether to become actively or passively involved. Active involvement implies that the nurse is prepared to support the patients and their families throughout the time of living with a terminal disease, the actual dying process and the immediate bereavement period, caring for the myriad communication needs. Passive involvement implies that the nurses feel, for whatever reasons, that communication needs are not their direct responsibility and, as a consequence, may avoid the issues entirely, but must actively pass on that aspect of care to other members of the caring team.

The multidisciplinary team

Who is the multidisciplinary team? Anyone who has involvement with the patients and their families should be included as a member of the team, whether it be the porters or ancillary staff, the receptionist, consultant or nurse, social worker, occupational therapist, physiotherapist – each has a unique contribution to make and should be valued and supported as such.

For true multidisciplinary palliative care to be effective, there needs to be an overlap, between the roles of team members. Distinct differences serve only to act as barriers in providing holistic care. It is important to acknowledge that the patients and their families are part of the team in the sphere of palliation there are few clear-cut best choices of care, the implication being that, where possible, the individual's own wishes are important treatment indicators. However, to include the patient in decision making requires clear and open communication among all members of the health team.

Role ambiguity. Often within the multidisciplinary team it is perceived that there is a doctor–nurse clique which isolates others and serves to undermine/ negate their contribution; also within nursing there is the qualified/unqualified gap, with qualified staff appearing to forget the trauma of death as a student nurse experiences it.

Further difficulties occur when either the policy for talking to patients or relatives is unclear, or there is an authoritarian relationship with medical staff in the multidisciplinary team, whereby interactions and communications are subordinate to the senior doctor's wishes. In the United States and some other countries, the patient's right to know is enshrined in law. However, in the UK it is still (theoretically) possible for senior doctors to forbid others to communicate about certain matters, particularly prognosis and dying, thus denying the nurse's active contribution in these areas. This is despite the Medical Records Act, 1991.

If the nurse's role among team members is regarded as equal, then the patients' interests are well served by a collaborative relationship. This is especially apparent if not all team members are informed, or there is no documentation as to the information given to terminally ill patients and their relatives about their illness. Obviously this situation makes further support uncertain and interactions unnecessarily problematic.

At present, what is happening in terms of the relationship primarily between doctor and nurse is that the nurse offers active input into the partnership. Sometimes that input is accepted, sometimes sought and encouraged, and sometimes discounted. This relationship is certainly one step onward from the traditional authoritative model. However, it is still a long way from open communication, which is necessary to meet the needs of the patients and families. Ideally, the collaborative model of multidisciplinary care does offer such open communication and is demonstrated by mutual decision making and respect for the integrity of all parties involved, patients, relatives and team members.

Field (1984) in his observational studies, states that it is still doctors who control the information nurses are allowed to give patients and relatives about diagnosis and prognosis. Wilkinson (1988) identifies stressful incidents as perceived by nurses and found 'nurse/doctor conflicts' to be the most stressful. These were rated far higher than the second and fourth on her list of stressors, which were 'the inability to communicate effectively with the patient' and 'difficulties in communicating with and supporting relatives'.

However, it cannot be overlooked that, in some instances, the responsibility for lack of communication may lie with the patients and/or relatives.

Team needs. Mutual advice, support and encouragement are among the benefits of good teamwork. Health professionals are often very isolated in their care of the dying, so team meetings and case conferences work as an effective bolster to improve performance, providing they are not excessively formal, monopolised by one or two members, or under the authoritarian influence of the medical staff. To be effective, they should be based on the mutual respect of all parties and work as a forum for improving patient care, updating education by increasing knowledge and skills in palliation, and increasing support by fostering self-disclosure and openness in discussing difficulties, triumphs and auditing of care.

Within the team concept it is important to recognise that it is unlikely that one person can cope with all the communication needs of the dying patient and family. Hence, sharing the situation improves support for the patients and relatives as well as for the team members. Occasionally there are communication needs within the multidisciplinary team. Some individuals need to act as arbiters, mutual supporters, ethicists or teachers, so that the team can learn and grow as a result of the care they are providing.

Patients and their families, as members of the team, have a part to play in aiding health professionals to communicate with them and each other; they are excellent teachers, often guiding the professional through difficult situations. Patients sometimes find it easier to talk with health-care professionals about particular emotional concerns. An example of the nurse and doctor sharing a 'breaking bad news' consultation is beneficial on many levels. It identifies weaknesses, improves skills through role modelling; provides support during a difficult encounter and enables one person to act as observer of verbal and non-verbal cues relating to distress, incomprehension, and to perhaps translate the medical jargon or to intervene if the consultation becomes problematic.

How to communicate: general guidelines for effective communication in palliative care

Setting the scene

Aim. To optimise the non-verbal quality of the communication, by appearing to take account of the vulnerability of the patient's relative's situation, preparing them for a difficult conversation, and returning some control of the interaction to them. This 'setting of the scene' should enable the professional to feel more comfortable (by using practical guidelines) with what follows and prepare them in switching to communication mode.

How to do it. The health-care professional needs to pay attention to the following.

* *Environment.* Creating a sense of privacy and quiet, e.g. drawing the curtains or using an office, preferably without a telephone.
* *Non-verbal behaviour.* Appearing unhurried, that time is not a problem (even though it probably is). The professional positioning him or herself well by sitting down, being on the same level or slightly lower than the patient with a comfortable distance between them, not too close or too far away. Ensuring that the patient is physically comfortable, e.g. not in pain or actively vomiting, otherwise these symptoms will act as a barrier to effective communication. Enabling the patient to be adequately dressed so that they do not feel intimidated.

Getting started. Particular skills – open questions

Aim. The purposes of this type of question are
* To find out how the individual is really feeling, not to confirm what the professional thinks he or she is feeling. In particular, what they are feeling at the time/moment of the conversation.
* To ensure that both professional and patient are on the same 'wavelength'.
* To discover if it is an appropriate time to embark on a deeper type of conversation: is the patient pain-free? Is the patient expecting visitors?
* To determine whether the relationship between the professional and the patient is good enough to cope with the ensuing conversation.

How to do it.
* Note that there must be congruence between questions and non-verbal behaviour.

- Elicit information precisely, e.g. 'How are you feeling today?' 'How were you feeling yesterday?'.
- Give the patient the opportunity to respond at a level at which they feel comfortable and in the way they choose, e.g. 'Not so well today, I seem to have a lot on my mind.' 'Surprisingly well, I really feel I'm getting so much better.'
- The patient is thus in control and guiding the subsequent conversation.
- It is important to be aware of the significance of the patient's non-verbal responses, e.g. do they look relaxed/anxious/tearful?

How not to do it.
- When using open questions the professional should not bias or prejudice responses for their own convenience or safety, e.g. 'You look really well today – how are you feeling?' Most patients would find it difficult to respond other than positively to such a question. The opposite may also be true, e.g. 'Gosh you do look exhausted – how are you sleeping?'
- Do not ask open questions:
  without setting the scene to deal with the responses
  whilst looking at your watch or looking busy and pre-occupied
  with a large number of other people present, mostly unknown to the patient, e.g. whilst taking visitors around the ward
  as 'throw away lines', e.g. asking 'How are you?' and either walking away before the patient can reply, or pre-empting the reply by automatic responses such as 'That's good', 'That's great'.

Asking unhelpful open questions will only serve to preclude the beneficial effect of appropriate open questioning by the patient being uncertain as to when the professional is willing to establish an effective communicating relationship.

Particular skills – conversation encouragers

These are, techniques of facilitating conversation by enabling and encouraging the patient to talk freely and feel comfortable with the health-care professional. They are extremely simple and may even seem obvious but are highly effective.

Aim.
- To keep the communication channels open for the benefit of the patient/relative by giving support and consequently easing their distress.

How to do it.
- *Non-verbal prompters.* For example nodding, smiling, touching a hand or arm (especially when the conversation is proving painful), maintaining/encouraging eye contact.
- *Verbal prompters.* Saying 'Yes', 'Yes, I see, do go on', 'hm mmm', 'Could you tell me more about that', 'Explain what you mean', 'Help me to understand what you mean'. Being comfortable with silence, not talking for the sake of talking or interrupting prematurely, but using it as an encourager, allowing people to think or to feel safe about their next words.
- *Repetition.* Occasionally repeating the last few key words of the patient's sentence encourages them and proves that the professional is actively listening.

However, if this skill is used too much it can sound like a learned rather than spontaneous response.

- *Reflecting/paraphrasing.* Repeating what the patient/relative has said using the professional's own words proves that the professional is understanding exactly what has been said.
- *Displaying warmth and empathy.* The professional can show that they understand how the patient/relative is feeling by moving closer if they become distressed, by showing that they are at ease with the patient's emotions and that they will stay with the patient. The professional should not respond to anger with anger, but should feel able to encourage the patient/relative to give vent to their feelings. (Responding to overt emotions is difficult for most people, but fear, anger and sadness are all normal reactions. Helping people to deal with them is beneficial to their emotional well-being.)
- *Talking about distress.* This can, in part, help to relieve it.
- *Encouraging the patient/relative to express their thoughts and emotions.* Thoughts and emotions that are repeatedly buried may eventually do harm, by increasing distress and the sense of isolation of the individual 'being alone with their dying'.
- *If a pause/silence is prolonged.* Encouragement may be helpful by saying, for example 'What are you thinking about?' 'Would it help to share what you are thinking about?' However, this should not be so powerful that it makes the patient feel forced to continue or precipitate withdrawal.
- *Slight hesitancy* on the part of the professional (not having the right words on the tip of your tongue) helps the patient/relative by making them feel that their situation is unique and personal and that the communication is not merely an academic exercise.

Specific areas relating to palliative care

- How much does the patient know?
- How much do they want to know?
- Sharing the news
- What next?

How much does the patient know?

This is an important part of the communication process as it enables the professional carer to establish a starting point on which to build. A patient's knowledge may not be the same as they have been *told* or what their family and friends believe they are aware of. Nurses and doctors are poor predictors of patients' levels of knowledge relating to life-threatening disease, and tend not to allow for the usual initial reaction of denial.

Professional carers have to accept at face value what the patient remembers and understands of what has been said previously relating to diagnosis and prognosis.

- Patients forget at least 40 per cent of what they hear in an interview, and this is likely to be much higher when the news is bad.
- Patients and relatives often state that after they hear key words like 'cancer', 'death', 'no further treatment' they cannot remember anything of the conversation that follows.

- The patients choice of words about their disease (malignant neoplasm, tumour, cancer, ulcer or growth) gives clues as to what has been said previously and how much jargon was used, how they have dealt with and interpreted the information and which word they are suggesting or insisting be used when talking to them.
- By eliciting the patient's level of knowledge it is possible to estimate the 'bad news gap' (Buckman, 1988), the gap between their expectations and reality.
- For the individual with advanced cancer their knowledge may not have been updated. Consequently they may be still expecting active, potentially curative treatment, or be angry or distressed by the lack of cure resulting from a variety of unpleasant treatments.
- It is important to understand that, in some circumstances patients and/or relatives need to apportion blame, for example to their previous professional carers. Ascertaining their level of knowledge may trigger expression of their emotions. This approach may also help in avoiding being drawn into blaming or excusing previous professional carers.

Possible useful questions.
'It would be helpful if you could tell me what the doctors looking after you before have told you about your illness?'
'I see, and what do you understand by that?'
'How does that information make you feel?'
'What did it all mean to you?'
'How did that information affect you?'
'Could you tell me what you have been told about your husband's/wife's illness?'

How much do they want to know?

By returning control to the patient it is possible to get a clear idea of how much they want to know; this gives permission to proceed and discuss the bad news in accordance with their wishes.

The nurse's professional responsibility, as outlined in the Code of Professional Conduct issued by the United Kingdom Central Council for Nursing, Midwifery and Health Visiting (1984), is primarily to the patient. At their request they are entitled to full knowledge about their medical condition, being assured that such information will be treated in strictest confidence. Any imparting of such information to family/friends will only occur after their permission is obtained and, if it is their decision, such information will be withheld.

The patient may ask directly for information, be it the results of the tests or whether their condition is serious.

Check.
- Are they prepared for bad news?
- Do they look relaxed, are they asking the questions calmly?
- How well do you know the patient relative?
- Are they anxious, asking the question without being prepared for the answer?
- Do they need some support (relatives/friend present) to cope with the news?

Before answering direct questions it may be helpful to ask the patient what they *think* is likely to be going on.

'Have you had any thoughts about what is wrong?'
'What sort type of thoughts?'

This enables the professional to gauge how seriously the patient is interpreting his or her symptoms. Some individuals do not ask for information because the possibility of their condition being serious has not occurred to them. This is especially true for the young and fit; for others, denying the seriousness may be appropriate if it reduces their anxiety.

Giving individuals an element of free choice over the information may prove beneficial. Prior to investigative procedures, or after receiving test results, they can be given control of decisions relating to their illness. Questions like 'if your condition turned out to be something serious would you like to know the full details?' can, for those who says 'yes', give a clear indication to proceed, showing that the patient is prepared for and is requesting information. In this way the health professional is enabling the patient to share in the decision making surrounding their illness and restoring a sense of personal autonomy.

When a patient says 'no' or 'no, I don't want to know', they should still be able to maintain their own strategies, for example denial for coping with the situation. Professionals must respect all different ways of coping. Whatever the patient's response, it is always important to maintain non-judgemental support following their decision, to be aware that communication needs may change as their disease progresses, and to be available to talk and/or listen whenever the patient is ready.

> 'Every dying patient needs some more information about his illness and prognosis if he is to make his own decisions. We have no right to withhold such information, but neither have we a right to force information on a patient that he cannot accept.' (Webster, 1986, p. 44).

Sharing the news

The patient is in control of the news, the knowledge is theirs by right although the professional carer has the key to it. The professional's role is to be their guide and supporter through the information sharing process and beyond.

What is bad news? Buckman (1988) states that bad news can be defined as: 'any news that materially alters the patient's view of his/her future'. In other words the 'badness' of bad news is the gap between the patients expectation of their future and the reality of the situation.

Maguire and Faulkner (1988) state that: 'You cannot soften the impact of bad news since it is still bad news however it is broken'.

The following points showed be remembered.

- Bad news can never sound good.
- The honesty of the message should never be changed to improve its acceptability.
- It is important to encourage and support hope realistic to a patient's particular circumstances, and to describe palliative care as an active treatment modality in its own right.

How to approach it? The key to breaking bad news, as stated in Maguire and Faulkner (1988) is 'to try to slow down the speed of the transition from a patient's perception of himself as being well to a realisation that he has a life threatening disease'. This can be facilitated by the following.

- The professional carer warning the patient's relative that they are going to be given serious information. This gives the patient relative time to psychologically prepare themselves rather than to switch off the communication channels. It also gives the communicator the opportunity to monitor non-verbal reactions as well as to respond to verbal responses, for example, do they want to continue or have they heard enough?
- Progressing along the 'bad news staircase' over a short period of time, allowing the patient/relative to adjust slowly to more serious levels of knowledge and leading to realisation at their own pace.
- When imparting news the communicator must avoid jargon, tailoring language and information to fit individual needs and levels of comprehension.
- The use of checking phrases like 'does that make sense?' and 'do you understand what I am saying?' allows the communicator to check that the message is being received and understood by facilitating two-way communication.
- Following the breaking of bad news, the patient's emotional and psychological well-being is influenced by the subsequent support by their family/friends and the health-care team.

What next?

After the breaking or confirming of bad news it is helpful to explore the person's feelings about the 'news', to discover their immediate fears and concerns, rather than predicting their responses. Concerns about dying may be influenced by past experiences, acceptance of myths and 'old wives' tales', the portrayal of death in the media, and our cultural sanitisation of death, with the desire to protect family and friends from unnecessary anguish (see Chapter 7).

Exploring feelings and concerns

Sister 'How do you feel about this news?'
Mrs P. 'Really quite shocked I think. It is frightening to have your fears confirmed. My mother died from cancer it was so horrible, she had such a bad time . . . just got so terribly thin and the pain oh . . . to see her suffer'. [Whilst saying this Mrs P. looked extremely distressed, was wringing her hands, avoiding eye contact and biting her lip.]
Sister [Picking up on the non-verbal as well as verbal responses] 'That experience must have been very difficult for you. I can see you're very distressed. Would you like to talk about it further'.

In the above example the Sister displays awareness of the immediate emotional and physical concerns and gives Mrs P. permission to continue.

The following points may assist in exploring a patient's feelings and concerns.
- One block to the effective sharing of information is if the patient has a large number of concerns on their mind. It is sometimes useful to obtain a 'shopping list' of anxieties and questions before attempting to answer them: if the patient's first question is answered immediately, thoughts about further questions may distract their attention from the answer.

- Sometimes an initial question may appear quite trivial but hide deeper concerns. If deeper concerns are suspected it may be worth trying to gently question the patient further. If there is no deeper problem such gentle questioning is unlikely to cause the patient any undue distress.
- Patients may ask an apparently simple question to test the professional carer's responses, enabling the patient to decide whether or not the professional can be trusted, or will cope with their deeper concerns.

Mrs A. [following her mastectomy] 'Do you think I'll be able to use my normal bra with the prosthesis or will it slip?'
Nurse 'I don't know, it might be alright.'

This nurse's response is unhelpful, unsupportive, uncaring and would stop or deter Mrs A. from asking this nurse any other questions.

Alternatively, the nurse might reply:

Nurse 'It seems as though you are a little worried about the prosthesis and how it will fit and will it be secure. Would it be helpful to have a look and perhaps discuss the matter further?'

This response displays a more caring attitude, that Mrs A.'s concerns are important and resolvable but also leaves room for Mrs A. to discuss more intimate concerns that she may have.

Dealing with feelings and concerns. Once the patient's feelings and concerns are established it is important to help him or her to deal with them. Some of their concerns are potentially resolvable:

Mr W. 'The thought that it is going to be painful worries me.'
Nurse 'Yes, that's understandable.'
Mr W. 'Can you do anything to help the pain?'
Nurse 'Yes, it is likely that we will be able to help with the pain. But it is important to let us know if you have any pain so that we can discuss with the doctors and get something sorted out for it.'

The nurse did not promise to eliminate the pain, as that might not be realistic bearing in mind the complex nature of pain, but offered help and support in attempting this. A more detailed description of helping strategies will be discussed in Chapter 18.

Offering on-going support. When the prognosis is poor and the patient has been told that no further treatment is possible, the patient is likely to be overwhelmed by the situation believing that nothing can be done to help him or her. In this circumstance it is realistic to indicate that palliative care can improve their quality of life, by controlling their symptoms and facilitating effective communication to help with their psychological, emotional and spiritual concerns. Indicating that support will continue through the ups and downs of the disease process and apparent non-medical concerns are acceptable areas of discussion. A more detailed description of helping strategies will be discussed in Chapter 18.

It is important to remember that, when sharing bad news with the patient and/or relative, they are left with further dilemmas.

- Who else to tell? Close/extended family? Friends?
- How and how much to tell them?
- When and where to tell them?

These decisions, and the control of them, are the patient's, but they may need non-judgemental support and guidance in imparting or concealing such knowledge.

Specific problem areas

Difficult questions

Patients and relatives may ask questions that are difficult to answer, but are important to them in coping with their limited future. Consequently, the health-care professional needs to explore and respond to them appropriately.

Treatment questions:

'Is it worth me having any more chemotherapy?'
'Will it do any good?'
'What are my chances?'

These questions are problematic in that often there are no clear-cut answers and it is unlikely that an individual's response to any treatment can be accurately predicted (see Chapter 2).

- Never make the decision for the patient (they will blame the professional if it works out badly) and encourage them not to be overly influenced by their relatives wishes because only they will experience the effects of the treatment.
- In the short term it is easier for the nurse or health-care professional to tell someone what to do, but that is always their decision, not the patient's.
- Aim to give the patient as much information about a particular treatment as possible in a way that they can understand. This enables them to make an informed decision themselves, although no decision can be truly informed in these situations.
- Be aware that it is appropriate to give patients the pros and cons of a particular treatment, to be realistic about potential side-effects as well as benefits.
- Make the patient aware that there are some questions for which 'I don't know' is the true answer.

Is it cancer? When communicating with patients who have cancer, most people dread being asked difficult questions, in particular: 'Is it cancer?' When such a question is asked it is difficult to predict what reply is wanted.

- Does the patient want reassurance that it isn't cancer (to help them deny the reality of their situation)?
- Does the patient want the truth?
- What are the patient's reasons for asking the question? Occasionally the way the question is asked may give clues in determining the response. However, the patient may partly want to know or be undecided as to how much/what they need to know.

'I haven't got cancer have I?' 'I'm sure its cancer', 'is it cancer?' gives little idea as to how to respond; therefore it is important to elicit further information as to the way the patient wishes to proceed. Stating that you are happy to answer the question but reflecting the question back, for example 'I am happy to answer your question but it would be helpful if I could ask you why you're asking me?' is useful in:

- preparing all parties for the ensuing conversation, giving them permission to continue or withdraw;
- and checking that professional and patient/relative are on the same 'wavelength';
- that the patient wants information about their condition and situation;
- how much the patient is aware of;
- what words have been and should be used; and
- the degree of matching between the verbal and non-verbal behaviour of the patient.

Questions relating to dying and prognosis.
'Am I dying?'
'I'm going to get better aren't I?'
'I'm dying aren't I?'
These questions can be dealt with in a similar way to those relating to a diagnosis of cancer but further exploratory questions may ensue, for example 'How long have I left to live?'

- It is essential to emphasise to patients and relatives that the nurse and/or doctor cannot predict how long someone has to live.
- Remember that giving a time limit, be it weeks, months, years, is useless, unreliable and inaccurate. Patients and relatives have to learn to live with uncertainty – and our role is to support them with it.
- Be aware that the patient/relative may selectively recall (however careful the nurse or doctor may be) a precise time limit out of context of the conversation.
- Ensure that the patient is offered continued support for however long they have to live, and that their relatives will be supported in bereavement.
- Acknowledge that pre-existing problems can be exacerbated or diminished by a life-threatening illness, and that the health professional is unlikely to be able to solve them. Relationships, likewise, can be enhanced or deteriorate according to the responses of patients/relatives/friends/health-care workers.
- For those with a limited life expectancy, realistic goal setting with regard to planning activities is useful in maximising quality of life so that individuals learn to 'live' rather than 'die' prematurely with their illness.
- Be aware that fear of the future may stop someone enjoying the present.

'What will my dying be like?' For most people their fears and anxieties can be divided into two groups: the fear of death, and fears associated with the process of dying.

The fear of death

This is a fear of the unknown, of the actual ways and means of dying; the event itself and what happens afterwards. Questions relating to these concerns are impossible to answer. Although spiritual support is helpful in easing the passage towards death, dying is inevitably a lonely business, accompanied by uncertainty and many unanswerable questions.

Fears associated with the process of dying

These fears include loss of control and dignity, fears associated with the symptoms of disease, regrets of what might have been, that is 'our potential'; how family and friends will cope. It is important to recognise that there is often a disparity between intellectual recognition and emotional responses; people may reach intellectual awareness before they reach emotional awareness.

Effective communication will enable individuals to make decisions about death, for example

- *where* one is likely to die – home/hospice/hospital – not *when*;
- legal and funeral arrangements;
- organ donation;
- decisions relating to physical symptoms and deterioration in their condition; and
- practising facing up to death by discussing dream experiences – sometimes this is a more acceptable way of exploring their own feelings and discovering other people's responses.

How can nurses help? This is a particularly difficult area of communication as *there are no precise answers.* Support can be offered by talking, listening and touching; trying to ensure the ease of physical symptoms; but no-one can predict how someone will die, whether it be peacefully or as a result of an emergency event.

As a nurse it is difficult not to be able to give definite answers, but, in this situation, 'I don't know' is the only true answer, with the assurance of continued support. If appropriate, it is possible to warn the patient and/or relatives of a deterioration in the patient's condition, a deterioration which is perhaps leading to death.

Difficult situations

Some emphatic relatives insist that information relating to diagnosis and prognosis should be withheld: 'My husband must be given the best possible treatment but must never be told what is wrong with him, he couldn't cope'.

What can be done in this situation?

- Explore the possible reasons for the request. Are the relatives anxious that the patient will not be able to cope when he or she is aware of the true situation? Do they have distressing past experiences regarding the death of friends/ relatives? Have they previously been given instructions about what their relative, the patient, would like to be told?

The relatives should be assured of the following.

- Such information would never be 'blurted out' with the patient being unprepared, and such information would usually be given in response to questions from the patient. Quite often the patient has guessed the true situation and is merely wanting his or her suspicions confirmed.

- Patient's imaginings are often worse and/or more disturbing than the known; opening up fears and anxieties allows them to be confronted and, in part, resolved.

The nurse should be aware of the following.

- The relatives burden of keeping the truth from the patient is very difficult, and can cause a barrier between them at a time when openness is crucial and may leave them with a sense of guilt in the bereavement period.
- If the relatives still insist that information be withheld the nurse must emphasise that his or her primary responsibility is to the patient and that, as a professional, the nurse will not lie to the patient.
- Where possible it is important not to alienate the relatives as they are part of the caring team and may need continuing support.

Telephone communication

Breaking bad news over the telephone is particularly difficult, especially if the news is unexpected or it is the middle of the night. All relatives of seriously ill patients should be asked, as a matter of routine, if they wish to be telephoned at night. In particular if they wish to be informed of a deterioration in the patient's condition or if they wish to be present as their loved one is dying. Relatives and friends must not be made to feel obliged to behave in a particular way to please the health–care professional, but should have free choice in their decisions.

Some elderly people find the telephone daunting. In these situations it may be helpful to have the telephone number of another member of the family for contact so that someone will be with the elderly person and pass on the news face to face.

The police are trained in and used to passing on bad news and they may be able to act as go–betweens from hospital to home should the health–care professional be worried about a particular family. Often, if needed, the police will accompany the relatives to hospital

However well prepared, the news of someone's death invariably comes as a shock; the health–care professional must be prepared for the relatives' responses to manifest themselves in a variety of different ways, and must support the relatives as needed.

Written communication

Nursing care plans placed at the end of the patients' beds or left in patients' houses must display a congruence with their known level of knowledge, since is well known that patients and relatives will avidly read them. The campaign for freedom of information and the potential Access to Health Care Records Bill will ensure a more honest relationship between health–care workers, patients and relatives, facilitating more open communication by allowing patients access to their own notes.

One of the most useful questions to ask is: 'do our notes aid communication with other health–care professionals?' That is their purpose and, if they do not aid communication they should be rewritten or updated. Their primary use is as an effective medium for the giving and receiving of information on behalf of, and for the benefit of, the patient.

Conclusion

Effective communication should improve the quality of life for the patients, their families and friends and increase their satisfaction with the care received and, as a consequence, increase the nurse's job satisfaction, lessen stress and improve relationships within the multidisciplinary team.

Communication is a delicate network of interaction between patients, relatives and staff. It is hoped that this chapter proves there is no mystique about it; the skills can be learnt, mastered and effectively used, providing the carers have the confidence to try, and are well supported with their interactions. For many patients, it is not the complexity of skills, or the depth of understanding but the fact that someone cares enough to try that is important.

A 'just be there' approach has been advocated strongly by many authors and workers in the palliative care field, and its role is summarised thus:

> 'Just standing and holding the hand of a patient who is struggling with physical deterioration and mental anguish can itself be a very rewarding experience, because of the comfort such companionship brings to that patient and nurse' (Charnock, 1983, p. 64).

Acknowledgements

My thanks to all who commented constructively on the first edition, to Ronnie for waiting with infinite patience for the second. To Eileen without whom it would be in scribbled unintelligible form and especially to Lisa Franklin, RGN, BN (Hons) for her skill in exploring and editing the literature review, and to Mel, whose 'bullying' and support was so positively enabling!

References

AGUILERA, D. (1967). Relationship between physical contact and verbal interaction between nurses and patients. *Journal of Psychiatric Nursing* 5, 5121.

BOND, S. (1978). Processes about communication in a radiotherapy department. Unpublished PhD thesis, University of Edinburgh.

BARTON, D. (1972). The need for including instruction on death and dying in the medical curriculum. *Journal of Medical Education* 47, 169–75.

BREWIN, T. B. (1977). The cancer patient: communication and morale. *British Medical Journal* 2, 1623–7.

BUCKMAN, R. (1984). Breaking bad news: why is it still so difficult? *British Medical Journal* 288, 1597–9.

BUCKMAN, R. (1988). *I Don't Know What to Say – How to Help and Support Someone Who is Dying.* Papermac, London.

CHARNOCK, A. (1983). Care of the dying. *Nursing Times* 79, 38, 64.

CITY AND GUILDS (1990). Health care: direct personal care. National Vocational Qualifications Level 2, City and Guilds, London.

DOYLE, D. (1987). *Domiciliary Terminal Care.* Churchill Livingstone, Edinburgh.

ENGLISH NATIONAL BOARD FOR NURSING, MIDWIFERY AND HEALTH VISITING (1989). Project 2000 – 'A new preparation for practice'; Guidelines and Criteria for Course Development and the Formulation of Collaborative

Links between Approved Training Institutions within the National Health Service and Centres of Higher Education. ENB, London.

FIELD, D. (1984). 'We didn't want him to die on his own' – nurses' accounts of nursing dying patients. *Journal of Advanced Nursing* 9, 59–70.

FIELDING, R. G. and LLEWELLYN, S. P. (1987). Communication training in nursing may damage your health and enthusiasm: some warnings. *Journal of Advanced Nursing* 12, 281–90.

FRANCIS, V. and MORRIS, M. (1969). Gaps in doctor–patient communication: patients' response to medical advice. *New England Journal of Medicine* 280, 535–40.

FRY, J. (1983). Deaths and dying. *Update* 15 December, 1706–7.

HENLEY, A. (1986). *Good Practice in Hospital Care for the Dying.* King's Fund Publishing Office, London.

HISCOCKS, S. (1994). Unpublished GRASP data. Unit 4, Llandough Hospital, Penarth, South Glamorgan.

HUGHES, J. (1987). *Cancer and Emotion.* John Wiley, Chichester.

LANGLAND, R. M. and PANNICCUCCI, C. L. (1982). Effects of touch on communication with elderly confused clients. *Journal of Gerontology Nursing* 8, 152–5.

MAGUIRE, P. (1985). Barriers to psychological care of the dying. *British Medical Journal* 291, 1711–13.

MAGUIRE, P. and FAULKNER, A. (1988). Communicate with cancer patients: 1. Handling bad news and difficult questions. *British Medical Journal* 297, 907–9.

MOY, C. (1981). Touch in the counselling relationship: an exploratory study. *Patient Counselling and Health Education* 3rd quarter, 89–95.

MULLIGAN, J. C. A. (1989). Dying at home – an evaluation of a specialist home care service. Unpublished PhD thesis, University of Wales.

PARKES, C. M. and PARKES, J. (1984). Hospice versus hospital care: re-evaluation after 10 years as seen by surviving spouse. *Postgraduate Medical Journal* 60, 120–4.

REISETTER, K. H. and THOMAS, B. (1986). Nursing care of the dying: its relationship to selected nurse characteristics. *International Journal of Nursing Studies* 23, 39–50.

STEDEFORD, A. (1981). Couples facing death. II. Unsatisfactory communication. *British Medical Journal* 283, 10,098–101.

STEDEFORD, A. (1984). *Facing Death: Patients, Families and Professionals.* Heinemann, London.

UNITED KINGDOM CENTRAL COUNCIL FOR NURSING, MIDWIFERY AND HEALTH VISITING (1989). Information on Post-registration Education and Practice Project (PREPP). UKCC, London.

UNITED KINGDOM CENTRAL COUNCIL FOR NURSING, MIDWIFERY AND HEALTH VISITING (1990). The Report of the Post-registration Education and Practice Project. UKCC, London.

UNITED KINGDOM CENTRAL COUNCIL FOR NURSING, MIDWIFERY AND HEALTH VISITING (1992). Code of Professional Conduct for the Nurse, Midwife and Health Visitor. UKCC, London.

VACHON, M. L. S. (1988). Counselling and psychotherapy in palliative or hospital care: a review. *Palliative Medicine* 2, 36–50.

WEBSTER, M. (1981). Communicating with dying patients. *Nursing Times* June, 999–1002.

WEBSTER, M. E. (1986). Easing emotional distress. *Nursing Times* 83, 45, 38.
WILKINSON, S. (1988). Identifying the major stressors in cancer nursing. In: PRITCHARD, P. (ed.), *Cancer Nursing: A Revolution in Care*, pp. 68–72. Scutari Press, London.
WILKINSON, S. (1991). Factors which influence how nurses communicate with cancer patients. *Journal of Advanced Nursing* 16, 677–88.

Further reading

General communication skills

BURNARD, P. (1989). *Counselling Skills for Health Professionals*. Chapman & Hall, London.

Specific areas of death and dying

BUCKMAN, R. (1991). *I Don't Know What to Say – How to Help and Support Someone Who is Dying*. Papermac, London.
DE BEAUVOIR, S. (1969). *A Very Easy Death*. Penguin, Harmondsworth (last reprint, 1987).
STEDEFORD, A. (1994). *Facing Death: Patients, Families and Professionals*. Heinemann, London.

Further viewing

'Why don't they talk to me?'. Parts 1–5. Dr Robert Buckman and Dr Peter Maguire. Available from Lindward Productions, Shepperton Studio Centre, Shepperton, Middlesex. An audio–visual communication aid – attempting to help improve skills when listening and talking to patients.

17

Caring for bereaved relatives

Jenny Penson

'A man's dying is more the survivor's affair than his own.'
                                        Thomas Mann (1875–1955)

The experience of being bereaved is as old as life, and death, itself. We are probably the only species that has an awareness of its own vulnerability and certain death. Although we all know that one day we will die, we tend not to live in the present but in the future, always looking ahead to the next day, the next week, the next year.

In our fast-moving modern society we are increasingly having to face loss and change. Although people may have had less to do with death than in the past, they are more likely to confront transitions which involve losses, losing one's friends and networks when moving for a job, for example, losing self-esteem as well as colleagues when being made redundant, is another. The increasing divorce rate brings with it the pain and guilt of a failed relationship which affects not only the couple themselves but also their children, their parents and other family and friends.

The experience of loss is, therefore, a common experience for many but the particular pain of the loss of a loved person through death is, arguably, the hardest to bear.

Death may be sudden or expected and may involve long periods of caring for an ill person. Death can even take place before birth, as with miscarriages, abortions and stillbirths. Whatever the circumstances, in society today attitudes to death and dying are undergoing change. Increased secularisation and what Illich (1976) refers to as the medicalisation of natural life events contribute to an attitude of denial. Death is seen by many as being a taboo subject although others point out that it frequently features in the media, not only in dramatic ways as on the news, but in documentaries and debates on television, in radio programmes and in articles in Sunday papers.

The palliative care movement has done much to bring issues of death and dying to the fore. It is part of its philosophy that care of the patient always includes care of the relatives. The Report of a Working Group on Terminal Care (Wilkes, 1980) suggested that support should be offered to relatives both before and after the death and that hospitals should have facilities for relatives of dying patients. Sometimes the phrases 'significant others' or 'key people' are used instead of 'relatives' to indicate that the person who is closest to the patient may not always be the conventional family member.

The provision of some kind of bereavement follow-up is always made although the ways in which this is done, varies widely. Contact with bereaved relatives after the death is most commonly made by the home care service, and this may be supplemented by systems of visits from ward-based and/or day care staff as appropriate or by various kinds of volunteer support. However this is done, it seems to be universal that some contact is made or offered although bereavement visiting may be low in the list of priorities.

Mourning is society's response to loss and, though behaviours and expectations vary greatly in different cultures, the pain of loss is something everyone can relate to. Our immediate culture governs what is seen to be appropriate ritual and behaviour. Sociologists describe many rites of passage that mark the change in status from wife to widow, from husband to widower.

Bereavement means 'to be robbed of something valued' and this word rob is a useful one because it indicates that this person has been wrongfully and forcibly taken from you. It implies the sense of injustice that many people express.

It is necessary to be able to say good-bye and to let go of the past if the individual is to be able to adjust to loss. A useful analogy here is that losing someone loved is like the amputation of a limb, part of yourself has gone and can never be replaced. Everything that was shared with that particular person, all the memories and hopes cannot be repeated with anyone else. The response is one of grief.

Grief begins from the moment that the relative or friend knows that their loved one is unlikely to recover from their illness, often referred to as 'anticipatory grief'. It is complex, confusing and highly stressful and comprises of a variety of emotions which include shock, anger, guilt, despair, sadness, restlessness and anxiety all of which render the individual vulnerable to illness and death. Usually these are accompanied by some physical sensations such as shortness of breath, palpitations, weakness, headaches, digestive disturbances – all manifestations of stress which are thought to be psychosomatic in origin. Research indicates that there is higher mortality and morbidity following a major bereavement, for example there is a higher rate of cancer amongst bereaved people within 3 years of the loss (LeShan, 1961).

Most health-care professionals are familiar with the main perspectives on bereavement. Freud (1957) pointed out that grief is a normal reaction to loss and, therefore, does not usually necessitate treatment. He went further and stated that interference with the process may actually be harmful. He points out the connection between grief, anger and depression and that self-reproach and guilt are part of that depression.

Bowlby's work on attachment and separation showed us that even a child under a year old, reacts to the loss of an attachment figure. The bond between them is biologically determined in order to ensure survival of the child. The child's response to separation is one of protest followed by despair and then detachment. This is mirrored in adult bereavement as is the need, in stress or danger, to be close to our attachment figure. Grief is seen as an adaptive process, adjusting to the fact that life can never be the same again (Bowlby, 1982).

Others, most notably Parkes (1993) see it as a psychosocial transition, the characteristics of which are that people have to undertake a major revision of their assumptions about their worlds, they are lasting rather than transient and they take place over a relatively short period of time so that there is little time to prepare. This grief work has to be done by the bereaved person before detachment can take place. In palliative care, the grief work may already have begun with the realisation that the loved one is not going to recover. He eloquently refers to bereavement as 'the cost of commitment'.

Worden (1984) takes an active stance, seeing mourning as a series of tasks which need to be accomplished before the individual is able to move on. Firstly bereaved people need to accept the reality of the loss then experience all the painful feelings of grief. Next they must adjust to a new way of life, deprived of all the roles played by the deceased person. Finally, they have to let go of the emotional energy devoted to the loved one so that it can be reinvested in new relationships and ways of living. Many bereaved people find that this last task seems like a betrayal of the loved one but Parkes and Weiss (1983), Worden (1984) and others agree that this last step is necessary if recovery from grief is to occur.

The consensus seems to be that the expression of grief, in whatever form, is essential in order to adjust to bereavement. This can be put off by the pressure of circumstances such as responsibility for others, financial or social worries, or by deliberate avoidance of facing the pain. The prescription of tranquillisers and anti-depresssants may also help to put off this difficult time but ultimately these emotions have to be faced. If they are not, then they may surface later on, sometimes many years afterwards as in the case of an adult who has, perhaps, a surprisingly extreme reaction to a crisis or loss and it is found that they are still carrying the pain of a bereavement from childhood.

Whether adjustment to loss is thought to be a process of habituation or of grief work it is considered to take at least 2 years to reach a resolution. This may be achieved when the bereaved reach a point where they feel that they have not really lost the person they loved, but have, in some way, become part of them, carrying them inside in their memory. They may feel that some kind of reparation may need to be made before they can let go of the past and regain some degree of trust in life, the letting go representing the ultimate pain of grief.

During this time there will be many highs and lows and there is some suggestion that the second year of bereavement may be more difficult than the first. It may hit the bereaved person particularly hard when they find they still feel a lot of pain and others appear to have forgotten. The expectations of the general public and, often, of bereaved people themselves, is that they will feel better when the first anniversaries have passed. Many find that this is not the case.

There are many factors which can affect the outcome of bereavement, some of which may have implications for nurses when caring for relatives, before the patient dies.

Before death

The relationship between nurses and relatives is an evolving one. It is not that many years ago that relatives were seen as a nuisance, an intrusion which interrupted the order of things on the hospital ward. Darbyshire (1987) points to a recurring theme in research that there is an unwillingness or inability of nurses to make the best use of relatives and families. Now, most nurses accept that the patient and his family are not two separate entities, each interacts with the other. Therefore, attention given to the needs of relatives may also help to meet the needs of the patient. Often their emotional states mirror each other. An example of this is provided by a study of cancer patients and their relatives which found a correlation between the scores for the patient/relative pairs, that is if the patient scored highly on anxiety or depression, then the relative was likely to do so as well (Cassileth *et al.*, 1983).

Robinson and Thorne (1984) describe a three-stage process in which this relationship can be viewed.

1. *Naive trusting.* Initially, relatives believe that their values and perspectives are the same as the staff. They then begin to find that professional health-care providers are orientated towards the disease state whilst the relatives are focused on the total experience of illness.

2. *Disenchantment.* When the stage of naive trusting is shaken, relatives may begin to develop a 'them and us' attitude. They may find themselves in the position of needing to be the advocate for the patient, against the perceived failures of the system. It is now that relatives and patients face the possibility of being labelled by nursing and other staff as 'demanding', 'neurotic', 'over-anxious', 'manipulative'.

3. *Guarded alliance.* At this stage, families may come round to acknowledging the strengths as well as the limitations of the health-care system and try to make the best of it by negotiating for care.

In this, their attitude may be one of ambivalence for they may wish to attack the health-care staff as a means of expressing love and protection of the patient, at the same time, they are reliant on the goodwill of the same staff in order to provide the help they need. A relationship based on mutual respect is what has to be worked towards and here it is nurses who must take the lead.

The family of the dying patient can be viewed as moving through multiple transitions which involve coping with uncertainty, changes in role, plans for an altered future and high levels of stress. This is often centred on the hope system of the individual, where both patient and relative have to adjust to its changing nature from hope for a cure, to hope for effective treatment, from hope for prolongation of life to hope for a peaceful death. Eliciting from patients and relatives what they hope for, is an important part of nursing care. Krieger (1981) points out that people can learn to live with an incurable illness but not with the thought that it is hopeless. Molter (1979) studied the needs of the family and found that their universal and strongest need was for hope. Nurses can help by setting short-term goals for the patient, for example a weekend at home, the visit to a favourite place, planning some special treat to share together. This also goes some way towards providing some happy memories to look back on. Reassurance, (providing it is based on reality) that the patient will not be allowed to suffer pain or great distress, that someone will be with them when they die, and that support is available after the death if they wish, are all significant to those for whom no hope of ultimate recovery can be given.

Ambivalence may also be present if relatives do not feel what they think they ought to feel or what they think is expected of them. Relationships are not, after all, perfect and there may be resentment felt by the relative for all the care and attention being given to the patient. There may be anticipation towards the death as a release from a difficult or unhappy relationship, where, for example, the patient has been ill for some time and needed a lot of care. There is likely to be guilt associated with these negative feelings and they may also be accompanied by a sense of failure.

This failure may also be associated with the circumstances of the death, for example if the patient died in hospital when they showed a preference for home or if the relatives were not present at the death and had wanted to be.

A well-known study by Hampe (1975) concerning the needs of spouses of patients who were terminally ill, found that the spouses wanted nurses to give them time and to be available to them. They wanted them to explain the daily care of the patient, including medications, tests, etc. They wanted nurses to listen to their worries and concerns.

However, they also wanted nurses, more than anything else, to be helpful to the dying person. As Kubler-Ross (1970) states 'We cannot help the terminally ill patient in a really meaningful way if we do not include his family.'

It also appears feasible that the way in which the relatives are supported when their loved one dies, will have an effect on the way they can adjust to bereavement. Here the nurse needs to be sensitive to their wishes, encouraging them to stay with the dying person by offering to be there with them, or to go in and out, or to leave them alone according to what they feel comfortable with. It can be helpful to suggest that sitting quietly with the dying patient holding their hand, is still doing something and something very important, and that people who appear to be unconscious may well be aware of their loving presence. What is aimed for is a sense of peace and of letting go.

Sometimes we can sense that the relatives are trying to keep the person alive for a little longer, as if by sheer effort of will they can postpone death. Our experience may tell us that only when the relative leaves the bedside will the patient be able to die. In this kind of situation, it may be helpful to explain, very gently, the need to let the loved person go and the relative can sometimes be helped to do this in their own way.

After the death, relatives may need support to sit with the dead person, to touch them and to say all the things they wish. If they were not present, they may still appreciate the chance of doing this but need encouragement. They may feel afraid of what they may see and of the strength and depth of their feelings. Offering to say a short prayer with them at the bedside is often appreciated and almost never refused by relatives no matter what their beliefs. It is both a sharing and an acknowledgement that their loved one has died.

Another, perhaps more controversial, way of helping some relatives at this time, is to suggest that they may like to assist with the laying out of the body. When the relatives can see that this is done with reverence, maybe still talking to the person who is being laid out, and touching them gently, and they can feel that this last expression of their love and care can be made, it can be a very good memory for any relative to take with them.

Because they may not have had previous experience of death, relatives often appear to look to nurses for knowledge of how to behave appropriately and what practical tasks have to be completed.

After death

Having emphasised the importance of the care of relatives both from the point of view of the patient and to help adjustment to bereavement, it is necessary to turn to the care of relatives after the death has taken place.

The follow-up of bereaved relatives is often haphazard with great variations in what is offered, if at all, depending on where they live, who their general practitioner is, whether there are any support groups (either professional or voluntary) available in their locality and whether they died in a specialist unit, institution or at home. Palliative care has pioneered bereavement services but even here, there seems to be a lack of consensus as to what can be offered, at what time, in what way, and how it can be measured. In spite of this, bereavement support is usually felt to be useful and almost always welcomed although a few people may reject this help, perhaps fearing the implied inadequacy and dependency inherent in the role of someone needing help.

It would appear that any kind of bereavement service has three main functions, one is to assess how the person is adjusting and to refer them on if necessary, another is to use counselling skills in order to help the expression of feelings and clarify options and the third is to act as a resource. In order to offer such a service safely (that is safe for both client and helper) it is obviously necessary for such helpers to receive training and to have supervision and support.

Assessment

Assessment starts with our knowledge of the relatives during the illness and at the time of death. This information will help to identify potential problems and alert the primary health-care team or any existing bereavement service. From this assessment they can prioritise their work.

The information which can be helpful includes the following.

The bereaved person

Their age and position in their family, including whether they have other people who are dependent on them. The nature of their relationship with the person who died and with other family members, for example situations where there is a homosexual relationship or one where there is both a wife and a mistress or where there are children from a previous marriage living elsewhere.

The quality of that relationship, with particular reference to ambivalence where one is more dependent and the other more dominant because the attachment can be stronger but more insecure. Their previous experience of illness and death or of other losses. Their usual state of health and any previous history of physical or mental ill health. Poor physical health is likely to lower emotional resilience, impair mobility and opportunities for social contact. Whether they have suffered any other losses, not only through death or separation, but through, for example, redundancy, moving house, illness or crises in other family members or close friends.

Mode of death

The patient's age at the time of the onset of illness and at death. An untimely loss, that is one where the person who died was young or in childhood is especially hard to grieve, the relationship between parents and child is very intense and the sense of unfairness very strong (see Chapter 14). This can also happen when the one who died was an adult but died before their parents.

The way in which they died, was it peaceful or troubled, anticipated or unexpected and was the bereaved person present, if they wished to be. Whether the death took place at home, hospital, hospice or nursing home, and if in a place which was known or amongst strangers. The bereaved person's reactions at the time of death and the quality of the support they received at this time.

Customs

The culture and rituals which were or were not performed and whether the wishes of the relatives were able to be carried out. The kind of funeral service envisaged, whether the patient had made known their wishes for this and whether they wanted to be buried or cremated. The possible support available from the funeral director and from the church. The belief system of the bereaved person and the one who died.

Social factors

The existence or otherwise of a primary support group, i.e. people known by the bereaved person for more than 5 years. The existence of social networks of neighbours, regular contacts and a sense of belonging to a community. The financial situation of the bereaved person and the kind and permanency of their accommodation. If they go out to work or not, and if this gives them a role that can go some way towards balancing the change of status that occurs in bereavement. Whether or not there are others they are responsible for, including pets. Their usual pastimes and hobbies and if they belong to clubs, attend classes or participate in sports.

When making an assessment, the helper also needs to be aware of groups which are considered to be particularly at risk during bereavement.

Risk factors

Sudden, unexpected death is agreed to be the biggest single risk factor. Here there has been no chance to anticipate the loss and the sense of disbelief and shock is likely to be very strong. Feelings of helplessness predominate as trust in life is severely undermined. This will be exacerbated if there were quarrels or deep conflicts prior to the death.

Social isolation is an obvious risk factor and is heightened where people have moved to a new area or have lost other important people within the last 2 years.

Another group which is considered to be at risk are what Parkes (1993) has referred to as image conscious individuals. By this he means people, usually professionals, who are used to taking on the role of helper in the community. They are accustomed to functioning as givers of help rather than receivers, and others expect this from them. This can make it particularly hard to seek out help for themselves, and others may not appreciate that support is wanted by them.

Children and adolescents are also at risk and their needs can get subsumed as the family rallies around the bereaved adult and they themselves may be too deeply affected by the death to be able to give attention to the child or teenager. Of course, this will depend on the quality and type of relationships within the family, prior to the death (see Chapter 14 on children and adolescents).

Home assessment

When visiting a bereaved person at home for the first time, the assessment will include most of the above plus information about what has happened since the death, whether the funeral service went as they wanted it to, if they have the support of family and friends. It is not unusual for there to be the re-emergence of family disagreements after the death (and, even sometimes before they have died) and this is often centred on the reading of the will. It may also focus on issues such as the choosing of an appropriate memorial, the disposal of personal belongings and conflicting ideas as to what the dead person would have wanted to be done.

The aim of the assessment is to judge whether the bereaved person is able to cope at the time and appears to be going to adjust to their loss in the longer term. This can be difficult because we have to bear in mind, as discussed earlier, the danger of categorising people and suggesting that they are only grieving appropriately if its fits in with some kind of model of normality we have inside our heads!

Timeliness is a factor of great importance when making such an assessment, because a reaction which may be entirely appropriate at one stage may become an indicator of risk if it continues for many months after that. See Fig 17.1 for an approximate timescale for the emotional reactions to loss.

Before the death	Time of death	Six weeks	Nine months	Two years
Shock Denial Anxiety Fear of the future Anticipatory grief	Shock Numbness Denial Yearning Withdrawal Hysterical behaviour	Anger, bitterness Blame Guilt Searching Lack of concentration Loneliness Indecision Physical symptoms (they may be similar to the person who died)	Sadness Depression Loss of status Feelings of being stigmatised Loneliness Aimlessness	Acceptance of reality Adjustment Recovery New patterns of living Personal growth Gradual hope

Fig. 17.1 Possible emotional reactions to bereavement. An approximate timescale.

Immediate and radical changes in lifestyle may, combined with the already high stress score for bereavement (Holmes and Rahe, 1967) make the bereaved person more at risk. These might include the formation of deep new relationships before grieving for the old one is completed, excessive idealisation of the person who died, or maintaining their environment exactly as if they were still alive. Each of these are ways of coping but they may indicate an avoidance of the grieving process.

Grief does indeed affect everyone but its affects them unequally. Some people are devastated whilst others take loss more in their stride. Again, for some it may actually be welcomed although this may make the bereaved person feel very guilty. The death that is a true release from an unhappy relationship may open up new opportunities for those who are left, referred to occasionally as 'God-given divorce'. In the same way, the death of a dependent, elderly person may give new life to the one who has been doing the caring. However, contrary to one might at first suppose, the end of a troubled relationship may cause some bereaved people great difficulties in adjustment. There is more anger, resentment and guilt and less happy memories to give comfort and provide a sense of completion.

Assessment is made by observing, by asking open questions and by the skills of active listening and empathy. Intuition is also needed. An assessment tool devised by Huber and Gibson (1990) could be useful. In their small study they were trying to find out if bereaved people had been helped by hospice interventions prior to the death of their loved one. They devised an analogue scale for self-assessment 'the 10-mile mourning bridge' to see if the responses indicated that these bereaved people had been helped to cross part of this bridge before the death (see Fig. 17.2) Their findings indicated that hospice interventions did seem to have helped bereaved people to have moved further along the bridge than those who had not had that support before the death of their loved one. This raises the question of whether anticipatory grieving is considered to be useful? Parkes and Weiss (1983) dispute this, observing that the anticipation of death intensified attachment to the dying person rather than bringing about detachment. Silverman (1974) concluded that talking about impending death was not, in fact, grieving in advance, this could only happen after the death had taken place.

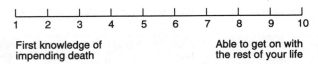

Fig. 17.2 'Ten-mile mourning bridge' (Huber and Gibson, 1990).

However, this kind of analogue scale could be a useful way of measuring progress over any period of the bereavement process and is more likely to be accurate as it is filled in by the bereaved person themselves.

Helping skills

The second function of the bereavement visitor is to use helping skills appropriately to facilitate the expression of thoughts and feelings, to enable the bereaved person to 'tell their story' (for more information about helping skills see Chapter 18). This is to help them, gently, to face the reality of their loss so that they can begin to adjust to it. Here it is necessary to avoid false hopes and condolences and, wherever possible, to know what happened near the time of death in order to offer explanations. This can be helpful for some people who may have misunderstandings about what happened or who need to release the feelings associated with that time. The helper needs to be willing to be the object of these emotions sometimes, an obvious example is being the target of the bereaved person's anger. The helper has to try to remain human and not hide behind a professional role, yet be non-reactive to the bereaved person's pain.

The helper also needs to be alert for signs that the bereaved person has become 'stuck' in some stage or in some role. Often this is to do with some kind of 'unfinished business', things left unsaid, conflicts left unresolved, visits not made. This may also happen if there have been several losses with no space to grieve.

The bereaved may react by, for example, trying substitution such as being overprotective of their children, or beginning a new close relationship before they have grieved for the one that has ended. Being over-dependent in another way of coping, allowing everyone to run round them and taking on the role of victim. Being irritable and rejecting of others is another way of expressing anger as is excessive self-blame. The helper may be able to explore these ways of coping, enabling the bereaved person to move forward.

Stroebe and Stroebe (1987) suggest that for many bereaved people it is sufficient to offer sympathetic company, reassurance, patient listening and to let the bereaved talk about their loss. They also point out that attempts to give advice, state opinions and to intervene is often resented and rejected by bereaved people. 'Ungenuine offers of help' and the absence of condolences from those who they expected to give them, were the behaviours most disliked by the bereaved.

By discussing the bereaved person's usual lifestyle, it may be possible to explore with them the times that may be most difficult and make some kind of contingency plans to help. Many people on their own find that the low points are Sundays and bank holidays as well as anniversaries which are unique to their family. One way round this was suggested by a very out-going elderly widow who organised a group of three widows and one widower to take turns in providing Sunday lunch for the others. This turned their Sundays into an occasion to look forward to rather than to dread, a complete change of attitude. Such an arrangement could be facilitated by a bereavement helper.

Attention to the physical health of the bereaved person can be useful for we know that physical fitness can assist in defusing all form of stress. This maybe about healthy eating or programmes of exercise (one man in his 40s considered that taking up jogging enabled him to 'jog away' his emotions) or about teaching ways of relaxation to combat stress and aid sleep. Teaching anxiety management techniques may be very helpful to bereaved people who experience panic attacks and other expressions of insecurity and fear. Keeping some kind of journal or notebook in which to express these feelings and reflect on progress can provide an outlet which is attractive because of its privacy.

An important aim is to encourage the bereaved person to feel secure in themselves and so it is important to avoid the temptation to become a prop. If in doubt it may be useful for the helper to ask themselves 'Who's needs am I meeting by continuing to visit this person?'

Resource

In acting as a resource to the bereaved family, the helper needs to be aware of the many kinds of support which are available in their locality. These will include self-help groups such as Cruse, church groups and groups related to other aspects of their situation such as Age Concern for elderly people or Gingerbread for one-parent families.

Many hospices and palliative care units have started their own groups, providing informal opportunities for recently bereaved people to come and meet others, or renew friendships which may have started on the ward. Here bereaved people meet to share experiences and information. Sometimes it may be felt that there is very little for such people in a particular area, and then the bereavement helper may be able to start such a group in a local village hall, health centre, etc. With both kinds of group the aim will be to facilitate it at the beginning and then to leave it for the members themselves to organise and run as they feel appropriate. It must always be realised that these groups will only appeal to a small number of people for many will always refuse to join something new, no matter how friendly, and some tell us that they do not want to mix with others in the same position as they perceive this as being morbid, or depressing.

The helper also needs to be aware of facilities for practical help in the community and to be able to direct the bereaved person to the appropriate place for financial and social problems and to the library and Health Promotion Unit for books, tapes, videos, leaflets etc., which can be used at home by those who would like this kind of information.

Supporting each other

When caring for dying patients and bereaved relatives, it needs to be acknowledged that loss and grief are part of our work. We can all remember patients or their relatives who became special to us during the time we knew them and when the death has taken place we really need to stop and to spend some quiet moments. These may be private or they may mean sharing a little of what we feel, with others in the team. We need to be sensitive to the needs of others, developing awareness of when they need support. When there have been several deaths in a short space of time or the death of a particularly popular patient it is essential to acknowledge this.

Sometimes the formation of a staff support group can be helpful although the problems of shift work, conflicting priorities and the differing expectations of members may make it difficult to achieve the trust and regular contact which is needed to make it viable.

Co-counselling, where two people make a contract to meet on a regular basis and to spend an equal amount of time on one sharing their problems whilst the other listens and then changing roles, is another way of supporting each other. (For further aspects of staff support, see Chapter 19.)

When involved in working with bereaved people we need to be aware that this will evoke memories of losses in our own lives. Sometimes we may feel so attached to a patient and family that we may need to attend the funeral or to visit the relatives at home in order to meet our own needs to say good-bye and let them go from us.

In spite of these considerations, it is important to point out that caring for bereaved people can be a very rewarding experience. Their struggles and their courage inspire us in our own. They remind us of our shared humanity and show us the importance of openness, being willing to share our thoughts and feelings and to build bridges, to those we love while we can do so.

References

BOWLBY, J. (1982). *Attachment and Loss: Volume 1: Attachment.* Penguin Harmondsworth.

CASSILETH, B. R. *et al.* (1983). A psychological analysis of cancer patients and their next of kin. *Cancer* 55, 72–5.

DARBYSHIRE, P. (1987). Sour grapes . . . the treatment of patients' relatives. *Nursing Times* 83, 23–5.

FREUD, S. (1957). *Mourning and Melancholia.* Hogarth Press, London

HAMPE, S. (1975). Needs of the grieving spouse in a hospital setting. *Nursing Research* 24, 20.

HOLMES, T. H. and RAHE, R. H. (1967). The social readjustment rating scale. *Journal of Psychosomatic Research* 2, 213–18.

HUBER, R. and GIBSON, J. W. (1990). New evidence for anticipatory grief. *The Hospice Journal* 6, 49–67.

ILLICH, I. (1976). *Limits to Medicine*. Penguin, Harmondsworth.

KRIEGER, D. (1981). *The Renaissance Nurse: Foundations of Holistic Health Practices*. J. B. Lippincott, Philadelphia.

KUBLER-ROSS, E. (1970). *Questions and Answers on Death and Dying*. Macmillan, London.

LeSHAN, L. (1961). In: STROEBE, W. and STROEB, M. S. (eds) (1987). *Bereavement and Health*. Cambridge University Press, Cambridge.

MOLTER, N. C. (1979). Needs of critically ill patients: a descriptive study. *Nursing Research* 8, 2.

PARKES, C. M. (1993). Bereavement as a psychosocial transition: processes of adaptation to change. In: DICKENSON, D. and JOHNSON, M. (eds), *Death, Dying and Bereavement*. Open University with Sage Publications, London.

PARKES C. M. and WEISS, R. (1983). *Recovery from Bereavement*. Basic Books, New York.

RAPHAEL, B. (1983). *Recovery from Bereavement*. Hutchinson, London.

ROBINSON, C. A. and THORNE, S. (1984). Strengthening family 'interference'. *Journal of Advanced Nursing* 9, 597–602.

SILVERMAN, P. (1974). Anticipatory grief from the perspective of widowhood. In: SCHOENBERG, CARR, KUTCHER *et al.* (eds), *Anticipatory Grief.* Columbia University Press, New York.

STROEBE, W. and STROEBE, M. S. (1987). *Bereavement and Health*. Cambridge University Press, Cambridge.

WILKES, E. (1980). Terminal Care: Report of a Working Group. Standing Medical Advisory Committee, Department of Health, London.

WORDEN, W. J. (1984). *Grief Counselling and Grief Therapy*. Tavistock, London.

Further reading

FAULKNER, A. (1993). Developments in bereavement services. In: CLARK, D. (ed.), *The Future for Palliative Care: Issues of Policy and Practice*. Open University Press, Buckingham.

PARKES, C. M. (1986). *Bereavement: Studies of Grief in Adult Life*, 2nd edn. Penguin, Harmondsworth.

PENSON, J. (1990). *Bereavement: A Guide for Nurses*. Chapman & Hall, London.

SANDERS, C. M. (1989). *Grief: The Mourning After: Dealing with Adult Bereavement*. John Wiley, New York.

VIOST, J. (1986). *Necessary Losses*. Simon & Schuster, New York.

18

Applying counselling to nursing care: a person-centred perspective

Morna C. Rutherford

> 'So when you are listening to somebody completely, attentively, then you are listening not only to the words, but also to the feeling of what is being conveyed, to the whole of it, not part of it.'
>
> *J. Krisknamurti*

Facing cancer involves many emotions. People with cancer confront daily the challenges of loss and change, affecting both themselves and the people to whom they matter. Chapter 7 describes the dynamics of change and some of the implications of loss. This chapter addresses nursing practice in relation to those individuals who require therapeutic support through the experience of loss and change. Nursing care requires a keen awareness of individual needs, however, this care is shapeless without human connection and communication. It is the promotion of this connection through counselling which forms the basis of this support, and thus nurses are called upon more and more to use counselling skills. The nurse who is offering the counselling is referred to here as 'the counsellor', and the person receiving counselling is called 'the client'. This chapter discusses counselling skills within the context of a person-centred philosophy of care.

What is counselling?

The aim of counselling is to provide a safe, supportive and caring atmosphere in which the client will be enabled to find strength and direction. 'Enabling' is defined as 'empowering' a person to take certain action (*Concise Oxford Dictionary*). Counselling is not an activity where the counsellor behaves powerfully to direct the client, but a process where he or she uses counselling skills to help the client find his or her own power and direction.

There is no place here for the counsellor to make judgements or to try to influence the client. Advice giving, if requested, may indeed be part of a helping relationship, but it is inappropriate within the context of counselling as defined above. Burnard (1987, p. 279) states that 'the counsellor who offers a lot of advice is asking for the client to become dependent'.

McLeod (1990, pp. 14–16) reviewed some recent research on what clients experience as helpful in counselling. It is interesting to note that 'advice from their counsellors . . . is highly valued, and the absence of advice is seen as unhelpful or uncaring'. It is necessary to know what clients mean by 'advice'. Clients may not be asking to be told what to do. Rather, they might be wanting to find personal clarity and direction through a system of problem-solving, and may need some guidance and support with this by taking one problem at a time. The locus of choice and responsibility for life lies firmly with the client, committing the counsellor with responsibility *to* clients, but not *for* them (Mearns and Thorne, 1988, p. 29).

Counselling is a journey of self-exploration and discovery involving challenges and hurdles on the way. It is, however, the client's personal journey, and the counsellor is a chosen companion. As such, the counsellor has no right to impose values or interpretations on the client. This is patronising and limits the client's ability to self-determination.

Emotional release is part of the healing process. It is therefore essential that the client's emotions are not ignored or smothered. Laura Allen (1990, p. 25) describes her experience of failure in counselling. When the counsellor tried to take her 'out' of her desperate crying with 'there, there, it will be alright', Laura stopped crying and became really 'stuck'. Blocking emotional release devalues the client and is certainly *not* helpful. There is no place in counselling for trying to stop the flow of emotions. Reassurance and encouragement do little to help people discover their strengths. For example, if a client expresses guilt it is basically *unhelpful* to discount the guilt by praising or 'reassuring' the client. The client's guilt will be stronger than the counsellor's platitude, and the client will remain saddled with the guilt. It is essential to acknowledge guilt in order to free the client to explore personal meaning.

Reid-Pionte (1992) discovered that the more skilled the primary nurse was in 'perceiving, feeling and listening', the more distress the patients experienced. She postulates that these skills encourage freer expression of distress. In discussion, she suggests that a teaching/information giving approach could be more distress-relieving, and this ties in with McLeod's (1990) observation on the value of advice. This notwithstanding, sensitivity to clients will enable determination of their need to express distress or control emotion. An essential component in this determination is the counsellor's ability to recognise in him or herself any need to either encourage or stem emotional flow.

In considering what is and what is not involved in counselling, it is important to know that the counselling relationship is not an arena within which the counsellor should attempt to satisfy personal needs. Nurse (1980, p. 41) describes the need to be needed. She states that 'the counsellor who feels unimportant or unnecessary in [his or] her personal life is especially vulnerable to seeking satisfaction for [his or] herself by keeping the client bound to and dependent upon [him or] her'. This will block the counsellor's ability to facilitate the client's growth. Moreover, as counselling aims to empower the client, a challenge is offered to any system of care which aims to control. Counselling can tie in beautifully with the ideal of individualised nursing care. The reality, however, is less than ideal when nurses are blocked by poor resources, limiting environment and personal needs. This notwithstanding, given the right conditions, it is possible for nurses to incorporate counselling into their care.

The relevance of counselling

In nursing, counselling is relevant in two senses: there is the pertinence of *counselling skills* in day-to-day communication, and the relevance also of more explicit *counselling contracts*. Counselling skills, such as listening and responding to another person, can be used at any time, whereas a counselling contract defines a more intense therapeutic partnership. The intention of a therapeutic partnership is well defined, with the client firstly making a *choice* to see a counsellor. The readiness of the client for counselling is a fundamental factor determining progress (Mearns and Thorne, 1988, p. 102). The contract will involve a negotiation on how and where the counsellor and client will work together and how much time they will initially spend on the issue at hand. This brings in the necessity of privacy and a discussion on confidentiality which must be explicit at the outset. If potential interruptions are prevented, both counsellor and client are assured the opportunity to work together without external inhibitions. Any evident limitations need to be defined as part of the contract which now creates the potential for a trusting relationship. More than the counsellor's skills are involved in a therapeutic partnership: the relationship itself becomes a therapeutic medium. Although the contract is usually informal, it is important to review the conditions of the relationship from time to time to check if the client's needs are being met. If the client experiences some kind of regularity in the commitment of the counsellor, then this regularity enables a safe, containing environment for the client. The therapeutic partnership is a potentially dynamic and potent area of care. Benefit, however, will only be achieved if the client is ready and willing to enter into a working relationship with the counsellor. Watson (1983) reviewed the data on the efficacy of psychosocial intervention programmes for patients with cancer. She found that provision of a support service for all patients is probably unnecessary. However, there should be improved methods of identifying those at risk so that selective support can then be offered with specific aims defined. Watson (1983) concludes that support may be needed over a long period.

Watson's (1983) study confirms the need to clarify the services offered to patients. Many nurses find it difficult enough to meet the basic physical needs of the people for whom they care. Consideration of the time and commitment needed for a counselling relationship may be beyond the scope of the nurse unless colleagues and management enable the redefinition of nursing priorities. With this support, the nurse can take the initiative in creating counselling opportunities. If time is short, the value of counselling skills should never be underestimated, as listening to and responding to a person may take just a few minutes and be all that is needed. Nevertheless, the nurse may be able to offer a more intense therapeutic relationship, if it is requested, by prioritising responsibilities so that time is created for the client's need.

This chapter will now explore counselling skills with relevance to nursing, then define a person-centred philosophy of care which enhances basic skills and creates the potential for therapeutic development.

Counselling skills

Any enabling interaction begins with counselling skills, and listening is the foundation of those skills. Burnard, (1987, p. 280) states that 'to really listen to another person is the most caring act of all, and takes skill and practice'. Nurse (1980, p. 70) describes the art of listening by saying, 'In counselling it is important to listen to what is said, how it is said, and also to listen to what is being implied behind the words'. This requires intensive use of the senses: hearing, watching, touching and smelling are all media of reception. Non-verbal processes can speak far louder than words, and may tell a very different tale. An example of this is given below.

Actions speak louder than words

John is in hospital for the results of his tests. He asks to see a nurse.
John [shaking hands with the nurse] 'Well, the doctor confirmed my suspicions. He told me the growth is cancer [voice breaks slightly]. But I don't mind [defiant stare]. I'm going to fight it if it's the last thing I do!'
   The nurse notices that John's hand is clammy when she shakes it. She hears the tremor in his voice when he mentions 'cancer'. She notices him shaking slightly. She also senses a mixture of emotions behind his defiant stare.

Effective listening requires concentration and focusing on the most important issue(s) presented. In order to focus on the client, the counsellor requires to develop an internal 'stillness' (Mearns and Thorne, 1988, p. 54), which is only possible if the counsellor can mentally set aside other concerns. Gendlin (1981, p. 71) calls this 'clearing a space' and describes a method of 'distancing' the self from personal troubles. This method can be practised and learned. Burnard (1991) states that attending to someone is attending to nothing else. Energy is focused entirely on the client.

Attention on the client is often facilitated by eye contact. Alternatively, some clients feel very self-conscious of constantly being held in the counsellor's gaze. The relative position of the counsellor is important in facilitating communication as some clients may need space between them and the counsellor, whereas others find closeness important: a table between the client and counsellor, for example, can feel like a barrier, and should be removed. Sensitivity to the client's need is built up through close awareness of his or her reactions.

If listening is the foundation of counselling skills, then clients need to know that they are *heard*. Acknowledging the importance of the client's communication and feelings is paramount, and Hodgson (1983) describes this as one of the factors which reduces fear and anxiety.

Acknowledgement can be conveyed by touch or facial expression and both are powerful means of communication. Marilyn Butcher (1988, p. 16) describes her fear when her cancer was diagnosed. As she talked to her anaesthetist, he held her hand, and 'that non-verbal reassurance reached and soothed the small child inside me who was frightened and alone'. She went on to say, 'I have learnt a lot about myself, but the most valuable thing of all is that a hand held is worth a million words'. Clearly, this was important for Marilyn. However, not every person can tolerate touch. It is important to be sensitive to intrusion or conveying unwanted sympathy. The meaning of non-verbal responses is not always evident to the client. Verbal acknowledgement of important issues, or responsive reflection to the client's experience offers immediate care and attention. A response the nurse might make to John following his statement in the example given above is illustrated below.

Response by counsellor

Nurse 'I hear how important fighting the cancer is to you. I also see that you are shaking' [reaches out and touches his arm].

This example of the nurse's response to John shows verbal acknowledgement of what he is saying. The nurse also shows verbal and non-verbal sensitivity to John's feelings. John may have a sense now that the counsellor is 'with' him and he has the opportunity to say more about how he feels. He also has the opportunity to deny his feelings if he wises to talk about his need to fight.

Response should flow naturally from the counsellor to the client and the counsellor should refrain from 'slipping in his [or her] interpretations' (Mearns, 1980) which might interfere with the client's process. Burnard (1987, p. 280) states that 'it is possible to pay so much attention to techniques that they impede listening and communicating', and McEvoy (1988, p. 458) supports this statement by describing failure in listening resulting from the counsellor concentrating on his or her own reply. Lamerton (1984, p. 583) suggests a way of transcending the counsellor's concern over his or her response. He states that 'there is no need to know what to say', and if the counsellor is focusing *fully* on the client, then his or her response will probably be appropriate. Lamerton (1984, p. 583) describes the 'trap' when no response comes to mind. However, this can be trusted also. If no reply is forthcoming, then we need not manufacture one' (Lamerton, 1984, p. 583): silence can be an important space for the client. Many counsellors feel the urge to fill this space. This urge is often precipitated by the counsellor's own discomfort. The value of silence can only be learned through experience and can be a very powerful way of 'being' with a client. However, if it feels right to do so, the counsellor may observe the silence by saying: 'We have been quiet for some time now and I am wondering if that's OK for you?'

Respect for the client is shown by the willingness of the counsellor to proceed at the client's own pace, with patience only being possible when the client's perspective is really valued. Simsen (1988, pp. 31–3) describes the need to 'stay with the person who is testing her [or his] own beliefs or struggling with questions of fear and faith'. This supportive presence does not need to be continual over 24 hours a day, as the client will need space to discover underlying strengths. Sensitive availability to the client may be all that is required.

A person-centred approach

Person-centred counselling exists as a distinct therapeutic approach through the work of Carl Rogers. He believed that an individual has sufficient insight and resources available for personal growth. Fundamental to Rogers' beliefs is that an actualising tendency is the primary motivating force in life. Barrett-Lennard (1988) contests that this principle is not necessarily a *sole* motivating force, but that it exists beside the tendency toward homoeostasis, balance and conservation. Life and behaviour, it seems, hinge on both growth and preservation forces. The person-centred approach encompasses both the impetus to develop, grow and transcend and the disposition to restore, recover and heal. Stevens (1967, p. 29) wrote, 'everything that I needed was right inside me'. This realisation embraces a unique approach which facilitates the client's self-awareness and inner strengths. Rogers' general hypothesis is:

> 'If I can provide a certain type of relationship, the other person will discover within [her or] himself the capacity to use that relationship for growth, and change and personal development will occur'.

This is an enormous claim. Inherent in the claim is a belief in the potential of the individual. It is one thing for the counsellor to believe in the client's potential, but it is quite another thing for the client if low self-esteem has destroyed all confidence in self. The task of counselling is to empower the client with self-belief, and the power of person-centred therapeutic relationship offers this possibility. This is a vital, dynamic approach offering the client the opportunity of seeing him or herself more clearly. Rogers (1961, p. 33) mentioned a 'certain type of relationship'. He defines this in terms of three core conditions:

* acceptance;
* empathy;
* realness.

If the counsellor can bring all three conditions to the relationship, and if the client can *experience* them, then, 'constructive personal development will invariably occur' (Rogers, 1961, p. 35).

Acceptance

There may be a great deal of fear involved in revealing innermost thoughts and feelings. So many values are imposed on an individual by society and significant others, and experience shows that exposing part of oneself leaves this part open to judgement. A client certainly will not risk sharing his or her vulnerabilities if he or she does not feel safe. The counsellor can build up a client's trust through warmth, valuing and respect. Rogers (1961, p. 47) describes this acceptance as 'unconditional positive regard'. Davies and Oberle (1990) found that valuing is the overarching concept that is both a pre- and co-requisite to care. This is a basic belief in the worth and capabilities of others beyond and together with apparent vulnerabilities. Mearns and Thorne (1988, p. 59) state that 'the counsellor who holds this attitude deeply values the humanity of [his or] her client and is not deflected in that valuing by any particular client behaviour. The attitude manifests itself in the counsellor's consistent acceptance of and enduring warmth towards [his or] her client'. It can be difficult to like a client who is angry, manipulative or withdrawn, or there may be particular aspects of the client's behaviour which are impossible to tolerate. Mearns and Thorne (1988, p. 59) suggest that 'it is possible to accept the client as a person of worth while still not liking some of the things he [or she] does'. It is important to look for and value the person *beyond* the behaviour. This allows the counsellor to have unconditional warm regard for the client while still not compromising person values. Offering acceptance of this calibre means that no judgements, assumptions or conditions are made on how the client 'should be'. This means accepting where the client is with their personal experience, accepting his or her place and relinquishing goals for the client's future. This attitude of acceptance is rarely found in health-care where plans are made daily without necessary consultation with the client involved, yet it is one of the fundamental conditions in a person-centred relationship, making it possible for the client to begin to find personal value.

Empathy

Empathy is a process of understanding how the client thinks, feels and experiences. This process involves perceptual skill and communicative ability involving an inter-active relationship between counsellor and client. Any preconceptions (for example, things which have helped other people in the past, or something which has helped the counsellor) may distort true understanding of the client's world. Empathy is not how the counsellor would feel in the client's position, nor is it how other people have felt in similar situations, it is understanding how this individual client is *experiencing* his or her reality here and now. Empathy involves setting aside personal values and experiences, and entering into the perceptual world of the client, 'as if' it were the counsellor's own world. Rogers (1961, pp. 62–3) emphasises the import-ance of the 'as if' quality. The counsellor needs to let go of personal philosophies and principles in order to understand fully and appreciate the client. The counsel-lor, however, must not let go of his or her *own* identity. If this does occur then the counsellor will be drawn into the client's world and will be unable to maintain the degree of separation which is required to be deeply empathic. Quilliam (1991) warns of the risk involved in being empathic. She describes the storing of distress which nurses pick up in the course of their work and how a patient's distress can trigger a nurse's personal unresolved issues. This emphasises the importance of support in enabling the nurse to realise his or her separate identity beyond the distress and the opportunity also to work with any unresolved issues.

It is possible to learn empathic skills (Reynolds, 1987). One way of under-standing empathy is envisaging the analogy of trying on the client's shoes in order to feel where they pinch. Just as foot size and shape differs individually, experi-encing someone else's world as they experience it is virtually impossible, yet the willingness to reach out and try can enable awareness and insight.

Communication of empathic understanding to the client is an essential part of the process of empathy. It is important for the counsellor to 'check out' what is being communicated. This can be done by focusing on an important statement from the client. The counsellor may use the phrase 'I'm hearing you saying . . .'. This is seen in the response by the counsellor given in the example on p. 286. Another kind of empathic response is illustrated below.

Reflecting on important issues

Client 'I've been spending so much time looking after Sheila that I don't seem to have much time left for anything else, let alone the children.'
Counsellor 'It seems like it's been really hard for you to have time for other things in your life – especially time for the children'.

This is a reflection of the client's statement, with the counsellor trying to get a sense of the client's perspective. If the counsellor's response is not quite accurate, the client has an opening to correct and 'help' the counsellor understand. In the above example, the client may well have replied: 'Well, yes, but my real concern is how to look after Sheila'. This 're-directs' the counsellor toward the client's concern, and gives the client the important opportunity to stop, clarify his position and determine his own understanding.

Reflecting on important statements may not be enough. It may be additionally important to reflect on any sense of underlying *feelings* the client may be experiencing. The counsellor above might have gone on to say: 'You seem really frustrated by that . . .'. All these responses can enable the client to say or feel more, if chosen. Nonetheless, the client may be needing more *depth* of empathy from the counsellor. The counsellor may have been able to offer that greater depth by saying: 'You seem really frustrated by that . . . but I sense something more . . . almost like a desperation?'

Truax and Carkhuff (1967, pp. 46–58) describe various degrees of empathy. These range from the inaccurate response through the reflection of surface statements and feelings to a 'depth reflection'. The depth reflection is described by Mearns and Thorne (1988, p. 42) as sensing deeper insight of which the client may not yet be aware. This may be facilitated by offering the client an opportunity to achieve this deeper sense without interpretation. An example is: 'I see that you are shaking . . . I wonder if there is something more happening inside you?'

Gilley (1988, p. 12) describes 'holding together knowing and not knowing'. There is regard here for the delicacy of a human being who is seeking support, yet who needs to discover a personal path.

Sensing the client's world as he or she is experiencing it, draws on the intuition and imagination of the counsellor. Burnard (1989, p. 52) describes intuition as 'knowledge beyond the senses' – it is an unexplained inner ability to 'know'. Mearns and Thorne (1988, p. 53) on the other hand, suggest that it is perfectly possible to explain this intuitive ability in terms of the vast experience gained through a lifetime of personal encounters. Trusting this sensitive ability will help enhance the counsellor's capacity to tune in to the multidimensional experience of the client.

Realness

The person-centred approach involves the person of the counsellor as much as the person of the client. While working with a client, the counsellor will experience various personal feelings. Some of these feelings will emanate from personal experience while others will be in response to the client. Being 'real' involves an awareness of the feelings which are related to the client, and a willingness to express them. There is little point in smiling at a client when deep down the counsellor feels anxious or shaken by what he or she is hearing. More often than not, the client will sense the counsellor's real feelings and this can lead to a confusion which is separate from the client's own dilemma. It is difficult for a client to trust a counsellor who is not genuine.

A counsellor who is 'willing to be fully present as a real, alive, relating human being who is not concealing' (Mearns and Thorne, 1988, p. 86) will risk sharing his or her personal feelings in response to me client. Rogers (1961, p. 61) describes this way of being as 'congruence'. The counsellor is 'genuine and without "front" or façade, openly being the feelings and attitudes which at that moment are flowing in him [or her]' (Rogers 1961, p. 61).

The counsellor may be confused by what the client is saying. Within the context, 'being real' means admitting to the client that there is a lack of understanding. For example: 'I must stop you just now, as I can't seem to grasp what you mean'. This allows the possibility of clarification. More important, it brings the counsellor back into the relationship. Effective relations with clients requires this kind of honesty and openness. Furthermore, the clarification may help clients to see ways in which they have been misleading themselves.

Another example of congruence is sharing a feeling which is persistent and seems to be related to the client. For example: 'I'm feeling really tense just now, and I'm not sure why that is. It's like I'm trying so hard to reach you, but there's some "barrier" in the way.' If there is significance to the client, he or she may be able to work with a new awareness. Has the client been putting up 'barriers' in relation to the counsellor? Is this something the client usually does in a relationship? In this way, the counsellor's realness in reflecting his or her experience of the client may help the client to make self-discoveries.

Being open in response to a client is different from self-disclosure. The counsellor's experience of life is never the same as the client's. It is not usually helpful in counselling to share life experiences with the client; 'even then the focus of attention would remain on the client rather than the counsellor' (Mearns and Thorne, 1988, p. 82). An example of this is: 'My son also left home when he was that age. I felt "lost" too. However, it sounds like you felt "abandoned" somehow . . . ?' This returns to the empathic response. Otherwise a common life experience can 'block' the counsellor's ability to be empathic.

Clearly, the three conditions of acceptance, empathy and realness are entwined and work together. For example, being real enhances the empathic response which is facilitated through valuing the client. Professional distancing or aloofness blocks the whole counselling process. This may be a necessary defence for some, yet it will never facilitate a true depth of caring. It is important for the counsellor to find a safe environment in which to explore any need for self-protection. Self-awareness at this level can free many defences.

Self-awareness and support

The counsellor's self-awareness is an essential prerequisite to effective counselling. Mearns and Thorne (1988, p. 23) states that, 'the relationship which the counsellor has with [him or] herself will, to a large extent, determine the quality of the work [he or] she is able to initiate with clients'. Self-knowledge helps distinguish between self-needs and empathic response. This knowledge is vital if the counsellor aims to enter fully into a counselling relationship. Self-awareness is enhanced and enabled by personal support and, without support, a counsellor may suffer undue stress (see Chapter 19). Alternatively, he or she may unconsciously protect him or herself by becoming complacent. Hodgson (1983, p. 65) describes complacency in staff. 'Someone who is sure he [or she] is doing everything right will not be really in touch with someone who is feeling all wrong'.

It is the counsellor's responsibility to seek support. This is an important part of personal value and work. However, Roberts and Fallowfield (1990) discovered that nearly half of their respondents providing oncology counselling were unsupported in their work. Support through personal supervision is an invaluable way of clarifying issues, discovering resources and moving forward. Support may be also found in group situations. The members can work together to share difficulties and enable insight. Implicit in any support is the need to trust the other person or people. As in counselling, trust is aided by drawing up a working contract and discussing confidentiality.

Confidentiality

If a person discloses something meaningful to another person, then the other person is being trusted with something personal. To pass this on to others might devalue this trust. With the importance attached to communication in nursing, confidentiality poses a dilemma. Support, however, is offered through the professional code of conduct for nurses, midwives and health visitors (United Kingdom Central Council for Nursing, Midwifery and Health Visiting, 1992) which clearly defines the nurse's position: as a registered nurse, midwife and health visitor you are personally accountable for your practice, and, in the exercise your professional accountability must:

> 'Protect all confidential information concerning patients and clients obtained in the course of professional practice and make disclosures only with consent, where required by the order of a court or where you can justify disclosure in the wider public interest.' (United Kingdom Central Council for Nursing, Midwifery and Health Visiting, 1992).

Within the context of counselling, whatever clients discover or reveal about themselves is their own. Except under exceptional circumstances, this should never be disclosed to another party. It is up to the client whether any personal information is to be shared.

If the counsellor feels there is something important to communicate with others, then it is essential that this is discussed firstly with the client. The counsellor has no right to share anything about the client with others, unless prior permission has been given. The value of the counselling relationship is dependent on the maintenance of this confidence.

Applying counselling in nursing care

Whether the nurse sets up an agreement to see a client regularly for counselling, so offering the opportunity of a therapeutic partnership, or whether he or she uses counselling skills in everyday communication, a person-centred approach offers a philosophy of care which facilitates the client's self-discovery. An example of counselling skills used with a client whom the author has been visiting is given below. The client has given permission for this material to be reproduced. The conversation described took less than 10 minutes, then the client moved on to discuss other matters.

Use of counselling skills

Client   [appearing really agitated] 'I just can't settle after seeing these two other women dying in the same room as me [referring to other patients] – I feel I've been forced to look at something I'm not ready for. You know, I *know* I'm going to die, and I'm not frightened of death – in fact I welcome it – but it was just *terrible* watching those women die.' [eyes wide]

Counsellor   [reaching to hold client's hand] 'I can feel you trembling and I sense your fear . . . I hear you saying that you're not frightened of death, yet I feel that there's something about dying which terrifies you'.

Client   [silence – shaking increases] 'It's the *process* of dying – involuntary sobs] – it's so undignified! [grips counsellor's hand tightly].

Counsellor. [silence] . . . 'I really hear the hear the *horror* in your voice . . . Keeping your dignity seems absolutely *vital* to you'

Client   [starts to relax a little – withdraws her hand] 'It's the idea of losing control over bodily functions – I just couldn't *bear* that' [starts shaking again].

Counsellor   'The thought of other people clearing up your mess seems really impossible for you to *allow*?'

Client   [looking directly at counsellor] 'Oh! I couldn't *possibly* accept it!'

Counsellor   'That really strikes me! – it's like it would be impossibly hard for you to let someone tend to you or care for you in a physical way'.

Client   [looks down] 'Yes you're right, I would be so embarrassed and ashamed.'

Counsellor   [quietly] 'There's something about these feelings you have . . . and I sense you don't want me to touch you right now . . . it's like you feel you're untouchable or maybe . . . not worth caring for?'

Client   [silence and tears] 'How can I be worth caring about?'

Counsellor   [silence] '. . . You sound so desolate, almost like you feel totally rejected.'

The client went on to talk for a short time about past events where she felt rejected by her father.

This counselling session is an example of the counsellor 'keeping track' with the client and not jumping to conclusions about the client's fear. When the client said, 'I've been forced to look at something I'm not ready for', the counsellor was aware of the fear and anxiety which the client had been carrying since the deaths of the other patients. In addition, the counsellor sensed that the client probably *was* ready to look at that 'something' but that a safe and supportive relationship would be necessary to help release the client's fear. The counsellor did not even try to reassure the client about her stated concern over incontinence, realising that this reassurance would have blocked the client at this point, preventing her from exploring the significance of her disgust. The counsellor had no idea what that significance was, and worked sensitively with empathic responses, so enabling the client to reach the depth of her troubles. By openly stating the sense that the client did not want to be touched, and yet by showing willingness to stay with and not back away from the client, the counsellor empowered the client to talk freely about painful past events. Once the client reached this very difficult area in her life, the counsellor was able to 'be with' and acknowledge the client's pain, and, most important, not reject or diminish the client in any way. This embodies the person-centred philosophy, offering acceptance, empathy and real presence with the counsellor's approach. The counsellor did not try to interpret the client's troubles: the client showed that she had the capacity to understand herself in her own way and in her own time. One week later, during another visit with the counsellor, the client said briefly: 'You know, I've been thinking a lot about my father recently, and I've actually forgiven him for what he did to me. I feel a warmth for him now, and that makes me feel better'. Only the client could reach inside herself and know what it is like to offer forgiveness and experience resultant warmth.

Rogers (1961, p. 357) states that 'the farmer cannot make the germ develop and sprout from the seed: he can only supply the nurturing conditions which will permit the seed to develop its own potentialities'. Clearly, the 'nurturing conditions' of the person–centred approach can free 'the natural healing capacity within the client' (Mearns and Thorne, 1988, p. 129), so enabling potential development. This development continues to be possible towards the end of life.

A client with cancer who is struggling with the attendant emotions brought by change and loss may present the counsellor with feelings such as fear, grief, anger and guilt (see Chapter 7). Initially, the counsellor may feel overwhelmed by these strong emotions. This notwithstanding, Mearns and Thorne (1988, p. 104) state that 'the very activity of empathic understanding often has the effect of defusing a crisis, of slowing down the pace and relieving to some extent the crippling sense of anxiety and dread which the client may be undergoing'. Slowing down the pace is one way of enhancing the quality of time, and offers an invaluable gift to the person whose lifetime is limited. This concept of 'being held in a moment of time' by empathic understanding is surely the ultimate connection in palliative care, offering human contact to those who are losing contact with life. Clearly, being with a client in a person–centred way is a powerful use of counselling in nursing care.

If people with cancer and members of their family can experience acceptance, depth of understanding and genuineness from health-care professionals, then they may be empowered by their own strengths and internal resources to live life to capacity and find meaning in the here and now. Through encountering life in all its painful dimensions, a process of discovery is launched which holds the dynamic potential for growth. Person-centred counselling can help release this potential through freeing the healing power of the individual, enabling creativity and increasing self-esteem.

> 'Perhaps there is more understanding and beauty in life when the glaring sunlight is softened by the patterns of shadows. Perhaps there is more depth in a relationship that has weathered some storms. Experience that never disappoints or saddens or stirs up feelings is a bland experience with little challenge or variation in colour. Perhaps when we experience confidence and faith and hope that we see materialize before our eyes this builds up within us a feeling of inner strength, courage, and security.
>
> We are all personalities that grow and develop as a result of all our experiences, relationships, thoughts and emotions. We are the sum total of all the parts that go into the making of a life.'
>
> Axline (1964, p. 194)

Acknowledgements

Thanks go to Professor Stuart Aitken, Department of Geography, San Diego State University; Diana Guthrie, Student Advisory and Counselling Service, University of Edinburgh; Elke Lambers and Dave Mearns, Co-Directors, Person Centred Therapy (Britain); Alison Shoemark, colleague and friend; and members of the Scottish PCT Supervision Group. The support and insight gained from all was invaluable. Special thanks also go to Mrs Arlene Ogston for typing, and to Sam for his unfailing patience and respect.

References

ALLEN, L. (1990). A client's experience of failure. In: MEARNS, D. and DRYDEN, W. (eds), *Experiences of Counselling in Action*, pp. 20–7. Sage, London.

AXLINE, V. M. (1964). *Dibs – In Search of Self*. Penguin, Harmondsworth.

BARRETT-LENNARD, G. T. (1988) Introducing the person centred approach to helping. Unpublished manuscript.

BURNARD, P. (1987). Counselling: basic principles in nursing. *The Professional Nurse* 2 June, 278–80.

BURNARD, P. (1989). The 'sixth sense'. *Nursing Times* 85, 52–3.

BUTCHER, M. (1988). The nightmare of the dreaded diagnosis. *The Independent* 18 October, 16.

UNITED KINGDOM CENTRAL COUNCIL FOR NURSING, MIDWIFERY AND HEALTH VISITING (1992) Code of Conduct for the Nurse, Midwife and Health Visitor. UKCC, London.

DAVIES, B. and OBERLE, K. (1990). Dimensions of the supportive role of the nurse in palliative care. *Oncology Nursing Forum* 17, 87–94.

GENDLIN, E. T. (1981). *Focusing*. Bantam, New York.

GILLEY, J. (1988). Intimacy and terminal care. *Journal of The Royal College of General Practitioners* 38, 121–2.

HODGSON, S. (1983). Enhancing patient–nurse communication. *Nursing Times, Occasional Papers* 79, 64–5.

LAMERTON, R. (1984). Communication with the dying patient. *The Practitioner* 228, 581–3.

MCEVOY, P. (1988). Introducing nurses to the counselling process. *The Professional Nurse* 3 August, 456–60.

MCLEOD, J. (1990). The client's experience of counselling and psychotherapy: a review of the research literature. In: MEARNS, D. and DRYDEN, W. (eds), *Experiences of Counselling in Action*, pp. 1–19. Sage, London.

MEARNS, D. (1980). The person centred approach to therapy. Unpublished paper produced for the Scottish Association for Counselling, 31 May.

MEARNS, D. and THORNE, B. (1988). *Person Centred Counselling in Action*. Sage, London.

NURSE, G. (1980). *Counselling and the Nurse*, 2nd edn. HM & M.

QUILLIAM, S. (1991). When empathy gets dangerous. *Practice Nurse* October, 305–6.

REID-POINTE, P. (1992). Distress in cancer patients and primary nurses' empathy skills. *Cancer Nursing* 15, 283–292.

REYNOLDS, W. J. (1987). Empathy: we know what we mean, but what do we teach? *Nurse Education Today* 7, 265–9.

ROBERTS, R. and FALLOWFIELD, L. (1990) Who supports the cancer counsellors? *Nursing Times* 86, 32–4.

ROGERS, C. R. (1961) *On Becoming a Person*. Constable, London.

SIMSEN, B. (1988) Nursing the spirit. *Nursing Times* 84, 31–3.

STEVENS, B. (1967). From my life 1. In: ROGERS, C. R. and STEVENS, B. (eds), *Person to Person: The Problem of Being Human*, pp. 29–40. Souvenir Press, London.

TRUAX, C. B. and CARKHUFF, R. R. (1967). *Towards Effective Counselling and Psychotherapy*. Aldine, Chicago.

WATSON, M. (1983). Psychosocial intervention with cancer patients: a review. *Psychological Medicine* 13, 839–46.

Further reading

BOND, M. (1986). *Stress and Self-awareness: A Guide for Nurses*. Heinemann Nursing, London.

BURNARD, P. (1985). *Learning Human Skills*. Heinemann Nursing, London.

DRYDEN, W. (ed.) (1984). *Individual Therapy in Britain*. Harper & Row. London.

GENDLIN, E. T. (1981). *Focusing*. Bantam, New York.

KAGAN, C., EVANS, J. and KAY, B. (1986). *A Manual of Interpersonal Skills for Nurses*. Harper & Row, London.

MEARNS, D. and DRYDEN, W. (eds) (1990). *Experiences of Counselling in Action*. Sage, London.

ROGERS, C. R. and STEVENS, B. (1967). *Person to Person: The Problem of Being Human*. Souvenir Press, London.

TSCHUDIN, V. (1987). *Counselling Skills for Nurses*, 2nd edn. Ballière-Tindall, London.

19

Learning to cope with the stress of palliative care

Pat Mathers

'The ultimate measure of man is not where he stands in moments of comfort and convenience but where he stands at times of challenge and controversy.'
Martin Luther King, Strength to Love (1963)

Introduction

The participants in the caring situation of a patient with advanced cancer are the patient, the family of the patient and the nurse. Flows of communication in the form of commitment of self take place between the nurse and family as they endeavour to maximise the quality of remaining life for the patient and the patient tries to ease any possible distress experienced by those around him or her. To understand some of the complexity of the flows of self, this chapter proposes a model in which care is identified with the energy and resource of the participants.

It is clear that the demand for energy and resource will be greatest for the nurse for it is the nurse who provides the specialist care for the patient and family and who also endeavours to maintain harmonious interrelationships between the participants of the model.

The role of the nurse then is that of a manager who determines whether or not the caring situation is maintained in a steady state. Such a role can be draining and exhausting for the nurse and some renewal of energy and resource is essential if this steady-state or homoeostasis of the model is to be achieved.

It is also a traumatic experience for the family and relatives who, confronted with the situation, pass from initial disbelief to great sadness as they see their loved one decline. They too require renewal and replenishment if they are to contribute to the care of the patient. Finally, the patient may still feel the shock of prognosis and be despairing about the future. Thus the balance between the positive and negative energy content of the model can easily be weighted to that of the negative end of the spectrum and it is important to identify how the stresses and strains within the palliative care model may be alleviated.

The literature has numerous accounts of the different forms of stress management (e.g. Cox, 1978; Greenberg, 1983) and it is sometimes difficult for the individual to make an appropriate choice. Each person feels stress in different ways and ideally stress management should be tailored to individual needs.

The classic examples are those of whole body relaxation and controlled breathing. These are the ones most widely adopted for they achieve mind and body links and the instructions for the methods are easy to use once they have been learnt.

A more unconscious form of stress management lies in the use of humour in the appropriate setting and point in time. It releases stress-related tension, provides emotional support for the patient and family and is an effective antidote to the dehumanising aspects of health care (Dugan, 1989; Gilligan, 1993). Humour and its associated smiles and laughter provide for the release of negative human feelings and yet have positive energising effects on the human spirit (Holden, 1994). In turn positive emotional state, as a consequence of humour, may enhance immune function (Dillon *et al.*, 1985; Martin and Dobbin, 1988). Tears, the opposite end of the laughter spectrum, also have a role to play in the model.

A description of the underlying psychophysiology of these stress management techniques appears at the end of this chapter.

The energy and resource model of care

The structure of the proposed conceptual model is shown in Fig. 19.1. Function in the model is based on the energy and resource flows between its participants. How it reacts and behaves is dependent on the energy and resources of the participants as well as the transactions within itself and the surrounding environment (Lazarus and Launier, 1977).

Each participant, whether patient, family or nurse, will bring those resources and energies to the model which are dependent on the stresses and strains they experience in its function. These latter may be external environmental stressors that develop in the social and interpersonal relationships of the model or they may come from within the participants themselves and be concerned with the need to counter the threat to security and control over the situation (Karasek, 1979). The scenario that embraces palliative care places the nurse as the key figure in the model. His or her task is to act both as a source of positive energy and resource as well as the recipient of negative flows of energy and resource.

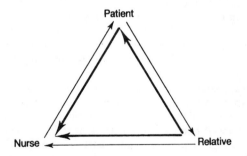

Fig. 19.1 A conceptual model of palliative care based on the energy and resource of the participants.

The speed of development of the model will be dependent on how quickly the ebbs and flows of energy and resource are established. Systems theory postulates that the slow development of function in a model makes for a smoother and more efficient adaptation over time (Beishon and Peters, 1972). Hence a hasty and hurried contact with the patient and his or her family in initial model development will not be conducive to the later stability of the model. Time and resource expended in building up relationships in the early stages will reap abundant dividends in the future with respect to the equable management of the model.

The tangible nature of these ebbs and flows of energy and resource in the model is evidenced in a number of ways. The efficacy of energy transfer through touch for the restoration of flagging patient energies has been documented by McCorkle (1974), Heidt (1981), Kreiger (1986), Le May (1986), Sims (1986, 1988) and Smith (1990). The value of laughter between nurse and patient as an antidote for negative emotions and a release of pent-up emotional energy has been described by a number of authors (Martin and Lefcourt, 1983; Dillon *et al.*, 1985; Bellert, 1989). Positive feedback from the patient and family with respect to nursing care can also act as a source of renewal of the energy and resource of the nurse his or herself (Adams, 1984). Positive emotional exchange of this type can tap inner strengths and enhance the psyche of the participants of the model.

By the same token negative flows of energy can disturb the smooth passage of the model. Such negative flows of energy take place when patients or relatives become anxious, angry or depressed. Perception of the potentially hopeless situation can trigger physiological and biochemical changes that will release resource and energy to cope with the lack of control they feel. This energy may be released slowly or it can result in random explosive outbursts of frustration and anger against those that are in the caring role. It is usually the nurse in palliative care who has to absorb these outflows of energy as well as provide those additional inputs of energy and resource to bring the model back into homoeostasis.

Strong emotional energies are seen as part of the inner flows of the model and are more effective in giving the model predictability. More peripheral are those flows of energy and communication utilised through the vision and hearing of the participants. The chemical energy of the food intake of the participants is translated into the mechanical energy of the posture and movement of non-verbal communication and in the completion of tasks essential in the purely physical process of caring. Energy is used to create the sound waves for hearing which are then re-translated back into the chemical and nervous energy of the receivers of the communication. In all such transfers there is a loss of some energy so time again is an essential resource if the maximum transfer of energy is to be achieved. Concentration of the flow of energy will ensure that it is focused on the recipient and will prevent the wastage that accompanies hasty communications and care.

Also included in the outer ring of the model are the coping strategies and skills of the participants themselves. These have been learned over time and represent small packets of information that can be utilised by the nurse in palliative care for the smoother function of the model. The strategy of stress monitoring in all the participants can alert the nurse to possible depletion of the energy stores of the model whilst the skills of reducing pain in the patient can add power to the model and prevent the energy drain that accompanies severe and continual pain.

Negative and stereotyped attitudes of the general public and health-care professionals towards cancer (Corner, 1988) may cause each participant to undergo

cycles of depression, guilt, despair and anxiety (Penson, 1979, 1984). These negative flows may cause an imbalance in the model and allow it to depart from the
bounds of a carrying capacity defined by its maximum and minimum energy and
resource content. The trajectory of the model will therefore be determined by the
balance of positive and negative flows prevailing at any one moment in time.

The passage of the model across the time continuum is illustrated in Fig. 19.2. In
homoeostasis the model will move and fluctuate between the boundaries of its upper
and lower limit of function (Appleby and Trumbull, 1986). If the energy and
resource input of one of the participants is low, perhaps due to fatigue, then the
model may move below the lower limit of function. Fatigue can reduce the personal
resources of the patient (Pickard-Holley, 1991) and influence the quality of care
given by the family, particularly if it has a significant impact on their daily routine
(Jensen and Given, 1991). In the palliative care nurse it will blur the perception of
the needs of the family, restrict the sensitivity and empathy required to handle
every day problems and reduce the time spent in the provision of support (Hull,
1991). The consequence may be that the model will drift below the points C and D
depicted in Fig. 19.2 unless some renewal can restore its function. Accessibility of
staff who are not tired and are willing to inform and explain can go some way to
bring the model back to the optimum level of function (Penson, 1984).

Similarly the sudden inputs of energy during a strong negative emotional
experience such as an outburst of anger or frustration can cause the model to
exceed the optimal boundaries of its function at E and F and become out of
control. A nurse who is knowledgeable, resourceful, decisive, warm and friendly
(Oskins, 1979) can do much to negate the despair of those concerned and hence
provide that input that will restore homoeostasis.

Acting as a source of energy and resource for the model can be demanding and
draining for the nurse and the need for renewal becomes paramount. The stresses
and strains experienced by nurses who care for the terminally ill are described well
by a number of authors (Kastenbaum, 1967; Knight and Field, 1981; Chiriboga *et
al.*, 1983; Conboy-Hill, 1986; Power and Sharp, 1988; Cathcart, 1989) and strategies
for coping are identified. These strategies are both cognitive and palliative in nature

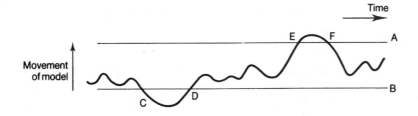

A – B represents the carrying capacity of the model. Movement within A and B
occurs when the model is in homeostasis.

C – D Drift into entropy due to energy and resource lack of the participants.

E – F Drift out of control due to explosive inputs of energy and resource
by the participants.

Fig. 19.2 Movement of the model of palliative care over a time continuum.

(Folkman, 1984), but do not really describe how the nurse may rebuild his or her strength which has been depleted in the caring process.

To understand how this replenishment may take place, it is necessary to know how the energy and resource is released as a response to the stress engendered by being part of the model.

Responses to stress

The early stages of the stress response are in response to the perception of a demand. Psychological processes are translated into physiological processes through the autonomic nervous system and the endocrine system. The response to the demand was described by Selye (1976) and it can take place through two pathways. The short term response to stress will take place through the hypothalamo–adrenal medullary component of the autonomic nervous system whilst the resources for the long-term response to stress are mobilised through the hypothalamo–pituitary–adrenal cortex axis of the endocrine system. The pathways do not occur in isolation but probably run in parallel with each other. Which one predominates is dependent on individual perception of the situation at the time. The details of the process are summarised in Fig. 19.3.

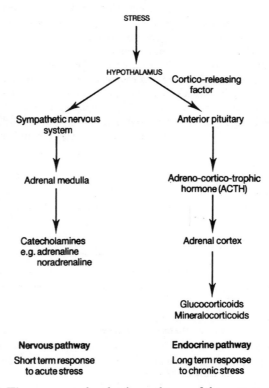

Fig. 19.3 The nervous and endocrine pathways of the response to stress.

The effect of the hormonal release is to change body stores of resource and energy into forms that can be used in the immediate and long-term response to the demands of the model. The changes are accompanied by certain signs and indicators of the psychological and physiological processes involved. Broadly these indicators can be categorised into emotional, behavioural and physiological factors and some examples of these categories are shown in Table 19.1 (Derogatis *et al.*, 1974; Selye, 1976).

In a recent survey of palliative care nurses on an international conference in Cambridge emotional and behavioural indicators were predominant with physiological indicators only accounting for 17 per cent of the recorded symptoms. This would seem to indicate that the behavioural techniques employed by the nurses were sufficient to prevent the breakthrough to the physiological spectrum. Highest on the list was the need to be alone and the urge to sleep leading to the conclusion that the nurses require time, rest and peace for a renewal of strength and purpose.

Hans Selye (1980) has described the finite nature of the stress response in the general adaptation syndrome. In the initial stages of alarm resources are mobilised quickly and for a time the body adapts and maintains levels of resources and energy sufficient to maintain the body in a state of homoeostasis. However, high continual use of these resources without rest results in rapid depletion of body stores and the individual can soon move into a state of exhaustion. It is clear that some of the nurses in the survey were beginning to be aware of those subtle changes that occur over time for exhaustion and depressed feelings received a high priority in the recording of symptoms.

Renewal of strength

How then can the participants in the palliative care model renew their strength and purpose and find sufficient energy to maintain optimal model function?

Laboratory experimentation indicates that subtle energy exchanges occur between an individual and their environment as a consequence of their emotions. Changes in the electrical conductance on the surface of the skin and varying heat energy losses to the surrounding air are examples of such activity (Dawson *et al.*, 1990).

In conceptual terms the energy field of an individual who is under stress, tired and exhausted is narrow and withdrawn. Smooth energy flow will be blocked by muscle tension and anxiety. Conservation of resources becomes paramount, attention span is reduced and the cognitive activities of memory and performance

Table 19.1 Emotional, behavioural and physiological indicators of stress

Emotional	Behavioural	Physiological
Exhaustion	Increased activity	Nausea
Exhilaration	Decreased activity	Constipation
Depressed feelings	Urge to sleep	Urinary frequency
Uneasy or anxious	Difficult to sleep	Palpitations
General tension	Urge to eat	Tremulousness
	Loss of appetite	Dizziness

will be impaired. Visually this is described in Fig. 19.4 which depicts the normal smooth energy flows in health compared to the distorted energy flow of the individual not in balance with the environment.

Human individuals subconsciously recognise these signs and a nurse or family relative with tenseness in their body posture will have a reciprocating effect on other participants in the model. The non-verbal communication of anxiety or worry of a family relative will not help the patient who may be unable to do anything about it.

How then may pschophysiological homoeostasis be restored? Relaxation and diaphragmatic breathing are two ways in which changed individual physiology can restore individual psychological balance while the use of humour in dyadic or group situations can operate at both individual and group level.

Relaxation

The physiology initiated through relaxation can have dramatic effects. Relaxation reduces muscle tension and lowers the level of blood lactate and hence the levels of anxiety induced by the build up of this metabolic by product of muscle biochemistry (Pitts, 1969). Heart rate, blood pressure and respiratory rate are lowered and the generalised vasodilation that occurs evens the heat energy field of the person under stress. The electrical energy field is also normalised through an increase in the alpha and theta activity of the EEG and the galvanic skin response (Pitts, 1969; Wallace and Benson, 1972; Luck, 1989). A summary of these changes appears in Fig. 19.5.

In progressive relaxation it is important to create optimum conditions of quiet, comfort and loose clothing. Details of the exact procedures are described by Jacobsen (1938) and Berstein and Borkovec (1973) and that of Jacobsen would seem to be the best method to adopt. In this method each muscle group is tensed (30 s) and relaxed (40–60 s) twice.

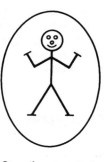
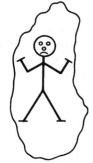

Smooth even energy
field of an individual in
homoeostasis

Uneven, distorted and
narrow energy field of an
individual under stress

Fig. 19.4 The energy fields of an individual in health and homoeostasis and an indiviual under stress.

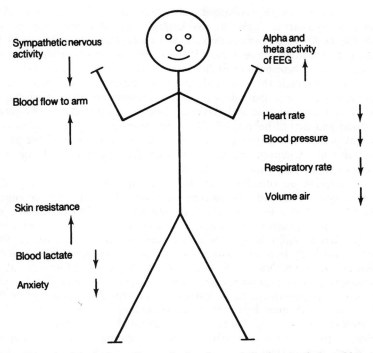

Sympathetic nervous
activity

Alpha and
theta activity
of EEG

Blood flow to arm

Heart rate

Blood pressure

Respiratory rate

Volume air

Skin resistance

Blood lactate

Anxiety

Fig. 19.5 The physiological correlates of relaxation and diaphragmatic breathing.

The rationale of the method requires the recognition of tension in the muscle and the ability to remember what it feels like to release tension from the muscle. Continual monitoring of the induced relaxation is essential to ensure that muscles once relaxed remain relaxed.

The exercises have to be repeated each day for several weeks for maximum benefit. Eventually the process becomes faster and it is possible to reach complete relaxation in a very short time.

Breathing techniques

Relaxation combined with a breathing technique can be even more beneficial (Bailey, 1985).

Each individual has their own pattern of breathing and breathing can vary with the state of mind. An anxious person tends to show a hasty and erratic pattern while intermittent gasps and sighs typify anger.

A person who is endeavouring to achieve the control of stress through breathing should aim for a slowing of the breathing pattern through slow and gentle prolonged exhalation followed by spontaneous inhalation at the end of each exhalation (Bailey, 1985).

The mild hyperventilation that may occur during prolonged exhalation may produce a slight tingling in the hands and feet. If this does occur then a temporary cessation of prolonged exhalation will rectify the physiological imbalance of hypocarbia. Theoretically however, the slow breathing pattern should allow the build up of carbon dioxide to replace that which has been lost in the prolonged exhalation. In this way there should be no disturbance to the carbon dioxide and acid base balance of the body.

Breathing through the nose induces warm feelings in the body and using the diaphragm stimulates the calming parasympathetic component of the autonomic nervous system. Thoracic and clavicular breathing contribute to heightened states of arousal and should be avoided. Breathing from the diaphragm also increases the depth of penetration of the air into the lungs. It is the base of the lungs that has the greater blood supply and it is here that the maximum exchange between the blood and respiratory gases can take place.

Concentration on breathing patterns frees the neuronal circuitry of the brain which is concerned with the anxiety of a situation. The higher centres of the brain cause muscles to tense automatically when demands are seen to outstrip coping. If these centres are occupied with control that is required for breathing patterns then muscle relaxation will be enhanced still further (Brown, 1978).

Mind and body become balanced and tension is reduced. The sensation is one of floating and complete freedom to ride on the wings of space and time. The experience of present existence produces a sense of personal identity and oneness with self. It is perhaps in these states of relaxation that the tenets of the Eastern philosophy of Zen and the art of pseudo-enlightenment are most nearly achieved, for fleeting moments of happiness are captured in moments of present time (Barker, 1989). Refreshment comes with the tapping of hidden energies and the gain of new perspectives.

Humour, laughter and tears

Humour used appropriately in the oncology setting can also have beneficial therapeutic effects (Dugan, 1989; Graham and Cates, 1989; Simon, 1989; Erdman, 1991; Radziewicz and Schneider, 1992; Davidhizar and Bowen, 1993; Gilligan, 1993). Laughter and the smiles which follow are a form of eustress (useful stress) which mobilises the energy and resource required to deal with a stressful situation. Crying and tears at the opposite end of the emotional spectrum eliminate the waste products of the stress hormones produced in stressful situations (Fry, 1989).

Both kinds of behaviour are followed by a feeling of being more in control of a situation and there is a discharge of pent-up tension.

Laughing and crying represent happiness and sadness and, although they can merge into each other they differ in the facial muscles which are used, their respiratory pattern (Bloch *et al.*, 1991) and their psychophysiology.

True smiles precede laughter and are accompanied by reflex lacrimation and pupil dilation. Crying causes pupils to constrict and the flow of tears is initiated by the parasympathetic nervous system. The feedback of the facial muscles used in either activity intensifies the perceived emotion (Marieb, 1989).

With respect to their respiratory pattern, sadness and crying are characterised by saccadic breathing movements on the inspiratory phase of the respiratory cycle (sob, sob) whilst laughing has superposed saccadic movements on the expiratory phase (ha, ha) (Bloch *et al.*, 1991).

A good belly laugh is a form of internal jogging. It involves whole body movement and encourages the blood supply to internal organs. It lowers blood pressure below baseline (Fry, 1986; Fry and Savin, 1988) and encourages residual air gas exchange (Fry and Stoft, 1971). Immune function is enhanced by increased production of salivary IgA (Dillon *et al.*, 1985; Martin and Dobbin, 1988), raised proliferation of lymphocytes and greater natural killer cell activity (Berk *et al.*, 1988).

Hormonal changes include lower levels of stress hormones in the blood, e.g. cortisol and the release of endorphins which help to alleviate pain (Cousins, 1979; Berk *et al.*, 1988, 1989a, b).

Psychologically, creative thinking, learning and memory are improved (Fry, 1986). Personal experience in the laboratory indicates that changes in mood state occur after laughter periods and graduate nurses become more untroubled, calm relaxed and happy than they were before the experimentation.

The benefits of laughter and crying therapy for all the participants of the model are clear to see. For the patient it is the relief of pain, enhancement of immune function and improved oxygen supply to the tissues. For the nurse it is the increase in positive mood and for the participants it relates the situation to normal everyday events. Perhaps it should be used more often in the oncology setting providing the time and place are appropriate.

Simon (1989) makes a number of suggestions for humour interventions which include the sharing of cartoons, jokes and funny stories, comedy videos, humour diaries and journals, humour rooms, etc. As Simon points out humour and laughter are contagious.

Laughter meditations as described by Sutorius at the Paris Conference of the International Stress Management Association in 1992 can be particularly effective in raising the energy levels of an individual.

Future research

The simultaneous use of any of these three stress management techniques by the nurse, patient and family has more beneficial effects on model behaviour than if there is asynchrony of their efforts.

Matrices which depict combinations of resource and energy levels of the participants will identify the unique character of each situation. They will of necessity be complex in nature but a setting out of the balances will enable an understanding of the processes that underline participant interaction .

Research is needed as to how the parameters of the model can be quantified and how they change over the course of time (Folkman and Lazarus, 1980, 1985; Folkman, 1984). There will be certain critical times when either conservation or extra effort is required. The identification of these critical times requires all the skills of the nurse and specialised training of nurses in palliative care is the only way the nurse will be able to make the appropriate decisions and choices (Barstow, 1980; Fisher, 1988; Manley, 1988).

References

ADAMS, J. (1984). A prescription for coping failure. *Nursing Forum* 21, 28–30.
APPLEY, M. H. and TRUMBULL, R. (eds) (1986). Dynamics of stress and its control. In: *Dynamics of Stress. Physiological, Psychological and Social Perspectives*, pp. 309–27. Plenum Press.

BAILEY, R. D. (1985). *Coping with Stress in Caring*. Blackwell Scientific.

BARKER, P. (1989). Zen and the art of pseudo-enlightenment. *Nursing Times* **85**, 30–2.

BARSTOW, J. (1980). Stress variance in hospice nursing. *Nursing Outlook* 751–4 (1984).

BEISHON, P. and PETERS, G. (1972). *Systems Behaviour*. Open University Press and Harper & Row.

BERK, L. S., TAN, S. A. and NEHLSEN-CANNARELLA, S. L. (1988). Humor associated laughter decreases cortisol and induces spontaneous lymphocyte blastogenesis. *Clinical Research* **36**, 435A.

BERK, L. S, TAN, S. A, NAPIER, B. J. and EBY, W. C. (1989a). Eustress of mirthful laughter modifies natural killer cell activity. *Clinical Research* **87**, 115A.

BERK, L. S., TAN, S. A., FRY, W. F., NAPIER B. J., LEE, J. W., HUBBARD R. W., LEWIS, J. E. and EBY, W. C. (1989b). Neuroendocrine and stress hormone changes during mirthful laughter. *American Journal of the Medical Sciences* **298**, 390–6.

BERSTEIN, D. and BORKOVEC, T. (1973). *Progressive Relaxation Training: A Manual for the Helping Professions*. Research Press, Chicago.

BELLERT, J. L. (1989). Humour. A therapeutic approach in oncology nursing. *Cancer Nursing* **12**, 65–70.

BLOCH, S., LEMEIGNAN, M. and AGUILERA, N. (1991). Specific respiratory patterns distinguish among human basic emotions. *International Journal of Psychophysiology* **11**, 141–54.

BROWN, B. B. (1978). *Stress and the Art of Biofeedback*. Bantam.

CATHCART, F. (1989). Coping with distress. *Nursing Times* **85**, 33–5.

CHIRIBOGA, D., JENKINS, G. and BAILEY, J. (1983). Stress and coping among hospice nurses: tests of an analytic model. *Nursing Research* **32**, 294–9.

CONBOY-HILL, S. (1986). Psychosocial aspects of terminal care. *International Nursing* **33**, 19–21.

CORNER, J. L. (1988). Assessment of nurses' attitudes towards cancer: a critical review of research methods. *Journal of Advanced Nursing* **13**, 640–8.

COUSINS, N. (1979). *Anatomy of an Illness*. Bantam.

COX, T. (1978). *Stress*. Macmillan Education.

DAVIDHIZAR, R. (1993). When nurses cry. *Todays Nurse* **15**, 36–9.

DAVIDHIZAR, R. and BOWEN, M. (1993). The dynamics of laughter. *Archives of Psychiatric Nursing* **VI**, 132–7.

DAWSON, M., SCHELL, A. and FILION, D. (1990). The electrodermal system. In: CACIOPPO, J. T. and TASSINARY, G. (eds), *Principles of Psychophysiology*, pp. 295–324. Cambridge University Press.

DEROGATIS, L. R., LIPMAN, R. S., RICKELS, K., UHLENHUTH, E. H. and COVI, L. (1974). The Hopkins Symptom Checklist (HSCL). In: PICHOT, P. (ed.), *Psychological Measurements in Psychopharmacology*. *Mod. Probl. Pharmacopsychiat*, Vol. 7, pp. 79–110. Karger, Basel.

DILLON, K. M., MINCHOFF, B. and BAKER, K. H. (1985). Positive emotional states and enhancement of the immune system. *International Journal of Psychiatry in Medicine*, **15**, 13–17.

DUGAN, D. O. (1989). Laughter and tears: best medicine for stress. *Nursing Forum* **XXIV**, 18–26.

ERDMAN, L. (1991). Laughter therapy for patients with cancer. *Oncology Nursing Forum* **18**, 1359–63.

FISHER, M. (1988). Hospice nursing. *Nursing* 3, 8–10.

FOLKMAN, S. (1984). Personal control and stress and coping processes. *Journal of Personality and Social Psychology*, 46, 839–52.

FOLKMAN, S. and LAZARUS, R. S. (1980). An analysis of coping in a middle aged community sample. *Journal of Health and Social Behaviour* 21, 219–39.

FOLKMAN, S. and LAZARUS, R. S. (1985). If it changes, it must be a process: study of emotion and coping during three stages of a college examination. *Journal of Personality and Social Psychology* 48, 150–70.

FRY, W. F. (1986). Humor, physiology and the aging process. In: NAHEMOW, L., McCLUSKEY-FAWCETT, K. A. and McGHEE, P. E. (eds), *Humor and Aging*, pp. 81–98. Academic Press.

FRY, W. F. (1989). Tears. BBC 1. QED programme, 8 March 1989, 21.30–22.00 hours.

FRY, W. F. and SAVIN, W. M. (1988). Mirthful laughter and blood pressure. *International Journal of Humor Research* 1, 49–62.

FRY, W. F. and STOFT, P. E. (1971). Mirth and oxygen saturation levels of peripheral blood. *Psychotherapy and Psychosomatics* 19, 76–84

Gilligan, B. (1993). A positive coping strategy. Humor in the oncology setting. *Professional Nurse* 8, 232–3.

GRAHAM, L. L. and CATES, J. A. (1989). Responding to the needs of the terminally ill through laughter and play. *American Journal of Hospice Care* 6, 29–30.

Greenberg, J. S. (1983). *Comprehensive Stress Management*. Wm. C. Brown.

HEIDT, P. (1981). Effect of therapeutic touch on anxiety level of hospitalised patients. *Nursing Research* 30, 32–7.

HOLDEN, R. (1993). *Laughter: The Best Medicine*. Thorsons.

HULL, M. H. (1991). Hospice nurses. Caring support for care giving families. *Cancer Nursing* 14, 63–70.

JACOBSON, E. (1938). *Progressive Relaxation*. University of Chicago Press, Chicago.

JENSEN, S. and GIVEN, B. A. (1991). Fatigue affecting family care givers of cancer patients. *Cancer Nursing* 14, 181–9.

KARASEK, R. A. (1979). Job demands, job decision latitude and mental strain: implications for job redesign. *Administrative Science Quarterly* 24, 285–311.

KASTENBAUM, R. (1967). Multiple perspectives on a geriatric death valley. *Community Mental Health Journal* 3, 21–9.

KNIGHT, M. and FIELD, D. (1981). A silent conspiracy: coping with dying cancer patients on an acute surgical ward. *Journal of Advanced Nursing* 6, 221–9.

KREIGER, D. (1986). *The Therapeutic Touch. How to Use Your Hands to Help or to Heal*. Prentice-Hall

LAZARUS, R. S. and LAUNIER, R. (1977). Stress related transactions between person and environment. In: PERVIN, L. A. and LEWIS, M. (eds), *Perspectives in International Psychology*, pp. 287–327. Plenum Press.

LE MAY, A. (1986). The human connection. *Nursing Times* 82, 28–30.

LUCK, N. A. (1989). Transcending stress. *Nursing Times* 85, 40–1.

MALLET, J. (1993). Use of humour and laughter in patient care. *British Journal of Nursing* 2, 172–5.

MANLEY, K. (1988). The needs and support of relatives. *Nursing* 32, 19–22.

MARIEB, E. (1989). *Human Anatomy and Physiology*. Benjamin Cummings.

MARTIN, R. A and DOBBIN, J. P. (1988). Sense of humor, hassles and immunoglobulin A. *International Journal of Psychiatry in Medicine* 18, 93–105.

MARTIN, R. A. and LEFCOURT, H. M. (1983). Sense of humour as a moderator of the relation between stressors and moods. *Journal of Personality and Social Psychology* 45, 1313–24.

McCORKLE, R (1974). Effects of touch on seriously ill patients. *Nursing Research* 23, 125–32.

OSKINS, S. L. (1979). Identification of situational stressors and coping methods by intensive care nurses. *Heart and Lung* 8, 953–60.

PENSON, J. M. (1979). Helping the bereaved. *Nursing Times* 5 April, 593–5.

PENSON, J. M. (1984). Helping relatives cope with cancer. *Nursing Times* 11 April, 24–6.

PICKARD-HOLLEY, S. (1991). Fatigue in cancer patients. *Cancer Nursing* 14, 13–19.

PITTS, F. N. (1969). The biochemistry of anxiety. *Scientific American* February, 69–75.

POWER, K. G. and SHARP, G. R. (1988). A comparison of sources of nursing stress and job satisfaction among mental handicap and hospice nursing staff. *Journal of Advanced Nursing* 13, 726–32.

RADZIEWICZ, R. M. and SCHNEIDER, S. M. (1992). Using diversional activity to enhance coping. *Cancer Nursing* 15, 293–8.

SELYE, H. (1974). *Stress without Distress*. Corgi.

SELYE, H. (1976). *Stress in Health and Disease*. Butterworths.

SELYE, H. (1980). The stress concept today. In: KUTASH, I. L. and SCHLESINGER, L. B. (eds), *Handbook on Stress and Anxiety*. Jossey Bass, San Francisco.

SIMON, J. (1989). Humor techniques for oncology nurses. *Oncology Nursing Forum* 16, 667–70.

SIMS, S. (1986). Slow stroke back massage for cancer patients. Occasional paper. *Nursing Times* 82, 47–50.

SIMS, S. (1988). The significance of touch in palliative care. *Palliative Medicine* 2, 58–61.

SMITH, M. (1990). Healing through touch. *Nursing Times* 86, 31–2.

SUTORIUS, D. (1992). The positive, transforming and healing force of laughter. Paper presented at the Conference of the International Stress Management Association, Paris.

WALLACE, R. K. and BENSON, H. (1972). The physiology of meditation. *Scientific American* February, 84–91.

Further reading

BOND, M. (1987). *Stress and Self-awareness: A Guide for Nurses*. Heinemann Nursing, London.

CHADDERTON, N. H. (1986). A stress adaption model in terminal care. In: KERSHAW, B. and SAVAGE, J. (eds), *Models fof Nursing*. John Wiley, Chichester.

MADDERS, J. (1981). *Stress and Relaxation*. Martin Dunitz, London.

MITCHELL, L. (1988). *Simple Relaxation. The Mitchell Method for Easing Tension*. John Murray, London.

WHICH BOOKS (1988). *Understanding Stress*. A Consumer Publication. Consumers Association.

20

Standard setting in palliative care

Hilary Salway

'I keep six honest serving-men
(They taught me all I knew);
Their names are What and Why and When
And How and Where and Who.'

Rudyard Kipling, Just So Stories (1902)

Introduction

The quality of nursing care, and the way in which the service is delivered, is attained by the standards nurses set out to achieve. We aim to give the best possible service to the patient and family during the palliative stage of the illness, and to follow this care through, after death, to the loved ones left behind.

This chapter sets out to consider the various implications of setting standards which meet the needs of the dying patient, ways of making the issue and setting the standards easier to understand, how to use them as a resource and how they can be reviewed.

We shall follow Kipling's words and consider the implications of the who, what, how, why and when of the philosophy.

What is a standard?

Standard setting is not a new concept. Florence Nightingale in *Notes on Nursing* (Nightingale, 1860) proposed the first standards of care, defining ones which enabled her to assess and evaluate the care given to military personnel. Standard setting is not peculiar only to nursing and medical care. Industry looks to its quality of production related to economic output, as a measure of success. Many supermarkets take pride in their well-deserved reputation of high standards and the quality of their service and provisions!

A standard may be defined as 'a cluster of variables related to the expected performance levels' (Hagan, 1976). The dictionary definition is more didactic and defines it as 'something established as a rule of basis of comparison in measuring or judging quality, value, and a usage that is practised, generally accepted or followed' (*Collins Concise English Dictionary*). We are considering the features of quality which make something what it is and its degree of excellence. Quality is how the patient views what is done for him or her or indeed, what is not done. But how does he or she perceive it? As a notion, an ideal? What is the patient measuring quality against? How do we, as nurses measure the patient's concept of the standards of care, against our own? Nurses caring for dying people enjoy a high reputation, but this statement can only be justified if the results of care are measured against identified levels – agreed levels of performance.

These standards appropriate to nursing in the palliative care setting must be professional and compassionate. The outcome is that the measured results improve both the effectiveness and efficiency of nursing and, as such, meet the total needs of the patient.

Why is the setting of nursing and health-care standards in palliative care necessary?

Scholfield (1990) has determined that what we must do is to 'raise care to the highest level'. However, that is only one of the elements involved. Dr Ronald Fisher, in his introduction to this book says, 'The term "palliative care" brings with it a hint of hope', so setting standards which are achievable can actually change the negative aspects of problems associated with such a momentous time in people's lives, towards a more positive, yet realistic approach. Setting standards encourages the nurse to meet goals, which can make this difficult time easier. There are no experts in dying, and an individual only dies once, therefore we only have one chance to get the process right for the patient. If we fail, that is what the family will remember for the rest of their lives (Elliott, 1994). Neither can we, as providers of the service, presume that it meets the needs of the patients or the profession.

However, let us consider why working towards standards is necessary, from a more systematic viewpoint. The Royal College of Nursing (RCN) Standards of Care Project – Quality Patient Care (Kitson, 1990) states that there are four reasons:

- personal;
- political;
- social; and
- professional.

Personal reasons

In the RCN paper Kitson says that 'nurses, and indeed other professionals, should bother to set standards' (Kitson, 1990). So why? You are the one having to undertake what can seem to be a mammoth, time-consuming task, which takes you away from your patient. Hardly a good move towards delivering high standards of care! But nobody wants to do a bad job and in palliative care, the job satisfaction comes from knowing that you have helped and cared for the patient and his or her family to the best possible standard. This in turn helps you to carry on with a demanding, emotional and draining role. Nurses and other professionals, working in different specialities have the joy of seeing patients get well again and go back into their community life in much better health. Palliative care workers have to ensure that the quality of life in the time remaining to the patient is as fulfilling as possible. Working towards a standard helps you to assess your own competences and can give you confidence in your work, because it helps you to measure your knowledge against a pre-determined level. This enables you to feel good about what you are doing. It also gives recognition to staff who work well, do a good job and are committed towards notable standards. As a qualified person you also have to accept accountability for what you do and how you conduct yourself, working within this framework gives you the necessary, supportive feedback.

Political reasons

To initiate, implement and measure quality control programmes, ensuring that the whole process works, the concept must be owned by those involved in the particular clinical area, those having contact with the patient.

If, as professionals, we do not address this issue, then it is probable that the programme will be enforced by personnel who do not understand the problems and nuances of palliative care. The introduction of quality assurance programmes has been determined by government and is rightly seen to be advantageous by senior management, so that most authorities have appointed facilitators for quality control for some time. It could be disadvantageous for nurses not to be involved with the policy making, having repercussions when determining staff levels. An example of this is the staff-to-patient ratio. The standard statement may determine that no patient dies alone. However a busy and demanding schedule, with low staffing numbers and nurses having heavy case loads may make this a difficult criterion to meet. A non-nurse manager, passing by a bed where the nurse is sitting holding an unconscious patient's hand could question the justification for it. A set standard will help to clarify the situation.

It can also be that, if standards cannot be met because of low staffing levels, the unit manager will be able to use the predetermined criterion as a tool to argue effectively, justifying necessary budgeting for manpower, to ensure correct staffing levels, and grades of staff, who have the appropriate experience for high-quality patient care.

Social reasons

The government of today has determined The Patient's Charter (Department of Health, 1991) which states on its front cover that it is 'raising the standard'. It outlines seven existing rights for patients with the delivery of care, one of which states that we always put the patient and his or her needs first, in a satisfying manner. As professionals we are governed by the law and have to work within these realms, once again being accountable for what we do. We also live in a society which is encouraged to challenge care, indicated by the increased number of legal actions. Working towards set standards quantifies what we attempt to achieve. The ethics of palliative care are complex and can be disturbing to those people delivering care. A standard which defines the management of pain control, for example, can remove any doubts over practised philosophy of euthanasia. A core standard statement may assert that all patients will have their symptoms recognised and controlled to a level which is acceptable to them, and which can be achieved by the multidisciplinary team. The process stage of the statement will have in its outline that for the nurse or other health-care professional to achieve this, they must work within the guidelines of their governing body; in the case of the nurse, the United Kingdom Central Council for Nursing, Midwifery and Health Visiting (1992). The process aspect of the standard will, of course also, determine other influencing factors.

Professional reasons

The quality of what we do needs to be measured, but it is difficult to measure palliative care, particularly if we do not have standards to use as a baseline. There are many arguments for their use which can be pinpointed succinctly without tedious descriptions. Quality management, incorporating standard setting, is necessary:

- For the provision of quality information, a yardstick for excellence, to be used as a foundation on which to improve patient care.
- As evaluated standards provide a warning of undetected problems, giving an overall reflection of the palliative care unit's achievements. They encourage reflective practice.
- Because although it enables nurses and others to assess the care they deliver, it can also have the benefit of removing the negative aspects of the professional's judgement. There is a collective approach which can enable the nurse and others identify aspects of the care given, that which is good as well as that which is poor, or needs improvement.
- As it improves management and determines clearly the valid use of resources; what is required and why. This can help ensure a cost-effective team unit.
- To help facilitate the patient's autonomy, not easy in the palliative care scene, but this will be strengthened with patient evaluation incorporated in the standard structure.
- Because it helps determine the core issues involved with the care of the dying patient. This can be a strong motivating force, be innovative and help determine progress made.
- As it enables the team to focus on what the unit is trying to achieve, provided the standards are structured on shared objectives.
- Because it is a document for accountability and facilitates staff appraisal.
- As a useful educational tool. Knowledge can be measured against them, identifying the particular needs of staff development, whether it is possible to apply research in particular areas, and indeed if a research programme is applicable.
- Because, although standard setting can be a hassle, in the end, it lessens such hassle. This is because it aids communication, which fosters the ability for the team to work constructively; the overall having a positive effect on the working relationship.
- In order to enable the nurse to act as the patient's advocate, which when considered with all the other reasons mentioned above, has the fundamental importance of improving patient care.

Who is involved with standard setting?

For the project to succeed the people involved must be motivated and enthusiastic, committed and willing to share ideas and expertise. Everyone working in the palliative care field has a valuable contribution to ensure the quality of the service, so ideally the working party would have a multidisciplinary input, with the executive management accepting responsibility for support towards implementation. However, it must be considered whether a multidisciplinary approach is appropriate if the standards to be set are for clinical nursing practice, but this will be discussed when we consider how to initiate the work.

The process needs to be a consultative one, incorporating all grades of staff, involving people who are instrumental in the direct care of the patient. The learner and the unqualified, will also have something to contribute; maybe the health-care assistant who has direct patient contact and who can articulate the patient's view. It is also worth considering if the patient should be involved. But, as the RCN has determined, standard setting needs to have the support of someone who has the authority to act (Quinn, 1981).

The role of the leader, usually the chair of the working party, is of fundamental importance. He or she requires skills which will keep the group working towards cohesive aims, working within time structures and constrictions, yet enabling the ideas and thoughts of those involved to be as creative and as appropriately innovative as is possible. It necessitates co-ordinating the many complexities and aspects of all involved, yet following shared objectives. The chair also needs to have influence, to ensure that conflict is dissolved when problems arise. It is a facilitative role, which in the true sense of the word, endeavours to make the work as easy as possible.

Who should be involved in the working party? The leader of the team, maybe the primary nurse, the senior social worker, the medical director, the senior nurse? Not necessarily, providing the individuals from each team communicates well with all her associates in his/her field and that there are correct and informative channels for feedback. The representative needs to ensure that the ideas of all staff supporting the patient's views are promoted.

There must be, however, clinical staff input, because if the professional is to implement and meet the standard he/she needs to feel involved. It has the benefit that all the feelings of ownership have. The support and contribution of the manager responsible for the unit cannot be underestimated, management must be involved.

So should the motivating force be structured from top to bottom or bottom to top of the hierarchy? The answer must take into consideration the points already raised, but it is important for there to be a collective team approach and that an atmosphere of trust and co-operation is fostered. Consider, too, the many people in the health-care structure who can contribute and guide, as this will ensure that the issues are being tackled from a sound professional standpoint following the structure adopted by the employing authority. It would be foolish to ignore the valuable contribution from the quality assurance staff member, who may not have palliative care experience, but does have tremendous experience with formulating standards, and can help to structure the model of standard setting which you will finally use.

Involving and organising a quality circle

Quality circles, a Japanese philosophy, are designed to promote creativity and commitment within a group effort. The meetings are a management approach, allowing the individual to become more fully involved and facilitates solving the job-related problems in an organised way. So quality circles are described as:

- active;
- productive;
- objective;
- effective.

It may be that a quality circle meeting is arranged to explore the interest and to elect members of the working party. The facilitator of the meeting acts as a catalyst, for example, a brain-storming session, encouraging those present to identify issues around the standards of care for the service, what is good and what needs improvement. These issues are then collated into areas of specific interest. Members of the team are given responsibilities and goals which are to be achieved before a given time. A standard setting working party is then arranged. The number should not be so large that it is unwieldy, but it has to be large enough to promote the team approach. Last, but not least, the work will need the invaluable help of clerical and secretarial back-up. The standard needs to be presented in a professional mode, and notes of meetings should be available to others not actually involved.

When should we be thinking of standard setting?

The simple answer is now; but of course it is more complicated than that. The employing authority needs to be keen and willing. The staff involved need to ensure that they have had the staff development which enables them to work in an informed way. This development also acts as a strong motivator! It must also be considered what else is happening in the unit: too many unfinished projects are destructive and can lower the morale of staff more than the actual stressful aspect of palliative care. There may be staffing problems or the unit may be going through a particularly harrowing and stressful period.

Thought needs to be given on the logistics of the project, where the meetings are to be held and their timings. Setting time limits encourages people to work towards deadlines; however if too little time is given for these to be met, the work can become confused and may give the impression of an ill-thought through project. The meetings should be held on a pre-determined basis, held regularly, often enough to ensure that motivation is not lost, yet allowing sufficient time for work to be done, say every three or four weeks. They should be held at a time which does not interrupt the activities of the patient's day too much: afternoons can be a good time. Staff also needs to know how long they are going to be away from the clinical area, so it is a useful concept to work towards a time limit for the meetings, perhaps one to one and a half hours. Once these considerations have been met, it is best not to prevaricate too long – standards are a tool which ensure quality and are therefore needed.

Where – in which clinical areas does standard setting apply?

The answer is simple. Standards need to be set for all aspects of care. Whether a multidisciplinary approach is taken depends upon all of the influencing factors.

How should the model of care be determined?

There is a rationale for this work. It is that the achievement of a qualitative, realistic method for determining standards of care is what all professionals want to achieve. But this work can be used as an evaluating tool, because within the structure there are clearly defined performance indicators.

Having decided that this is going to be the next unit's project, having a good skill mix of informed people willing to give their time and energy towards making this professional step a success, a quality circle meeting is held to determine what is to be achieved. A brain-storming session will help to determine pertinent issues.

An overall philosophy which can be aimed at the differing aspects of the service must be determined. This will include inpatient care, day care, community care, bereavement support, spiritual support, support for staff working in clinical and educational areas. It must be considered where and how others involved are incorporated, e.g. management and clerical staff.

It must be understood that the standard setting exercise is a continuous process, where the needs are identified, ensuring that these are appropriate and are focused realistically. It is too time consuming to be a hypothetical exercise! The process adopts a model long since used by the nursing profession of identifying the need, planning the structure, working through a quota of it and then utilising an accepted method of evaluation. This identifies what has been achieved and what needs to be done in the future, improving and resolving any anomalies.

For the purpose of this chapter the model of the Michigan Emeritus Professor of Public Health, Avedis Donabedian is used. His name has long been equated with quality assurance. His method asks for the rationale of the particular statement to be considered (this is sometimes called the mission statement or standard statement); the structure of what is to be achieved, the process of how this is to be accomplished and the criteria which helps to determine the outcome (Donabedian, 1966).

- The standard statement – this asks for it to state, quite briefly, what the outcome and the quality of the care should be.
- The structure criteria – the available resources and those needed to ensure the standard can be met must be taken into consideration. This will entail thinking of the organisation structure, policies, rules and regulations, the staff, their experience and knowledge, communication and information channels, equipment and the environment.
- The process criteria – the pre-requisite is to assess what needs to be achieved, what should be included in the plan, whether it is possible to include and demonstrates the model of nursing used in the unit, the values and beliefs which are in practice, the method of intervention and how the whole is to be implemented. It must also include a structure for reflection and reviewing and how to evaluate the level of competences of the staff carrying out the role.
- The outcome criteria – this shows the results of the care and whether or not the desired standard has been achieved. Documentation should be in a measurable form, saying how the patient feels, how the nurse sees the patient, and the manner of care. The aim should be to accomplish this objectively, using any available indicators such as measurement tools. An example of this is outlined in Table 20.1.

However, if we try to determine all aspects of care which the patient and his or her family will require we may get into the difficult situation of setting standards for all professional behaviour. This is far too cumbersome and would indeed be almost unattainable. The Trent Hospice Audit Group have overcome this problem by setting six core standards which consider the overall palliative care service. These are determined as:

Standard 1 – collaboration with other agencies
Standard 2 – symptom control
Standard 3 – patient/carer information
Standard 4 – emotional support
Standard 5 – bereavement care and support
Standard 6 – specialist education/training for staff (Trent Hospice Audit Group, 1992).

However, the standards of care for specific areas may be the structure which can follow the work undertaken by Luthert and Robinson at The Royal Marsden Hospital. This has evolved over the last few years, to include standard setting and audits for clinical procedures and has excellent examples on how to determine quality assurance for such problems as the care of patients experiencing fatigue, fungating and ulcerating malignant lesions, care of patients experiencing constipation, etc. (Luthert and Robinson, 1993). Their book is designed to be cross-referenced with The Royal Marsden Manual of Nursing Policies and Procedures (Pritchard and Walker, 1984). So it is a feasible proposition if the quality circle considers core standards in the first instance and then works towards specific standards. It is an evolving process.

Evaluating the standards

When writing standards it is important to remember that if they are to be effective, they must be written in terms which can be measured. Much is written about audit and measurement tools. An interpretation of audit by some nurses is that subjective measurement can determine whether the standard statement has been met. Others were concerned with measuring the outcome criteria (Kitson, 1990). What is being asked is the examination, on a regular, formal basis, the care

Table 20.1 The standard statement

Symptom control: all patients will have their symptoms controlled to a level which is acceptable to them, and which can be achieved by the multidisciplinary team.

Structure criteria	Process criteria	Outcome criteria
The patient will be able to discuss his or her symptoms with an identified member of the team.	The multidisciplinary team will assess the symptoms, implementing changes with the patient's consent	The patient will confirm that his problems are controlled to an acceptable level
The multidisciplinary team will be knowledge-able to enable symptom control	The patient/relative will be informed of possible choices	Documentation will show how the multi-disciplinary team were involved
	Documentation will record change with a review date	

given against pre-determined standards. How regularly this occurs depends on the unit's resources. One idea is to evaluate all the standards in one full sweep, taking two or three days to do so. An easier option is to consider a standard every month, or two months. This is not too demanding on the staff, an on-going account of what is happening is available and feedback can be given to the team on a regular basis. It also means that any problem is recognised earlier, so that measures can be made to rectify it.

The methods utilized for this purpose can vary, namely

- checking against written statements;
- verification with patient's notes/documentation;
- examining nursing care plans.

There are also various types of audits – clinical and nursing, medical, prospective audits – where the standards and measures are agreed at the start, and retrospective audits, looking back at the care of the patient, using either clinical notes and/or extracting information by asking the families (Higginson, 1993). These can be measured against defined questionnaires, checklists, by face-to-face interviewing or using specific audit checking documentation. The documentation is related to the standard using words which state the behaviour, e.g. the patient *will* say if the pain is controlled or relieved. The relatives *have confirmed* that the procedure was explained. Table 20.2 is an example.

During the evaluation the statement and structure must be considered to ensure that necessary resources have been available and that staff are working within the unit's guidelines and policies, rules and regulations. Auditing the process means examining if what is stated has happened, whilst auditing the outcome ensures that what has happened is both necessary and effective.

The whole process needs to be kept as simple as possible causing the least disruption to the patient, the staff and the unit. The aim is to make good practice common practice, constantly reviewing and improving care, with the overall aim of seeing if change is necessary. Obviously it would not be appropriate for all members of the working party to undertake the evaluation. Two people are ample, a senior member of the team and someone involved in clinical care. It is important to include the patient and relatives. Griffiths (1984) described the consumer as a legitimate judge of quality. The work can also be undertaken by an outside agency or can be kept internal to those who set the standard.

An ethical, professional, confidential approach is essential. Feedback must be given as soon as possible, followed by written confirmation. Staff tend to find the process stressful, so the results must be discussed with all staff, with an identified person taking responsibility to ensure that any necessary action is taken. A follow-up review at a determined date is arranged.

There is so much written which raises questions on the feasibility of standard setting. The answer is to ensure that the concept is accepted by all staff, and that language avoids ambiguity, but as Higginson states, you say what you mean and you mean what you say (Higginson, 1993). The results will then give excellent feedback on the standard of the service, which goes towards ensuring quality assurance and patient satisfaction.

Table 20.2 Core standard evaluation

Symptom control					
Outcome audit	Yes	No	Process audit	Yes	No
1. The patient will confirm that the symptoms have been controlled to his or her satisfaction	☐	☐	1. Did the multi-disciplinary team assess symptoms and implement necessary change	☐	☐
2. There is evidence that a multiteam approach, involving the patient/carer	☐	☐	2. Was the patient's/carer's agreement sought and, where appropriate, were other agencies involved	☐	☐
			3. There is documented evidence of the patient's/carer's involvement	☐	☐
			4. There is written evidence that the patient's symptoms were reviewed and necessary changes made	☐	☐

Comments ....
....
....
....

Recommendation ....
....
....
....

Signature/s ....
....
....

Review date ....

Acknowledgements

Ms Jenny Penson, for her support and encouragement. Dr Ronnie Fisher for his mentorship. Dr Malcolm Bottomley, my husband, for his patience, for his critique of my work and his enthusiasm.

References

DONABEDIAN, A. (1966). Evaluation in the quality of medical care. *Milbank Memorial Fund Quarterly* **XLIV**, No. 3, Part 2, 166–203.

ELLIOTT, H. (1994). *Palliative Care Manual*. Southmead Health Services, Bristol.

GRIFFITHS, R. (1984). National Health Service Management Inquiry Report. HMSO London.

HAGAN, E. (1976). Conceptual issues in appraising quality of nursing care. Unpublished paper, Columbia University Teacher's College, New York City.

HIGGINSON, I. (1993). *Clinical Audit in Palliative Care*. Radcliffe Medical Press.

KITSON, A. (1990). Royal College of Nursing Standards of Care Project. Quality Patient Care. The Dynamic Standard Setting System (DySSSy). The Royal College of Nursing.

LUTHERT, J. and ROBINSON, L. (1993). The Royal Marsden Hospital. *Manual of Standards of Care*. Blackwells.

NIGHTINGALE, F. (1860). *Notes on Nursing: What It Is, And What It Is Not*, 2nd edn. Harrison.

PRITCHARD, A. and WALKER, V.-A. (1984). *Manual of Clinical Nursing Policies and Procedures*. Harper & Row.

QUINN, S. (1981). Towards Standards. A Discussion Document. The Royal College of Nursing.

SCHOFIELD, J. (1990). Practical standards. *Nursing Times* **86**, 31–3.

TRENT HOSPICE AUDIT GROUP (1992). Palliative Core Standards. A Multi-disciplinary Approach. Trent Hospice Audit Group, Derbyshire Royal Infirmary.

DEPARTMENT OF HEALTH (1991). The Patient's Charter. Raising the Standard. HMSO.

UNITED KINGDOM CENTRAL COUNCIL FOR NURSING, MIDWIFERY AND HEALTH VISITING (1992). *Code of Professional Conduct*. UKCC, London.

Further reading

HIGGINSON, I. (1993). *Clinical Audit in Palliative Care*. Radcliffe Medical Press.

KITSON, A. (1990). Royal College of Nursing Standards of Care Project. Quality Patient Care. The Dynamic Standard Setting System (DySSSy). The Royal College of Nursing.

LUTHERT, J. and ROBINSON, L. (1993). The Royal Marsden Hospital. *Manual of Standards of Care*. Blackwells.

TRENT HOSPICE AUDIT GROUP (1992). Palliative Core Standards. A Multi-disciplinary Approach. Trent Hospice Audit Group. The Derbyshire Royal Infirmary.

THE ROYAL COLLEGE OF NURSING PALLIATIVE NURSING GROUP AND HOSPICE NURSE MANAGERS FORUM (1993). Standards of Care for Palliative Nursing. The Royal College of Nursing.

21

Reflections

Olga M. Craig

> 'In the case of a friendless foreigner dying in a Public Hospital who was brought here, the most dreadful kind of death was at least at intervals freed from pain and even a smile from time to time rewarded those who were around her – to whom, when assured of their sympathy, she was able to express her thoughts and feelings.'
>
> *Reports to the governors of her nursing home (1853–1854), Florence Nightingale*

When I look back through many years of being privileged to share closely with people life's problems, some incidents stay in my memory, and later I can see that they were really pointers in illuminating something profound, even if at the time I did not fully realise the significance.

I believe the practice of social work to be a creative art: social workers have no drugs, no syringe, nothing to offer but themselves, their own self-awareness and experience. In their training they learn to look at themselves, their thoughts and feelings, their potential. They try to understand why they react in certain ways, why they may react to situations with anger, hostility, fear, withdrawal, aggression and, in looking at this human motivation, they try better to understand how patients and their relatives feel, to help them to face themselves and, in sharing, transmute their feelings. The patients and their relatives are facing the impact of cancer, possibly death, and the fear of this; and the fear of something is often more destructive than the thing itself. In expressing their fears the space between the patient, relatives and the carer, be they a social worker or a nurse, can be filled with something more positive and bearable, and many of the anxieties dissolve.

I remember the words of a philosopher: 'What you are speaks so loudly, I cannot hear what you say to the contrary.'

When you approach this type of caring you bring not only your professional self, but the person that you really are, the things you have achieved, your failures, your ideals, your total personality, and it is all this and more that you share with your patients, their families and your colleagues. I see patients as living, not dying, and my work is concerned with the living – not the length of time, but the quality of life in the period that they are still in this world. If we share with them closely, honestly, and compassionately, that time can sometimes be the most meaningful of their lives.

Some years ago I read, in a social work journal, a review of some of the works of Martin Buber, the Jewish philosopher. I do not know which were the words of Buber and which were those of the reviewer, but the following made sense to me.

'For this thinker the quality of the relationship between people is what brings about the healing process. For Buber, the therapist must be ready to be surprised by his patient and to be guided by what the patient brings him. The way to achieve this is by "obedient listening". It is much easier to impose oneself on the patient than it is to use the whole force of one's soul to leave the patient to himself and not to touch him. The real master responds to uniqueness. The kind of healing Buber has in mind takes place through the meeting of one person with another rather than through insight and analysis. A situation is transformed when something in the other person comes alive in me.'

What we are trying to do with our patients and families is not new and not just related to cancer. It is to do with the sharing with anyone who is facing a deep, profound life experience because, in my view, illness is an experience, just as are birth, marriage, loss and love. It is what you make of the experience, how you learn about yourself and life, and how you can grow through it that is important, not the experience itself.

I completed my midwifery training, because that was the thing to do, and during that training I had some time working in the community. As I walked out of the gate of the hospital I realised that, for the first time, I was free to work as an individual and not as an adjunct to others. That was the final experience which led me to move into the social work field. For many years I worked in child care, with families, marriage problems, delinquency, children, and all the common traumas of life. However, when it all became too bureaucratic with too many people telling me what to do, I moved into medical social work where this intense need to work as an individual and in a free way was still possible. However, soon this field was taken over by the same bureaucratic set-up. At that time, 'out of the blue', the first Macmillan unit was being built nearby. I was fortunate in being appointed as the only social worker and, as it was a pioneering venture, I felt I would be free to work creatively, face to face, with the patients. With much perseverance and 'battling' I succeeded.

As the unit, at that time, was the first under the National Health Service, it was seen to be different and controversial. We were prepared to face problems which, before, were often pushed under the carpet, or perhaps more correctly, behind the screens on many a ward round I have seen the retinue pass the rejected patient with 'terminal cancer' with hardly a word except to ask if I could hurry up the discharge. Although things are now different prejudice is still found, often born of fear, within many professional workers – they too need help.

From my diary of experiences I have recalled a few examples which you may meet from time to time.

Most of us end up with titles and qualifications, but these are just labels and we should perhaps be wary of 'labels'. There is a danger that we and our patients will turn into our 'labels'. He has cancer, he is terminal, hasn't long to live, I give him six months, he is difficult, uncooperative, daft as a brush, gone to the fairies, he has cerebral secondaries. I have seen many patients with the last label become quite rational and normal when someone spent time penetrating the barrier of fear. I remember a patient who had 'an ulcer that was leaking'. She was very depressed and was still running a temperature. I was asked to see her and I listened to her life story. She had always been the strength of the home and was now fearful for the future. She wept, and weeping for the right reason can be a marvellous release. 'You see', she said, 'the nurses and doctors keep telling me about my ulcer, that it is drying-up, getting smaller and so on. Sometimes I feel I am becoming a leaking abscess'. When we have to cope with the physical body it is very important that we do not forget the human being within.

I trained as a nurse just before the advent of antibiotics. Patients were often in hospital for months, not days. We had time to get to know them, and because we couldn't just treat them with drugs, which remove the symptoms but not always the cause, we had to use our imagination and traditional bedside nursing to treat and 'comfort' our patients. When I see someone in hospital who is ill, I do not see a patient, but a unique human being with a unique life history of which the illness is only a part.

As a second-year nurse I came on duty one night to be told by the Sister that one of my patients, an elderly woman from the east end of London who had advanced cancer, was dying and unlikely to survive the night. The relatives were round the bed and the curtains were drawn. The night wore on and I looked frequently at my patient, with drips in her nose, and in her arms and hardly breathing. Some relatives were crying. At one point I sent them away to have a cup of tea and a rest, and tidied up and washed the old lady's face. About a half an hour later, as I passed the bed, I looked in astonishment as somehow she had hooked her spectacles over the tubes and her eyes were open. I leaned over, and in a broad Cockney accent, she said clearly, 'I want a cup of tea, nurse!' Many weeks later she walked out of the ward. Of course it caused quite a commotion, when someone who should have died recovered, both for the staff and the relatives.

I remember another night with this same patient, as she was getting better, talking to her about her remarkable recovery. I did not understand then what I do now, but she looked me straight in the eye and said, 'I saw them all standing round my bed, wishing me away and dividing up my money and I thought, not yet you don't!' Now, one is aware that many factors apart from our care, are working to affect our patients. Perhaps not always for the best of reasons, but a shift in outlook can often change the course of an illness.

I can recall another significant happening. I was a staff nurse on a medical ward, at that time, an experiment was being tried of placing a few psychiatric patients in the ward. I was given the main charge of these patients. The psychiatrist was very good and explained everything fully to me. It was a new experience, because all the social aspects were discussed, and then I began to feel I wanted to work with people before they were admitted, and I'm sure this is what ultimately led me to social work. One of the patients was a girl of limited intelligence who had a paralysed arm. She had had all the usual tests, and X-rays which showed nothing abnormal. In my presence the psychiatrist hypnotised the girl, and while under hypnosis at his suggestion the arm became completely relaxed. However, he did now allow the arm to remain like this and when she woke, he explained that whatever trauma was causing it, must be found first or worse symptoms could follow. It was after many more sessions before, on one occasion, she became very disturbed and eventually admitted that her brother had raped her.

With each of the patients and families who come for our help, we feel like part of an extended family. It is perhaps the most profound experience of living to be facing the possibility of death, and experience of people in this dimension reminds me of when I was a midwife, and later when involved in placing babies for adoption, both emotive happenings, and in the case of adoption actually bringing the baby to the couple. I felt part of the whole family unit during the period that I was involved. It would seem the same with our patients with cancer, perhaps facing death.

Many patients and their families feel guilty and inadequate, and often react with aggression and project their uncomfortable feelings on others, including staff. As the woman who placed her feelings about rape into her arm because it was too awful to face it in reality, so people will blame others for their distress. We have to remember it is no help being sentimental in this work, empathy not sympathy is needed. A young woman about whom I shall say more later, said to me one day 'Don't pity me, it is degrading, when I cry with pain you all go soft on me, it's no help'. I also remember her on another occasion. When I came on duty the staff said she had had a bad night in pain and very angry. I passed her bed, and seeing her expression I almost went past without stopping! However, I sat beside her and she said, 'What can you know about my pain, and you are only here because it is your job'. 'No', I replied 'I can never know your pain, it is yours alone, but I can sit beside you while you swear at me if it will help'. We sat together and talked, and after a time the pain eased. You see, pain of the body is often pain of the heart.

Relatives do not always feel loving towards themselves or the patient. For example, a daughter who had resentfully looked after her demanding elderly mother and sometimes 'wished her dead'. Now the mother is dying and the daughter is filled with guilt. Being able to voice these feelings before the death is the beginning of help towards the bereavement period.

The woman who refused to have her husband around when she was dying, 'He will only mess it up, as he has messed everything else up in my life'. When I saw the husband he wept, and admitted he was impotent and had never been able to satisfy his wife who despised him.

It is of value to a person to be able to voice these thoughts with someone who can accept but not necessarily condone – 'acceptance' is one of the social worker's prime casework principles. So this I found was part of my role, as someone a little outside the dependency role, to whom people can voice their true feelings. To be able to sit with someone and look into their eyes, so that they can bring out what is in their heart, not what they think you want to hear.

Remember that because of the 'image' of a doctor, nurse, minister, or social worker, some people will only say what they think we expect. I came on a ward one day in my capacity as a social worker, and the Ward Sister said, 'You will have to see Mrs Smith, she has been restless all night, and refusing to go to another hospital for tests. I've told her that a bed will be kept for her here, and the doctor has assured her the tests will not hurt, but she refuses to budge until she sees the social worker'. Needless to say, Sister was not too pleased! As soon as Mrs Smith saw me, she said, 'I'm not going in that ambulance without my knickers on, it isn't decent with them ambulance men, but I couldn't tell Sister, 'er being what she is.' She was a very good Sister, but she thought the patient was worried about her bed, the doctor thought she was afraid the tests would be painful. I am not quite sure what it makes me, but there has to be someone around to whom you can literally or metaphorically talk about your 'knickers'. Like the husband of a woman whose face was slowly disintegrating and she had a long spell in our unit. He did not like to ask if there was a room where he could make love to her; 'I thought you might think it "dirty".' Of course we found a room without a glass panel. The spinster aged 60 years who, with great distress, told me her father had sexually abused her as a child, the shame was still deep within her and she had not told anyone until she became ill.

So often, when faced with something serious and profound, people find a need to bring out the hurts, disappointments and frustrations of their life which may have been bottled up for years. The illegitimate child, the wife he never really loved, the fact that someone was homosexual. The wife and mistress both in a man's life, and he wants both to visit him. The soldier who, in the last war, was a prisoner of the Japanese, had worked on the infamous railway and seen his comrades shot when they collapsed. Luckily, he had told me all this, and when one night he fell out of bed and was a little confused, he tried to strangle a nurse, but was distressed afterwards and said to me, 'I thought I was back on the track and the Japs would kill me'. At least this knowledge saved him from being considered a psychiatric case.

In social work we have always to look at the total person – physically, mentally, spiritually, emotionally, the home, work situation, family interaction, hobbies, the marriage, the children. The patients and family sense this and the kind of questions we ask seem to make them feel we are interested in them as people not patients. This results in comments like 'I've never spoken to anyone like this before, now I don't have to pretend, I feel so at ease now I have told you this'. With the bringing out of these deep-seated things which laid hidden there often comes a release, with the release comes a lessening of tension which is sometimes followed by an easing of symptoms and consequently the ability to reduce drugs – it is like a human tranquilliser. One woman, after admitting that she had dreaded making love to her husband all her married life, took her hands and said 'This fear has sat like a hard lump here', and where she put her hands was just where the cancer had appeared. 'Now', she said, 'it is as if a cloud has been lifted'. Difficulties occur when professionals contemplate telling patients 'the truth'. What the professional carer thinks and what the patients think are often very different. A man who had worked in the police service was admitted and sat silently in the entrance of the ward for several days. Eventually he asked a Staff Nurse who had tried to talk to him to wheel him into the grounds, and then he point-blank asked, 'Have I got cancer?' The nurse had never before told this to a patient, but she did on this occasion. She felt completely shaken and, because I knew her well, she came to talk to me. She said. 'I feel I cannot continue with this work, by telling him he has cancer I feel I have given him the disease'.

The nurse felt that the actuality of knowing would hasten the disease. In fact, the next day, there was a knock at my door and in came this man saying 'Well, I've at last been told I've got cancer, I knew something was up, because they are so damned kind here. Now we can get to grips with things, and I can do what has to be done'. I made sure that the nurse followed through with me what transpired next. The patient was an intelligent man, he wanted to see his employer, his minister and, most of all, he said 'Now my wife and I can discuss the future honestly'. He wanted to put his affairs in order, talk to his children, and a great deal of good positive work was done which, without the initial 'telling', might not have happened. And so the nurse saw that her act, far from being destructive, was the opening to something better.

There was an educated woman who had been a concert pianist. She had travel-led the world, and now she was admitted because there was no-one at home to look after her. I went to see her soon after admission and she said, 'Have I got cancer?' As I did not know much about her I suggested she might like to see the doctor. Three times the doctor saw her, and tried to give her an opening to talk, but she did not ask. Then one day I again saw her and she said, 'No-one will tell me I have cancer, and I know I have, because I have read my notes!' I said, 'Do you want me to tell you that you have cancer', 'Oh no dear', she replied, 'I am a single woman, I have always had to plan my own life, and I want to know whether I should get my solicitor in and make my will, or should I buy a local paper and start looking for a flat.' I suggested she should put her affairs in order, as by now she was very ill. And she did this and died soon after.

A rough, tough man who had been a docker in Glasgow was admitted. At first, staff thought he was a bit 'peculiar', but I found he spoke with a broad Scottish dialect full of swear words, and hated being fussed over by all the nurses. As I came from his country I understood him, and tried to help him adjust. Eventually I traced a long lost daughter and grandchildren in Australia, and they all wrote to him. One day when he was near the end, he said to me, 'I'm not going to get better am I?' I knew he had been told 'the truth' by a doctor in a previous hospital, so I said, 'I think you know that you have cancer, and were told that before you came here'. 'Yes', he said, 'but I'm no having a young chit of a girl telling me something as serious as that, I don't mind you telling me, as you are a good woman' – by that he meant an old woman! But there is a time for telling, and there has sometimes to be a re-telling, when the patient is ready to face the full import.

There was also the young mother who was going to die. Her husband was a kind but uneducated man, who had been brought up in children's homes. 'I haven't got a way with words', he told me. He had told the elder daughter the truth, but couldn't tell his young son, as he had always been the mother's favourite. At first he asked me to tell him, but I helped him to see that this would solve nothing. When at last he plucked up courage and told him, he was shattered when the lad said, 'Oh, I've known mother was going to "pop off" for ages, can I go and play now'. One can rarely hide the truth from children, they have their own radar system.

Communication is indeed an art. To be able to communicate not only in words but by look, touch and physical contact, is most important. When I was involved with foster children, often rejected and separated from their families, tiny children right up to teenage, they were so distressed, lonely and afraid they could not hear what you said. You had to hold them tight, so that they felt your thoughts and love. To be able to sit quietly relaxed, without fear, with a patient or relative, to stroke their forehead, hold their hands, and say nothing – they so often need this tangible expression of acceptance and understanding when they face this lonely journey. I remember, on a ward round, an elderly woman who had just lost her husband before being admitted, and she was particularly vulnerable. When the doctor put out his hand, her eyes lit up, and she put out her hands to his. It was pushed aside with 'Let us see her abdomen, sister' and I can still see that arm slowly fall and the head droop.

Through all that nurses and social workers try to do there runs this special alchemy called *love*, which nurses in particular, with their frequent intimate contact with people can evoke, sometimes without being aware of it. If it cannot always turn a person from sickness to health, then certainly it can turn them from distress to peace.

A man who had lost weight was admitted to a medical ward. He had all the tests including an interview with a psychiatrist, but with no results. As a last resort he was referred to me. After we had got to know one another he told me his only daughter had married a man he did not approve of, 7 years ago. He told her he did not want to see her again, and in fact he never did because she died of cancer a year later. His guilt and distress were so deep he had not been able to share the event with his wife. The houseman on the ward was particularly sensitive and I suggested he follow up my talk, and the man again poured out his feelings. It was very therapeutic and eventually he was due to be discharged. I arranged for him to talk about his diet with the dietician and because he liked porridge, I suggested he sprinkle some wheatgerm on it. Good for the nerves I said. Three months later I was walking through the out-patients department when this same man rushed up with bright eyes, and colour in his cheeks. 'Miss Craig, that wheatgerm is marvellous, from the first mouthful I felt better!' Well, you can see, it was only a vehicle into which he projected what he felt was the love and understanding experienced in the hospital. But it worked.

A sad little spinster of uncertain years came in, she had no visitors and no family. She ultimately told me she had always 'missed' everything in life. She lost her job, she never had a boy-friend, and even her grandmother called her 'Miss one too many' when she was young. 'I never felt I belonged'. I shared this with all the staff, who in their own special way gave her lot of TLC (tender loving care). After some months when the end was near, I brought some flowers to her which had been given to me. She looked up at me and said, 'All my life I have been looking for somewhere and someone who would love me for myself. Now that I have found it with you all, it does not matter any more whether I die'. She smiled, and I never saw her again.

Staff often have to spend a great deal of time dealing with unpleasant and distressing physical symptoms. One can get caught up and submerged in this. I have always shared and encouraged staff to see the very positive and happy things that may be occurring within the family while the body is being eaten away. The woman whose face was ultimately just a cavity, but she remained mentally intact to the end. She told me that she and her husband had become closer since the illness, than in all married life, and were able to share their real feelings. The husband who had never been very capable found he could cope with the children and home, and his self-confidence improved.

When someone becomes seriously ill, close members of the family are affected in different ways, but all feel that they have a right to participate in the experience. A young woman who is dying, has a husband, parents, in-laws, children, brothers or sisters, and all have a part to play. The parents may blame the son-in-law for the illness, there may be squabbling as to who is going to look after the children. A young father may feel inadequate and be glad of help while his wife is ill, but later may want to care for the children himself, and be afraid he will offend the parents or in-laws if he insists. A young man was dying and his mother refused to come and visit him because she did not want to watch him die, and he felt she had rejected him. Three daughters and a grand-daughter arguing and rowing over the unconscious mother, and all the years of past jealousy and friction spilling out – perhaps it was no wonder the mother remained unconscious, sometimes death may be a blessed escape.

However, all these various people need to air their mixed feelings and often, with help, resolve many of the destructive consequences. This, again, is the start of bereavement process.

A pending death can precipitate past memories and hurts. I remember a daughter whose father was dying – she poured out a flood of resentment against him. 'He always made use of me, and was always criticising me, and yet my brother was his favourite and could do no wrong'. But now the brother couldn't find time to come and see his father. The bitterness poured out and although she was 40 years of age, she wept and even spoke like a hurt young child again.

There are difficulties when a family is prepared for someone to die and the patient improves. If a person is 'set' for bereavement it can be traumatic to have to switch their feelings again.

What of the children themselves? Special thought is required to help parents prepare their children for loss: the right word and moment is needed, and this depends on the ages of the children. Some children react to difficulties by becoming aggressive, or ignoring them, some become silent and withdrawn and take their tears to their pillow. If the truth is not spoken and shared with them they can build up a fantasy picture and fears which may be worse than is actually the case. Parents absorbed in their own grief may have little time or emotion left for the children and an aunt, grandparent or good friend can share the burden.

A young father who had a great deal of pain and discomfort sometimes shouted at his children when they were being noisy at home. One day he was sitting in his bedroom and heard one of his sons say, 'I wish daddy would die soon, I don't like him any more'. A single mother took a great deal of trouble to make sure that her daughter would have legal guardians after her death, and be protected from any argument as to who would look after her. These are just a few of the dilemmas which can occur.

Now, one or two of the more practical aspects of our patients care.

When someone becomes ill or they are admitted to hospital, they leave behind many worries and responsibilities. With patients who may die, it is especially important that they are helped to remain as involved as possible in their lives. Relatives or staff who try to shield patients from dealing with their affairs can make the patient feel that they have already been pushed aside. The patient is often more concerned that they will lose their mental faculties than about the physical symptoms. The professional career must be there to offer help, but self determination, another case work principle, is most important for both patient and relatives.

Help may be needed to arrange care for dependants left at home. Children may need the support of relatives, friends, schools or social services. Financial matters loom large. Assistance may be required in contacting a patient's employer regarding benefits, early retirement, pension schemes, etc., and finding sources of grants which might be appropriate. As I had a good knowledge of community resources, staff used me as a reservoir of information as to where to go and who to contact for help with a particular problem. Links with all people involved with a family should be maintained so that there is no overlapping and maximum efficient help and support can be offered.

Patients may wish to make or remake their will, or wish to cut somebody out of their will, and they do not always want the relatives involved. Hence there is a need for sensitive solicitors. One 'gentleman of the road' had nothing to leave but a wristwatch, but felt if he was going to die he should make a will. A very special solicitor spent an hour with him doing all that was necessary. Now, that is an example of what this word 'dignity' is all about.

Many people want to plan their own funeral. A patient who had had little peace in her life asked for the rose called 'Peace' to be planted in the garden. Many relatives have never been involved with a funeral and want to discuss all the details before the patient dies – the cost, how to pay, insurance, and whether burial or cremation. Some patients come from abroad, different religions, and special arrangements may be needed. Tactful talking about all these matters can relieve a great deal of anxiety when the patient actually dies.

Patients whose health improves may need alternative accommodation, some may need help to move to other parts of the country to be near relatives, or even to another country. Then there is the question of tracing relatives often out of the picture for years. This may also be a time for reconciliation. I remember a man who was admitted from a hostel for the homeless. I was told he had no next of kin, only a mate in the hostel. I saw the patient, and because I so often get an intuitive feeling about someone, I asked about himself. Eventually he admitted that he had a sister somewhere, but as he had been a 'black sheep' and had done nothing for her, he did not feel it was fair to bother her. After some persuasion, he agreed that I could try and trace her. This I did with the help of the Salvation Army. I found not only the sister, but three brothers, an ex-wife, a daughter, and a grand-daughter he had never seen! They all came to see him, and the loose threads were gathered together, even if they did not all get on with one another!

We are not always successful – a young man longed to meet his real father before he died. Although we traced the father he would not come because he felt it would be too upsetting.

I will conclude with the story of a remarkable, courageous and special woman in her early 20s, who came under our care. She had been the rounds of several hospitals, had had many forms of treatment, and, eventually, had been sent home to the care of her parents because 'nothing' more could be done. She had lived apart from her family for some years, and it was not easy for either side to deal with the situation. She was not expected to live long, but in fact she lived 2 years. During that time she found her creative centre, perhaps because she could no longer avoid facing herself by being continually on the move. She taught us all a great deal.

When she was first admitted she was angry and resentful, and could see no point in living if it meant being in a wheel chair. She had many of the usual problems of a normal young woman, including a boy-friend who had let her down, and all these were as important to her as the illness. It was a long hard battle, and that is a story in itself. Suffice it to say that when she began to become close to her family and ourselves, she decided to write about her experiences, in order to help others. We sent her on a writing course, where the staff were marvellous and put a bed in the classroom. Her article was accepted by a magazine and she received her fee!

About this time, when she started to 'give of herself' to others (and when this happens it is often the beginning of true healing, not physical but healing of the soul), she pushed the following poem into my hands. When later I asked if I could use it for teaching she looked at me very directly – she was a very direct woman – and said, 'Yes, by all means use it, actually you ought to, you lot are just talking about it. I'm in it.'

Although it is addressed to me, it is written to all of us who try to help by taking a step into this other dimension into which many of our patients eventually move.

To Miss Craig – who always cared

A patient's feelings about her social worker

On my back, lying flat,
Looking up and staring at the ceiling.
You, your white coat, painted smile,
Thought you'd just drop by a while.
Do you know what I am feeling?

I'm a number in your book,
Come on have a damn good look,
Another problem to be solved
Better not get too involved.
Put me neatly in the filing.
Sorry I don't feel like smiling.

Do you want to know my name
No – you lot, you're all the same
Helping me to know my rights?
Oh, my head, these bloody lights.
Disabled Persons pension schemes?
Bet it isn't all it seems.
You might think that I am thick,
To hell with it, you make me sick

Oh Hi! again, thought I'd seen
The last of you when you had been.
Always want it all my way,
But glad you came again to-day,
And you gave me food
for thought

Sorry I was rude.
I ought
to hold my tongue
I know you're only here to try
To help me out by and by,
To get back among Society.
Won't you stay and have some tea?

Want to have a heart to heart
God, I don't know where to start
Can't express how I feel,
All this pain, it can't be real.
The doctor says he'll do what's best
Take the pills and lots of rest.
Most of all I need some hope,
Please be the one to help me cope.

Now I'm home and so much better
Thought I'd write this little letter,
Just to wish you all the best,
Thanks a lot and all the rest
You know, you helped me very much
I'd like to try to keep in touch,
You helped me win this long hard fight,
And sometimes in the dead of night,
I lay back and think a while
Those things I said, that 'painted smile'
Knowing now that from the start,
It really did come from the heart
Thanks again, and though I've cried
Please file me under 'satisfied'.

© Olga M. Craig

Useful addresses

There are many groups which offer help to people affected by cancer either as a patient, or the family and friends of a patient. The following national groups will provide information and advice, as well as support and practical help. All the groups listed try to work alongside the health service professionals, and offer help other than medical advice and treatment.

The authors are grateful to the Cancer Relief Macmillan Fund for permission to reproduce this information which is included in their leaflet, *Help is There*. Also to Hospice Information Service, St Christopher's Hospice.

AIDS

ACET (AIDS Care, Education and Training)
Medical Director: Dr P. Dixon
Education Director: Mrs J. Clemence
P.O. Box 3693
London SW15 2BQ
Tel: 0181-780 0400 Fax: 0181-780 0450.
A national and international AIDS charity providing home care support throughout the UK and Ireland. Overseas offices are located in: Romania, Uganda, New Zealand and Thailand. Also offers education and training for schools.

National AIDS Helpline
P.O. Box LB400
London WC2B 6JG
Tel: 0800 567123 (24-h helpline)
Tel: 0800 555777 literature line (also for health professionals).
Provides a free and confidential telephone advisory service for people who are worried about HIV or AIDS. Information covers all aspects of HIV and AIDS ranging from where to get tested to drug trials and hospital and hospice information.

The Terrence Higgins Trust
52–54 Gray's Inn Road
London WC1X 8JU
Tel: 0171-831 0330 (administration) Fax: 0171-242 0121
Tel: 0171-242 1010 (helpline)
Tel: 0171-405 2381 (legal line).
Provides information, advice and help to all those concerned about AIDS and HIV infection. Practical help includes 'buddies' for people with AIDS; welfare and legal advice; counselling; support groups.

Lesbian & Gay Bereavement Project
Vaughan M. Williams Centre
Colindale Hospital
London NW9 5GH

Tel: 0181-455 8894 (helpline)
Tel: 0181-200 0511 (administration) (15.00–18.00 weekdays).
Telephone counselling for lesbians and gay men bereaved by the loss of a same-sex partner, or otherwise affected by bereavement; a member is on duty from 19.00 to midnight. Publishes will form, and can often find suitable clergy or secular officiants for funerals. Also offers speakers and discussion leaders for any group concerned with death or dying.

Cancer

BACUP
3 Bath Place
Rivington St
London EC2A 3JR
Tel: 0171-608 1661
0800 181199 outside London (information linkline).
Helps patients, their families and friends, cope with cancer. Trained cancer nurses provide information, emotional support and practical advice by telephone or letter. A range of free publications and a newspaper are available. One-to-one counselling service in greater London.

Breast Care and Mastectomy Association of Great Britain (BCMA)
26a Harrison Street
Kings Cross
London WC1H 8JG
Tel: 0171-837 0908.
A free service of practical advice, information and support to women concerned about breast cancer. Volunteers who have had breast cancer themselves assist the staff in providing emotional support, nation-wide. The BCMA complements medical and nursing care.

British Association for Counselling
1 Regent Place, Rugby
Warks CV21 2PJ
Tel: 01788 78328.
BAC members are individuals and organisations concerned with counselling in a variety of settings. The information office publishes directories listing counselling services and will refer enquirers to an experienced local counsellor, free of charge. Please send SAE with enquiries.

British Colostomy Association
38-39 Eccleston Square
London SW1V 1PB
Tel: 0171-828 5175.
An information and advisory service, giving comfort, reassurance and encourage-ment to patients to return to their previous active lifestyle. Emotional support is given on a personal and confidential basis by helpers who have long experience in living with a colostomy. Free leaflets and list of local contacts available. Can arrange visits in hospital or at home on request.

Useful addresses

er Aftercare and Rehabilitation Society (CARE)
,etland Road
land, Bristol BS6 7AH
Tel: 0117-942 7419.
An organisation of cancer patients formed into self-help groups who offer advice and support. Forty-seven branches and contacts throughout the country provide social outlets as well as informative activities.

Cancer Link
17 Britannia Street
London WC1X 9JN
Tel: 0171-833 2451.
Provides emotional support and information in response to telephone and letter enquiries on all aspects of cancer, from people with cancer, families and friends and professionals working with them. Resource to over 300 cancer support and self-help groups throughout Britain and helps people who set up new groups. Various free publications available.

Cancer Relief Macmillan Fund
Anchor House, 15/19 Britten Street
London SW3 3TZ
Tel: 0171-351 7811.
Supports and develops services to provide skilled care for people with cancer and their families. Macmillan nurses; Macmillan units for in-patient and day care; financial help through grants. Services usually part of the NHS. Information on Macmillan services available on request. Grant applications through community nurses, hospital or local authority social workers.

Carer's National Association
29 Chilworth Mews
London W2 3RG
Tel: 0171-724 7776.
Offers information and advice, including contacts for local groups, and links carers with each other. Encourages self-help and lobbies government, both local and national on behalf of carers.

Clic UK
Clic House, 11/12 Freemantle Square,
Cotham, Bristol BS6 5TL
Tel: 0117-924 4333.
Aims to help young people under 21 years who have any form of cancer or leukaemia, and their families. Provides free 'home from home' accommodation adjacent to paediatric oncology units (nine homes at present). Supports home care nursing team in the south-west and provides welfare grants.

The Compassionate Friends
53 North Street
Bedminster, Bristol BS3 1EN
Tel: 0117-953 9639 (helpline)

Tel: 0117-966 5202 (administration).
A self-help group of parents who have lost a son or daughter of any age, including adult. Quarterly newsletter, postal library, range of leaflets. Personal and group support, rather than counselling.

CRUSE
Bereavement Care
Cruse House, 126 Sheen Road
Richmond, Surrey TW9 1UR
Tel: 0181-940 4818.
Helps any bereaved person by providing counselling individually and in groups by trained counsellors. Advice and information on practical problems, and social contact. Training courses for professionals and counselling. Publications list available.

Asian Family Counselling Service
74 The Avenue, West Ealing
London W13 8LB
Tel: 0181-997 5749.
Offers individual and marital counselling service; also bereavement counselling.

Headway – National Head Injuries Association Ltd
200 Mansfield Road
Nottingham NG1 3HX
Tel: 0115-962 2382.
Provides help, advice and support for patients who suffer the devastating effects of head injury, and their families. The aim is to help them come to terms with the enormous responsibilities of home care and rehabilitation.

Hodgkin's Disease Association
P.O. Box 275, Haddenham
Aylesbury, Bucks HP17 8JJ
Tel: 01844 291500.
Provides information and emotional support for lymphoma (Hodgkin's disease and non-Hodgkin's lymphoma) patients and their families. Literature and video available. National network of helpers with experience of the disease, with whom enquiries may be linked, usually by telephone.

Hospice Information Service
Information Officers: Avril Jackson and Ann Eve
St Christopher's Hospice
51 Lawrie Park Road
Sydenham, London SE26 6DZ
Tel: 0181-778 9252 Fax: 0181-659 8680.
A world-wide network and resource for members of the public and health professionals interested in hospices and palliative care services. Publications include: annual survey of hospice activities, directories of hospices in the UK and overseas, fact sheets on hospice planning and organisation, *Choices* a nation-wide listing of courses and conferences on palliative care and bereavement and a quarterly newsletter, the *Hospice Bulletin*. Telephoned and written enquiries welcomed.

Help the Hospices
Chief Executive: Mr Terry Taylor
34–44 Britannia Street
London WClX 9JG
Tel: 0171-278 5668 Fax: 0171-278 1021.
Will fund specific projects, equipment, education and research in the field of
terminal care. It runs or supports management policy, counselling and family
therapy workshops and clinical courses in this field. It does not support major
construction work or the routine running costs of established units.

Hysterectomy Support
c/o WHRIC
52 Featherstone Street
London EC1Y 8RT
Tel: 0171-251 6332/6580 (11.00–17.00 Mon., Wed.–Fri.)
Refers women (and family or partners) concerned about hysterectomy to former
patients in their area, who will provide encouragement advice and support
through the informal sharing of experiences and information. Membership of local
support groups (details from above). Contact by letter, over the telephone, or
through group meetings. Booklet available.

Institute for Complementary Medicine
21 Portland Place
London WlN 3AF.
Can supply names of reliable practitioners of various kinds of complementary medicine, such as homoeopathy, relaxation techniques, and osteopathy. Also has contact
with other support groups. Please send SAE for information, stating area of interest.

Institute of Family Therapy
43 New Cavendish Street
London WlM 7RG
Tel: 0171-935 1651.
The institute's Elizabeth Raven Memorial Fund offers free counselling to recently
bereaved families, or those with seriously ill family members. Works with the
whole family. While the service is free, voluntary donations to the Fund are
welcomed to help other families.

Let's Face It
Christine Piff
10 Wood End, Crowthorne,
Berks RG11 6DO
Tel: 01344 774405.
A contact point for people of any age coping with facial disfigurement. Provides a
link for people with similar experiences. Telephone and letter contact; meetings
for self-help or social contact.

Leukaemia Care Society
P.O. Box 82, Exeter
Devon EX2 5DP

Tel: 01392 218514.
Promotes the welfare of people with leukaemia and allied blood disorders. Offers family caravan holidays and friendship and support via unpaid area secretaries throughout Great Britain. Limited financial assistance. Membership is free.

The Malcolm Sargent Cancer Fund for Children
14 Abingdon Road
London W8 6AF
Tel: 0171-937 4548.
Can provide cash grants for parents of children up to the age of 21 with cancer, to help pay for clothing, equipment travel, fuel bills etc. Apply through a hospital social worker anywhere in the UK who will fill in a form on patients' behalf.

Marie Curie Cancer Care
28 Belgrave Square
London SW1X 8QG
Tel: 0171-235 3325.
Nursing care available in 11 Marie Curie homes throughout the UK. Admission details through the individual Matrons. Day and night nursing can be provided in patients' home through the community nursing service, administered by the appropriate local health authority. Welfare grant schemes; applications through the district nursing service.

National Association of Laryngectomee Clubs
4th Floor, 39 Eccleston Square
London SW1V 1PB
Tel: 0171-834 2857.
Promotes the welfare of laryngectomees within the British Isles. Encourages the formation of clubs with objective of assisting rehabilitation through speech therapy, social support and monthly meetings. Advises on speech aids and medical supplies. Offers referral service.

The Neuroblastoma Society
Neville and Janet Oldridge
Woodlands, Ordsall Park Road
Retford, Notts DN2 7PJ
Tel: 01777 709238.
Information and advice by telephone or letter for patients and their families. Provides contact where possible with others who have experienced the illness in the family, for mutual support.

Oesophageal Patients' Association
16 Whitefields Crescent
Solihull, W. Midlands B91 3NU
Tel: 0121-704 9860.
Leaflets, telephone advice and support, before and during treatment. Visits, where possible by former patients to people with oesophageal cancer.

Retinoblastoma Society
Mrs Kaye Balmforth
c/o Children's Department
Moorfields Eye Hospital
City Road, London EC1V 2PD
Tel: 0171-253 3411 ext. 2345.
Links families in the same situation and area, to give moral support and practical help. Creates an opportunity for parents to exchange information and share experiences.

Save Our Sons (SOS)
Shirley Wilcox
Tides Reach, 1 Kite Hill
Wooton Bridge
Isle of Wight PO33 4LA
Tel: 01983 882876 (evenings preferred).
Information and emotional support for men with testicular cancer. Advice given by qualified nurse, who will listen and offer help where possible. Leaflet on self-examination techniques available.

The Sue Ryder Foundation
Cavendish, Sudbury
Suffolk CO10 8AY
Tel: 01787 280252.
Six Sue Ryder Homes in England specialise in cancer care. Visiting nurses care for patients in their own homes. Advice and bereavement counselling.

Urostomy Association
(Central Office)
'Buckland', Beaumont Park
Danbury, Essex CM3 4DE
Tel: 01245 414294.
Assists patients before and after surgery with counselling on appliances, housing, work situations or marital problems. Helps them to resume as full a life as possible with confidence. Branch and house meetings held. Can also arrange hospital and home visits by former patients on request.

Other organisations

Samaritans
For telephone number look in your local phone book under 'S' or on the emergency page. Offer emotional support and befriending to the suicidal and despairing.

British Red Cross Medical Loans Service
For the address and telephone number look in your local phone book (under British Red Cross). All branches provide medical equipment on loan for short periods for patients living at home. This includes wheelchairs and commodes.

Buddhist Hospice Trust
P.O. Box 123
Ashford
Kent TN24 9TF
Tel: 0181-789 6170 to request an Ananda network volunteer.
Provides emotional support and spiritual care for those who are dying or bereaved from within a Buddhist perspective; publishes a bi-annual journal and offers seminars and study weekends. Also offers a nation-wide network of Buddhist volunteers, the Ananda network who will visit the dying and bereaved.

British Association for Counselling
1 Regent Place
Rugby
Warwickshire CV21 2PJ
Tel: 01788 578328 Fax: 01788 562189.
A membership organisation for counsellors and those involved in counselling which also provides a counselling and psychotherapy information service for the general public. An A5 stamped addressed envelope should accompany requests for information.

National Association of Bereavement Services
20 Norton Folgate
London E1 6DB
Tel: 0171-247 0617 administration
Tel: 0171-247 1080 referrals.
A support organisation for bereavement services, and a referral agency to put bereaved and grieving people in touch with their appropriate local service. Promotes networking, training and professional standards through the regional representatives, quarterly newsletter and annual training conference. Publishes the *National Directory of Bereavement and Loss Services*, and guidelines for setting up and running a bereavement counselling or support group.

Day care

National Association of Hospice/Palliative Day Care Leaders
Luton and South Beds Hospice
Great Bramingham Lane
Streatley
Luton LU3 3NT
Tel: 01582 492339.
Secretary: Linda Watts, Thames Valley Hospice
Tel: 01753 842121.
Provides a network for day care leaders, both locally and nationally, through education and support and promotes good practice within the membership. Organises an annual meeting and produces a newsletter.

Complementary therapies

Cancer Help Centre
Grove House
Cornwallis Grove
Clifton, Bristol BS8 4PG
Tel: 0117-974 3216 Fax: 0117-923 9184.
Offers a holistic-dealing with the whole person-healing programme (to comple-ment medical treatment) including relation, counselling, healing, nutrition and meditation. Patients can attend for one day or a residential week. Education programmes for health professionals.

Complementary Cancer Care Programme
The Royal Homoeopathic Hospital NHS Trust
Great Ormond Street
London WC1N 3HR
Tel: 0171-837 8833.
Macmillan clinical nurse specialist: Caroline Stevenson.
Medical consultant: Dr Anne Clover.
Offers a programme of homoeopathy and other complementary therapies to support well-being and quality of life which may be used in conjunction with conventional cancer treatments. Referral for outpatient or inpatient care via patient's general practitioner. General enquiries from health professionals and members of the public are welcomed and an education programme is being developed.

Complementary Therapies in Nursing Forum – Special Interest Group
Royal College of Nursing
20 Cavendish Square
London W1M 0AB
Tel: 0171-409 3333.

Centre for Complementary Health Studies
University of Exeter
Rennes Drive
Exeter EX4 4PU
Tel: 01392 433828.

The Didsbury Trust (Therapeutic touch)
Jean Sayre-Adams
Sherbourne Cottage
Litton, nr. Bath
Avon BA3 4PS
Tel: 01761 241640.

PAT Dogs (Pets as Therapy)
National Head Office: Rocky Bank
4 New Road, Ditton
Maidstone, Kent ME20 6AD
Tel: 01732 848499.

TENDA
The European Nursing Development Agency,
Tameside General Hospital,
Ashton–under–Lyne
Lancs OL6 9RW
Tel: 0161-339 5535.

The arts

Hospice Arts
The Forbes Trust
9 Artillery Lane
London E1 7LP
Tel: 0171-377 8484.
A national charity established by the Forbes Trust and Help the Hospices to
develop creative and therapeutic arts activities for hospice patients in the UK.
Offers advice, information and contacts to any Hospice organisation wishing to
establish or develop an arts programme. Also arranges seminars and evaluations,
and publishes reports of arts projects. Small pump-priming grants sometimes
available, but Hospice Arts is unable to support ongoing revenue expenditure.
Correspondence should be addressed to the Director.

National Music and Disability Information Service
Director: Laura Crichton
Foxhole, Dartington
Totnes, Devon TQ9 6EB
Tel: 01803 866701.
Provides information and advice on all music and music related matters
concerning disabled people. Publishes resource papers, reports and a quarterly
newsletter, *Music News*.

Voices for Hospices
Chairman: Mrs Sheila Hurton
P.O. Box 171
Cobham
Surrey KT11 2YL
Tel: 01932 860719 Fax: 01932 860719.
National Coordinator: Mrs Alexandra White, Tel: 01483 34481.

Council for Music in Hospitals
Director: Mrs Pam Smith
74 Queen's Road
Hersham
Surrey KT12 5LW
Tel: 01932 252809/252811 Fax: 01932 252966.
Provides live concerts given by carefully selected professional musicians in
hospitals, homes and hospices throughout the UK. The hospice concerts may take
place in a variety of venues, e.g. the day room or chapel and, if requested, at
individual bedsides.

Professional associations
Doctors

Association for Palliative Medicine
Secretary: Sheila Richards
11 Westwood Road
Southampton SO2 1DL
Tel: 01703 672888.
The association encourages the principles of good palliative medicine to promote education, research and self audit in the specialty. It also advises on career and medical staffing matters. The association is open to all doctors.

Fund-raisers

National Association for Hospice Fundraisers
71 Portsmouth Road
Guildford
Surrey GU2 5BS
Tel: 01483 69920.
A national association supporting the role of hospice fund-raisers and to improve standards and efficiency in fund-raising. Regular regional meetings are held and education and training are available.

Volunteer co-ordinators

Association of Hospice Voluntary Service Co-ordinators
Secretary: Pam Warn
St Leonard's Hospice
185 Tadcaster Road
York YO2 2QL
Tel: 01904 708553 Fax: 01904 704337.
Membership secretary: Glenda Leach
St Giles Hospice
Tel: 01543 432031.
The association aims to represent and support nationally all voluntary service co-ordinators who are engaged in organising and coordinating volunteers in hospice and palliative services.

Chaplains

Association of Hospice Chaplains
Secretary: The Revd Stuart Coates
Strathcarron Hospice
Randolph Hill
Denny
Stirling FK6 5HJ
Tel: 01324 826222 Fax: 01324 824576.
Chairman: The Revd Len Lunn
St Christopher's Hospice.
Tel: 0181-778 9252.

Children

ACT Association for Children with Life-threatening or Terminal Conditions & Their Families
Director: Stella Elston
65 St Michael's Hill
Bristol BS2 8DZ
Tel: 0117-922 1556 Fax: 0115-925 5051.
A national resource and information service for families and health-care professionals involved in caring for children with life-threatening and terminal illness. ACT is concerned with representing the needs of children and families and with promoting models of good care throughout the UK and has a multi-disciplinary membership.

Architecture and building

Cancer Relief Macmillan Fund Planning Department
Spadesbourne House
184 Worcester Road
Bromsgrove Worcestershire B61 7AZ
Tel: 01527 872948 Fax: 01527 579214
Consultant planning adviser: Derek P. Spooner.
Provides a comprehensive capital development service embracing design, construction and fund-raising. Projects considered include in-patient and day patient palliative care units and improvements to patient facilities in oncology and radiotherapy departments. Projects undertaken in collaboration with an NHS authority or trust or with another charity. Enquiries welcomed.

Health Building Design Consultancy
Lawrence & Wrightson
Voysey House
Barley Mow Passage
London W4 4PN
Tel: 0181-994 2288 Fax: 0181-747 5013
Contacts: Clive Hicks and Christopher Richards.
A division of Lawrence Wrightson, Architects, offering advice and services relating to all aspects of medical building, particularly Hospices and palliative care day centres. The service extends from simple advice to construction procurement. Initial consultation is free of charge and without obligation. *Building a New Hospice*, by Clive Hicks is available from the Hospice Information Service or the consultancy.

Northern Ireland

The Ulster Cancer Foundation
40–42 Eglantine Avenue
Belfast BT9 6DX
Tel: 01232 663281/2/3
Helpline: 01232 663439 (09.30–12.30 weekdays).
Involved in many aspects of cancer, from prevention to patient support. Operates an

information helpline for cancer-related queries for patients and their families, staffed by experienced cancer nurses, who can arrange counselling by personal appointment at the centre. Rehabilitation support services include: mastectomy advice (volunteer visiting by former patients); laryngectomee club (monthly activities, support in hospitals and at home); lymphoma support (patient and family link-up).

Republic of Ireland

Irish Cancer Society
5 Northumberland Road
Dublin 4
Tel: 00 353 1668 1855 or dial 10 and ask for 'Freefone Cancer' (Ireland only).
Information on all aspects of cancer from nurses via Freefone service. Funds home care and rehabilitation programmes run by voluntary groups, for all cancer patients. Support groups for mastectomy, colostomy and laryngectomy patients, and Hodgkin's disease advice. Home night nursing service available on request of patient's doctor or public health nurse.

Scotland

Breast Care and Mastectomy Association
Cancer Relief Macmillan Fund
Cancer Link
9 Castle Terrace
Edinburgh EH1 2DP
Tel: 0131-228 6715 (BCMA)
Tel: 0131-229 3276 (CRMF)
Tel: 0131-228 5557 (Cancer Link).
Details for these associations are given above.

Tak Tent
Cancer Support Organisation Scotland
Block 20, Western Court
100 University Place
Glasgow G12 6SQ
Tel: 0141-211 1930.
Gives emotional support, counselling and information on cancers and treatments. Has support groups throughout Scotland, plus a one-to-one counselling service at centre by appointment. Runs various 'coping with cancer' courses.

Wales

Tenovus Cancer Information Centre
College Buildings, Courtenay Road
Splott
Cardiff CF1 1SA
Tel: 01222 497700.
Although the primary concern is prevention, the centre provides information and

advice on all cancer-related concerns. Contact by telephone, letter, or personal visit.

World Health Organization

Cancer and Palliative Care Unit
1211 Geneva 27
Switzerland
Tel: 0041 22 791 3477 Fax: 0041 22 791 0746.
Chief, Cancer and Palliative Care Unit: Dr Jan Stjernsward. Assists the WHO's member states in the areas of cancer and palliative care; coordinates palliative care and cancer activities world-wide.

Index